Governors State University
Library Hours:
Monday thru Thursday 8:00 to 10:30
Friday 8:00 to 5:00
Saturday 8:30 to 5:00
Sunday 1:00 to 5:00 (Fall
and Winter Trimester Only)

The Auditory Steady-State Response

GENERATION, RECORDING, AND CLINICAL APPLICATION

The Auditory Steady-State Response

GENERATION, RECORDING, AND CLINICAL APPLICATION

Edited by

Gary Rance, PhD

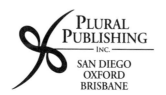

PLURAL
PUBLISHING
INC.
SAN DIEGO
OXFORD
BRISBANE

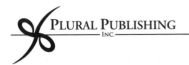

5521 Ruffin Road
San Diego, CA 92123

e-mail: info@pluralpublishing.com
Web site: http://www.pluralpublishing.com

49 Bath Street
Abingdon, Oxfordshire OX14 1EA
United Kingdom

ISBN-13: 1-59756-161-4
ISBN-10: 978-1-59756-161-7
Library of Congress Cataloging-in-Publication Data:

Contents

Foreword by James W. Hall III, PhD   vii
Preface   ix
Acknowledgments   x
Contributors   xi

Chapter One: **Auditory Steady-State Responses: From the Beginning**   1
Field W. Rickards

Chapter Two: **Introduction to Technical Principles of Auditory Steady-State Response Testing**   11
M. Sasha John and David W. Purcell

Chapter Three: **The Stimulus-Response Relationship in Auditory Steady-State Response Testing**   55
David W. Purcell and Hilmi R. Dajani

Chapter Four: **Neural Generators of the Auditory Steady-State Response**   83
Andrew Dimitrijevic and Bernhard Ross

Chapter Five: **Subject Variables in Auditory Steady-State Response Testing: State, Anesthesia, Age, and Attention**   109
Barbara Cone-Wesson

Chapter Six: **Clinical Application of Auditory Steady-State Responses**   119
Gary Rance and Barbara Cone-Wesson

Chapter Seven: **Behavioural Threshold Estimation for Auditory Steady-State Response Testing**   125
Kathy Vander Werff, Tiffany Johnson, and Carolyn Brown

Chapter Eight: **The 80-Hz Auditory Steady-State Response Compared with Other Auditory Evoked Potentials** 149
David R. Stapells

Chapter Nine: **Auditory Steady-State Responses in Neonates and Infants** 161
Gary Rance

Chapter Ten: **Auditory Steady-State Responses and Hearing Screening** 185
Guillermo Savio and Maria Cecilia Perez-Abalo

Chapter Eleven: **Bone Conduction Auditory Steady-State Responses** 201
Susan Small and David Stapells

Chapter Twelve: **Auditory Steady-State Responses and Suprathreshold Tests of Auditory Ability** 229
Andrew Dimitrijevic and Barbara Cone-Wesson

Chapter Thirteen: **Auditory Steady-State Responses and Hearing Device Fitting**

Part A—The Role of Auditory Steady-State Responses in Fitting Hearing Aids 241
Franz Zenker-Castro and José Juan Barajas de Prat

Part B—Fitting Cochlear Implants Using Electrically Evoked Auditory Steady-State Responses 259
Barbara Cone-Wesson

Chapter Fourteen: **Case Studies in Application of Auditory Steady-State Response Testing** 265
Gary Rance, Heleen Luts, Barbara Cone-Wesson, Anna Van Maanen, and Alison King

Chapter Fifteen: **Summary and Future Directions** 319
Gary Rance and Sasha John

Appendix 325
Index 329

Foreword

Dr. Field Rickards, who was among the earliest investigators of the auditory steady-state response (ASSR), has noted that "periodic potentials" were first recorded from human subjects close to 40 years ago, and that the ASSR has been applied clinically at several centers in Australia and Canada for more than 20 years. However, because devices approved by government agencies for use with patients were lacking until the past decade, particularly in the United States, audiologists tend to view the ASSR as a new technique for auditory assessment. Without doubt, one measure of the acceptance of a clinical technique in audiology is a publication of a book devoted entirely to the technique. Those of us who have been practicing audiology for over 30 years all remember the excitement surrounding publication in 1975 of the *Handbook of Clinical Impedance Audiometry*, edited by James Jerger. Aural immittance (then impedance techniques), subsequently became a regular and invaluable component of the clinical audiology armamentarium. The same clinical phenomenon was repeated 10 years later with the appearance of *The Auditory Brainstem Response*, edited by John Jacobson. Toward the end of the 1990s, two books were published that focused exclusively on otoacoustic emissions—*Otoacoustic Emissions: Clinical Applications*, edited by Martin Robinette and Theodore Glattke, and the *Handbook of Otoacoustic Emissions*, written by James W. Hall III.

The books were written, in large part, in response to growing demand by audiologists for more information on this latest addition to the clinical test battery.

Confirming the essential role of the ASSR in the assessment of auditory function, especially in children, *The Auditory Steady-State Response: Generation, Recording, and Clinical Application*, edited by Gary Rance, will now take its place among the collection of thorough treatises on important clinical procedures in audiology. As will be apparent from a perusal of the table of contents, the book includes chapters by many of the best-known names associated with basic and applied research on the ASSR.

Understanding anatomical origins and physiological mechanisms is critical for recording, and maximum clinical exploitation, of any auditory electrophysiological response. Three early chapters of the book are set aside for rather rigorous discussion of the "basic science" and "technical concepts" underlying the ASSR. Of course, despite extensive research efforts, our understanding of the neural origins of the ASSR remains incomplete. The information represented in this book, however, describes what is known at this time. The book next presents a number of chapters on clinical application of the ASSR and topics, such as nonpathologic factors, that must always be considered for meaningful analysis and interpretation of an electrophysiological response. The assignment of entire chapters to selected clinical applications of the ASSR —among them estimation of behavioral auditory thresholds for air and bone conduction signals, infant hearing screening, and the use of ASSR in hearing aid fitting —attests to the clinical value of the ASSR, and to the wealth of practical information now available to the audiologist. The book concludes with a chapter containing eight case studies that illustrate various applications of the ASSR and, in addition, serve to reinforce the concepts and technical points noted elsewhere in the book, followed by a look to the future.

With the emergence of any new clinical technique, there is a tendency among audiologists to question the relevance of preexisting procedures, or to pose the unanswerable question of which technique is "better." Some audiologists may even wonder whether, with the availability of ASSR, there is still a role for the auditory brainstem response (ABR) and, especially, frequency-specific (tone-burst)

ABR measurement. Within the rather brief history of clinical audiology, it has been repeatedly confirmed that new clinical techniques do not supplant older techniques; rather, new techniques complement the existing techniques. Put simply, the audiologic test battery gets bigger and better. The diagnostic power of the latest auditory electrophysiology technique—in this context, the ASSR—is wholly dependent on its consistent clinical inclusion within a test battery, and on its clinical interpretation with the context or the pattern of other audiologic findings. With the publication of *The Auditory Steady-State Response: Generation, Recording, and Clinical Application*, we have the first comprehensive review of a the clinical technique. I predict that accumulated clinical experience will, in time, reveal additional diagnostic applications of the ASSR in clinical audiology and that the full ASSR story will unfold in later editions of this book.

James W. Hall III, PhD
University of Florida
Gainesville

Preface

This book is the first publication dedicated entirely to the subject of the auditory steady-state response (ASSR). Its emergence in monograph form is a reflection of the weight of fundamental research and patient data that have accumulated over more than a quarter of a century. Although it is premature to suggest that the field has reached "maturity," investigators who have worked in this area over an extended period will recognize that ASSR-based research has moved from the periphery to somewhere near the mainstream of auditory science. One personal observation reflecting this change in emphasis involves the organization of scientific meetings—usually a good indicator of trends in research and clinical thinking. In the early 1990s, when I began presenting my group's clinical findings, ASSR papers were viewed as something of a curiosity, and were not viewed by many (as they were typically relegated to the "graveyard shift"). In complete contrast, the trend in recent international (audiological) symposia has been to dedicate entire sessions (if not days) to the field, reflecting the fact that ASSR-based assessment has now become one of the foundations of clinical practice.

This book presents a solid theoretical background on ASSR generation and recording technique and offers an overview of current (and future) clinical and research applications for the response. Accordingly, it should be of interest to researchers, audiologists, and students alike.

Chapters 1 to 5 focus on the fundamental research underlying the current understanding of the auditory steady-state response. In particular, these initial chapters define what the ASSR is (and how it differs from the more familiar transient auditory potentials), and discuss how the response is generated and optimally recorded.

Chapters 6 to 14 address the clinical application of the ASSR. These sections consider the various issues that arise when a technology moves from the laboratory to the clinic, and outline the degree to which these challenges have been met. In particular, the focus of these chapters is the ability of ASSR-based procedures to provide estimates of the behavioral audiogram in both normal and hearing-impaired subjects of all ages. Normative data for various subject populations are presented, along with a series of detailed case studies demonstrating the ways in which this information can inform the clinical assessment process.

Acknowledgments

Over the 12 months it took to prepare this book, the project has enjoyed the support of many colleagues and friends, who have lent their considerable energy and expertise. In particular, mention should be made of the authors, many of whom, in addition to preparing their own sections, have helped review the work of their peers. Special thanks to Sasha John and Barbara Cone-Wesson, who were a great help in this regard. One of the strengths of this book is that it contains input from leaders in a diverse range of disciplines including physics, engineering, auditory physiology, medicine, education, speech pathology, and clinical audiology. I am grateful to them all for their collegiality and contribution.

Thanks also to Dr. Sadanand Singh, Dr. Brad Stach, and the editorial team at Plural Publishing, who provided the original impetus for the project and exhibited laudable patience as it slowly took shape and to Jay Hall for his introductory comments.

Finally, special thanks to the research subjects, clinical patients, and their families who have taught us so much and to the Barker Charitable Foundation for its ongoing support.

Gary Rance
Melbourne, Australia

Contributors

Brad Stach, PhD, Editor-in-Chief for Audiology

Dr. José Juan Barajas de Prat
Associate Professor
Department of Educational,
    Developmental Psychology and
    Psychobiology
La Laguna University
Canary Islands, Spain
Chapter 13

Carolyn Brown, PhD
Professor
Department of Speech Pathology and
    Audiology and Department of
    Otolaryngology-Head and Neck
    Surgery
University of Iowa Hospitals and
    Clinics/University of Iowa
Iowa City, Iowa
Chapter 7

Barbara Cone-Wesson, PhD, CCC-A
Associate Professor
Department of Speech, Language and
    Hearing Sciences
University of Arizona
Tucson, Arizona
Chapters 5, 6, 12, 13, and 14

Hilmi R. Dajani, PhD
Assistant Professor
School of Information, Technology and
    Engineering
University of Ottawa
Ottawa, Canada
Chapter 3

Andrew Dimitrijevic, PhD
Postdoctoral Fellow
Department of Neurology
University of California, Irvine, School
    of Medicine
Irvine, California
Chapters 4 and 12

M. Sasha John, PhD
Research Associate
Rotman Research Institute at Baycrest
Toronto, Ontario, Canada
Chapters 2 and 15

Tiffany Johnson, PhD, CCC-A
Assistant Professor
Speech-Language-Hearing Sciences and
    Disorders
Dole Human Development Center
University of Kansas
Lawrence, Kansas
Chapter 7

Alison King
Australian Hearing Service
Melbourne, Australia
Chapter 14

Heleen Luts, PhD
ExpORL, Department of Neurosciences
University of Leuven
Leuven, Belgium
Chapter 14

Maria Cecilia Perez-Abalo, MD, PhD
Senior Researcher
Head, Phono-Audiology Department
Department of Language and Hearing
    Sciences
Cuban Neuroscience Center
Habana, Cuba
Chapter 10

David W. Purcell, PhD
Assistant Professor
National Centre for Audiology
School of Communication Sciences and
    Disorders
Faculty of Health Sciences
University of Western Ontario
Toronto, Ontario, Canada
Chapters 2 and 3

Gary Rance, PhD
Associate Professor
Wagstaff Research Fellow in
    Otolaryngology
The University of Melbourne
Melbourne, Australia
Chapters 6, 9, 14, and 15

Field W. Rickards, PhD
Dean
Faculty of Education
The University of Melbourne
Melbourne, Australia
Chapter 1

Bernhard Ross, PhD
Senior Scientist
Rotman Research Institute at Baycrest
    Centre, Toronto
Assistant Professor
Department for Medical Biophysics
University of Toronto
Toronto, Ontario, Canada
Chapter 4

Guillermo Savio, MD, PhD
Associate Researcher
Phono-Audiology Department
Department of Language and Hearing
    Sciences
Cuban Neuroscience Center
Habana, Cuba
Chapter 10

Susan Small, PhD
Assistant Professor
School of Audiology and Speech
    Sciences
University of British Columbia
Vancouver, British Columbia, Canada
Chapter 11

David R. Stapells, PhD
Professor
School of Audiology and Speech
    Sciences
University of British Columbia
Vancouver, British Columbia, Canada
Chapters 8 and 11

Kathy Vander Werff, PhD
Assistant Professor
Communication Sciences and Disorders
Syracuse University
Syracuse, New York
Chapter 7

Anna Van Maanen, AuD
Clinical Assistant Professor
University of British Columbia
Vancouver, British Columbia, Canada
Chapter 14

Franz Zenker-Castro
Head of Audiology Services
Audiology and Hearing Aid Department
Clinica Barajas
Canary Islands, Spain
Chapter 13

CHAPTER 1

The Auditory Steady-State Response: From the Beginning

FIELD W. RICKARDS

Utter originality is, of course, out of the question.
Ezra Pound

The *auditory steady-state response* (ASSR) is a periodic electrical response from the brain evoked by a periodically varying continuous acoustic signal, typically a sinusoidally modulated tone. The response is a complex waveform with the same periodicity as that of the acoustic signal. The constituent frequency (Fourier) components of the ASSR remain constant in amplitude and phase over a long period of time (Rickards, 1983). This is also true for the visual system (Regan, 1972, 1989). This is in contrast with recording a transient response, when the brain resumes its resting state, or an approximation of it, before a subsequent stimulus is applied. Beginning in the 1990s, the ASSR has gained considerable attention in clinical pediatric audiology settings as an electrophysiological measure of hearing in newborns and young infants. This clinical application of the ASSR builds largely on the foundational research of the 1980s, principally in Australia (e.g., Cohen, Rickards, & Clark, 1991; Rickards & Clark, 1984), Canada (e.g., Linden, Campbell, Hamel, & Picton, 1985; Stapells, Galambos, Costello, & Markeig, 1988; Stapells, Linden, Suffield, Hamel, & Picton, 1984), the United States (Galambos, Makeig, & Talmachoff, 1981; Kuwada, Batra, & Maher, 1986), and the United Kingdom (Rees, Green, & Kay, 1986), although earlier reports also have described the ASSR

1

(Campbell, Atkinson, Francis, & Green, 1977; Geisler, 1960).

This chapter provides a historical perspective on the development of the ASSR as a clinical and research tool, presented as a personal view from Down Under, with particular reference to relevant work in the Department of Otolaryngology at the University of Melbourne. In the interest of clarity and completeness, the ASSR is discussed in the context of the broader field of evoked potentials and auditory processing.

In 1971, the newly established Department of Otolaryngology, under the leadership of Graeme Clark, had two research foci. The first concerned the electrical stimulation of the auditory nerve, which in time led to the development of the Cochlear multichannel cochlear implant, and the second was improvement of diagnostic techniques for patients with hearing loss and communication disorders using auditory evoked potentials (AEPs). As a result of the work on electrical auditory nerve stimulation, more than 100,000 people worldwide now benefit from the cochlear multichannel implant. For the second focus of research, electrophysiological correlates of complex signals, were recorded using sounds of changing amplitude and changing frequency. The ultimate aim of this research was the development of improved methods for diagnosis of auditory processing disorders. Amplitude and frequency changes are acoustic characteristics which are important in speech perception. An important outcome of this research has been the development of a diagnostic tool that has been used extensively in Melbourne since 1990 for the preoperative evaluation of children being considered for cochlear implantation, and as part of a diagnostic audiological test battery for babies and infants at risk for hearing loss—a much narrower application than that originally envisaged. Since the mid-1990s, use of the ASSR as a clinical and research tool has expanded around the world as commercial systems were developed, based both on the Melbourne research and on the research of others.

In the early 1970s, the "state of the art" in work with AEPs was summarized nicely by Picton, Hillyard, Kraus, and Galambos (1974). These researchers classified AEPs into three types: transient responses, sustained responses, and perceptual responses. *Transient responses* are evoked by a reasonably rapid change in the auditory stimulus. This may be the turning on of a sound, a sound offset, a change in frequency, or a change in amplitude. The classification of the transient response has been according to poststimulus latency, for which three classes are recognized: early (0 to 10 ms), middle (10 to 50 ms), and late (50 to 250 ms) responses. The early category may be divided into cochlear and brainstem potentials. *Sustained responses* are in response to a continuance of the auditory stimulus. These responses are the cochlear microphonic, the summating potential, the frequency following response (FFR), and the sustained cortical negative potential occurring during a prolonged sound. *Perceptual responses* are those responses that are related to the significance and meaning of the sound, rather than its physical characteristics, such as frequency and sound pressure level (SPL). These include the contingent negative variation (CNV) and the late positive component, with a latency between 250 and 500 ms, sometimes called the P3, P300, or P350 wave. The CNV can be elicited by an auditory warning stimulus requiring some perceptual or motor response. The late positive wave follows a stimulus in any modality that has a particular significance for the subject. This may be achieved by demanding a discrimination or requiring a specific task to be performed.

At that time, published work on the ASSR was scarce. By contrast, steady-state evoked potentials were being recorded in the visual and somatosensory systems (Namerow, Sclebassi, & Enns, 1974; Regan, 1972). Like the ASSR, the visual and somatosensory steady-state potentials are long trains of repetitive waves that are elicited by repeating stimuli, and which remain constant in amplitude and phase with time. Regan (1972), who had done extensive work in the visual field with evoked potentials, had obtained steady-state potentials recorded in response to both spatially structured and unstructured visual fields. In both cases, the stimulus is repetitive. The unstructured stimulus may be sinusoidally modulated, amplitude-modulated (AM) light producing a flicker, and the structured stimulus may be a reversing checkerboard. Regan found that the amplitude and phase of the response were highly dependent on many variables, such as the repetition frequency, the type of stimulus used, the color, and so on. For flickering light, he found three regions of response: low frequency (less than 10 Hz), medium frequency (13 to 25 Hz), and high frequency (40 to 60 Hz) (Regan, 1966, 1968, 1972). He also found that the high-frequency evoked potentials had properties that were quite different from those in the medium- or low-frequency range, which seemed to come from different parts of the cortex and to have different color properties and different relationships to intensity. Quite a different pattern is seen for pattern reversal. Moreover, not only do steady-state potentials in the visual system have a component at the stimulus frequency, but higher harmonics may be present as well (Spekreijse, 1966).

Physiological systems such as the auditory and visual systems are nonlinear. The steady-state description of a linear system is given by amplitude versus frequency and phase versus frequency. This is equivalent to the description of the system by its impulse (transient) response of amplitude versus time. In nonlinear systems, the situation is quite different when no generally valid relationship exists between transient and steady-state responses. The transient response may contain information that cannot be obtained by the steady-state description, and vice versa. Many reasons for nonlinearity exist. Regan (1972) observed that the visual system (and the auditory system as well) is rich in neural organizations that preferentially respond to only a few stimulus features, or to only one such feature. In neurophysiology, these neural groupings often are called *feature detectors*, and in psychophysics, *information-processing channels*. Unless stimulated appropriately, a particular feature detector will not respond optimally. An inappropriate stimulus (a flash or a click) is likely to reveal little of the brain's information processing capabilities. Moreover, steady-state evoked potentials are less prone to change under the influence of psychological variables such as attention, so psychological investigations with evoked potentials should be limited to transient responses. The benefits of looking at both transient and steady-state responses in the visual system has been extensively studied by Regan and others, and these benefits have been summarized in detail by Regan (1977) and Hillyard, Picton, and Regan (1978).

The auditory work by the University of Melbourne's Department of Otolaryngology investigators has had both clinical and research foci. In the early 1970s, these investigators were using the late cortical transient response elicited by tones for clinical studies, but their research was focused on transient responses to complex tones. Typically, bursts of five cycles of a modulated tone were presented and and then averaged in the conventional way. In this early work, the investigators were recording near-field potentials from the brainstem of the cat in response to AM and frequency-modulated (FM) tones. Figure 1–1 shows potentials from the cochlear nucleus and the inferior colliculus of the anesthetized cat. The responses consist of an onset response, followed by a periodic component that has the same periodicity as that of the modulation waveform. The two responses have different waveforms, probably showing the effect of different processing in the two brain centers. The onset response is the transient response, which dies away, and

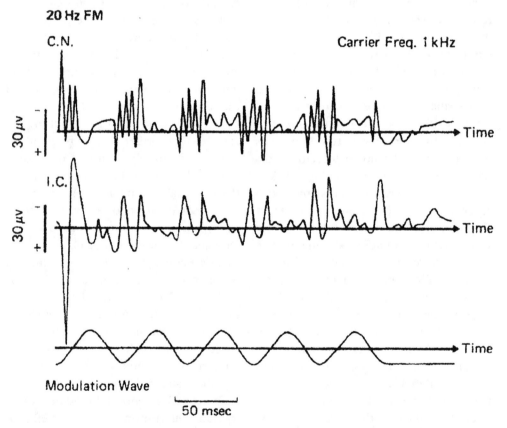

Figure 1–1. Field potentials from the cochlear nucleus (C.N., *upper trace*) and inferior colliculus (I.C., *lower trace*) of the cat in response to five-cycle bursts of a 1-kHz tone frequency-modulated (FM) at 20 Hz with an intensity of 70 dBSPL. Rising and falling edges of the modulation wave produce rising and falling frequencies. (From Rickards & Clark, 1972.)

the periodic component is the steady-state response, which continues to repeat with each cycle of modulation.

The University of Melbourne investigators first recorded this periodic component from the scalp in humans in 1973. They used bursts of five cycles of amplitude modulation or frequency modulation and observed an onset response and periodic pattern similar to those shown in Figure 1–1. Some of this early work intersected with that of the team at Oxford, whose researchers were studying auditory processing of AM and FM stimuli; this research included evoked potential studies (Green & Kay, 1973, 1974; Green, Kay, & Rees, 1979; Kay & Matthews, 1972).

In 1979 the Melbourne group designed a computer system to extract the steady-state component of the evoked potential. They therefore used the modulation waveform to "phase lock" the computer. The computer sampled electroencephalogram (EEG) segments exactly equivalent to four cycles of modulation of a continuous modulated tone and averaged the EEG segments. Because the tone was continuous, the transient component would quickly die away.

In an extensive study by Rickards and Clark (1984), AEPs recorded in response to AM tones were investigated in adult subjects of normal hearing. Figure 1–2 shows the response when 1000 EEG segments are averaged. In this instance, the stimulus was a 250-Hz tone modulated at 11 Hz and presented at 90 dB SPL. The duration of each sweep was 363.6 ms, so this recording took a little over 6 minutes. The response is a complex waveform, and the amplitude spectrum highlights the presence of the first four harmonics of this response—consistent with the nonlinear nature of the auditory system.

In this study, Rickards and Clark (1984) focused only on the first harmonic. Quantifying the amplitude and phase of the first harmonic was found to be sufficient for describing the broad characteristics of the response. By investigating the amplitude and phase characteristics, the researchers concluded that the ASSR to AM tones could be recorded over a wide range of modulation frequencies (less than 10 Hz to greater than 150 Hz); responses could be recorded at near-threshold levels; responses were largest near 40-Hz modulation in awake adults; and apparent latency–group delay estimates, using phase plotted against modulation frequency, suggested that latencies equivalent to the AEP transient peaks could be obtained using the ASSR procedure under certain stimulus conditions. Like Regan (1972) in the visual system, Rickards and Clark found that high-frequency ASSRs had properties that were quite different from medium- or low-frequency ranges, and that the frequency regions came from different parts of the brain. It was of particular interest that the apparent latency in these adults was in the range of 12 to 15 ms when the modulation frequency was between 60 and 140 Hz. The large ASSR in awake adults at 40 Hz is consistent with the middle latency response referred to as the 40-Hz event-related potential (ERP) (Galambos et al., 1981). At that time, the Melbourne group used the term *auditory steady-state evoked potential* (ASSEP). Over the years, other terms have been used, including the envelope following response (EFR) and the amplitude-modulated frequency response (AMFR), before universal acceptance of the designation *auditory steady-state response*.

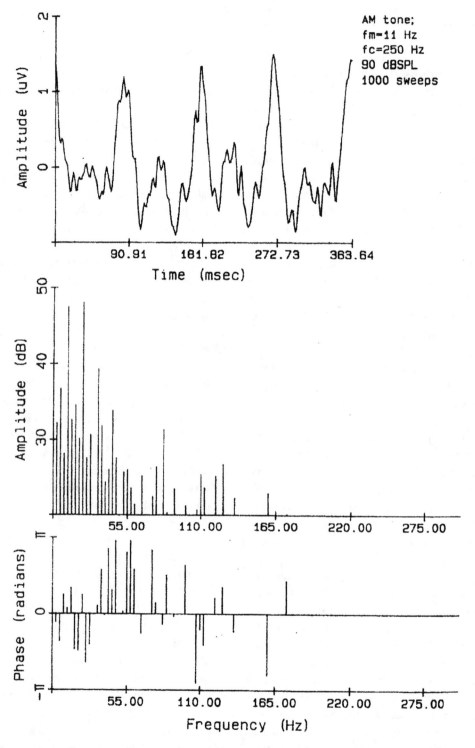

Figure 1–2. Steady-state evoked potentials with amplitude and phase spectra from an adult subject with normal hearing, in response to a 90-dBSPL, 250-Hz AM tone with a modulation frequency of 11 Hz. AM, amplitude modulation; fc, carrier frequency (Hz); fm, modulation frequency (Hz). (From Rickards, 1983.)

To expand the Melbourne research team's capacity to properly investigate the ASSR and its properties, a real-time system needed to be developed. Up until this time, responses were averaged and the Fourier analysis was performed off-line. This was time-consuming and did not allow the investigator to respond appropriately in an experimental setting. By 1985, a new system with unique capabilities had been developed (Figure 1–3)— thanks largely to the contributions of Laurie Cohen, who had joined the research team as a PhD student in the early 1980s. This system was used for scientific and clinical research and clinical assessments from 1985 until 1996. Phase coherence was used as the detection algorithm; technical details can be found in the report by Cohen and associates (1991).

Having developed a real-time system, the Melbourne investigators were eager to investigate use of the ASSR as an objective test for difficult-to-test children, particularly babies and young infants. This research focus stemmed in part from the success of the cochlear implant in adults with acquired hearing loss, leading to a desire to research the implant's application in children with acquired and congenital hearing loss (e.g., Busby et al. 1989) and also by the need for an objective test in the existing two-tiered statewide screening program in Victoria (Australia). Accordingly, these investigators identified three key questions:

- Could the ASSR be recorded from sleeping subjects?

- Could the ASSR be recorded in newborns?

- What is the relationship between ASSR and behavioural thresholds?

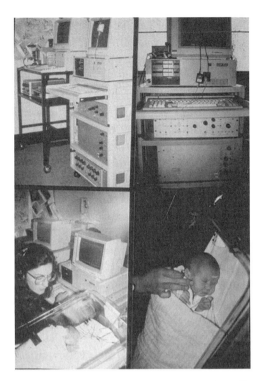

Figure 1–3. Prototype automated auditory steady-state response detection device, designed and built in 1985 by Laurie Cohen and Field Rickards. *Clockwise from upper left:* real time system for recording and analysis of ASSRs developed in 1985 (*foreground*); real time ASSR system with recording and analysis section (*bottom*) under the stimulus section (*top*); newborn being prepared for testing; Oriole Wilson recording ASSR from sleeping newborn.

In addressing the first question, the investigators found that when modulation rates were greater than 70 Hz, efficient ASSRs could be recorded from sleeping subjects (Cohen et al., 1991). It appeared that the ASSR was dominated by brainstem activity at these higher rates, which is broadly unaffected by sleep. Moreover, the background EEG noise at these spectral frequencies was significantly suppressed by sleep. In addition, combinations of amplitude and frequency modulation could enhance the signal strength.

The work with newborns—the focus of the second question—was driven in part by the international push for universal newborn hearing screening (UNHS). In a study conducted in newborn infants, aged 1 to 7 days, sleeping in a hospital nursery, Oriole Wilson and Lesley Tan tested 245 well babies at three frequencies (500, 1500, and 4000 Hz) (Rickards, Tan, Cohen, Wilson, Drew, & Clark, 1994). These researchers found that consistent responses could be obtained from newborns; the best modulation rates in newborns were greater than 60 Hz; the mean minimum response levels were 25 to 40 dBHL; the equivalent latencies generally were between 11 and 15 ms.

To address the third question, on the nature of the relationship between ASSR and behavioural thresholds, Rance and colleagues studied 60 subjects, both children and adults, with hearing ranging from normal to profound deafness, during sleep (Rance, Rickards, & Cohen, 1995). These investigators concluded that regression formulas could be used to predict behavioural thresholds. Predictive errors were greatest for the low frequencies with mild hearing loss, and smallest for greater hearing loss in the high frequencies.

Research focusing on clinical application of the ASSR has gathered pace since the mid-1990s, and a number of the prerequisites for successful transition from the laboratory to the clinic have now been addressed. Some of these issues include determining the reliability of the ASSR in persons of different ages,

optimizing test parameters for different subject groups and different test conditions, and establishing the effect of factors such as degree and type of hearing loss on the response. Detailed discussion of this work can be found in Chapters 5 and 6.

Encouraged by their early results, the University of Melbourne group of investigators took the step to develop a commercial ASSR recording system. ERA Systems P/L, Melbourne, Australia, began production of a device designed specifically for clinical use in July 1997. Since that time, a number of other products have been developed, including the AUDERA (GSI/VIASYS, Madison, Wisconsin), which evolved from the Melbourne ERA device; the AUDIX (Neuronic S.A.); the M.A.S.T.E.R. (Biologic); and the SmartEP (intelligent Hearing). A summary of these systems is presented in the Appendix at the end of the book.

It is now approaching 40 years since the Melbourne researchers first recorded periodic potentials from the scalp in humans, and more than 20 years since these investigators, and others in Canada and elsewhere, commenced clinical research using the ASSR technique. The ASSR has now become an important component of the test battery for evaluating babies and young infants who have hearing impairment. No doubt many children already have benefited from an earlier and more accurate measurement of their hearing, leading to more appropriate medical, audiological, and educational intervention. Although most of the international research generally has focused on the application of the ASSR as a hearing test, many exciting opportunities remain to extend ASSR research in audiology and other fields.

References

Busby, P. A., Tong, Y. C., Roberts, S. A., Altidis, P. M., Dettman, S. J., Blamey, P. J., et al. (1989). Results for two children using a multiple-electrode intracochlear implant. *Journal of the Acoustical Society of America, 86*, 2088-2102.

Campbell, F. W., Atkinson, J., Francis, M.R., & Green, D. M. (1977). Estimation of auditory thresholds using evoked potentials. A clinical screening test. *Progress in Clinical Neurophysiology, 2*, 68-78.

Cohen, L. T., Rickards F. W., & Clark, G. M. (1991). A comparison of steady-state evoked potentials to modulated tones in awake and sleeping humans. *Journal of the Acoustical Society of America, 90*, 2467-2479.

Galambos, R., Makeig, S., & Talmachoff, P. (1981). A 40-Hz auditory potential recorded from the human scalp. *Proceedings of the National Academy of Science of the United States of America, 78*(4), 2643-2647.

Geisler, C. D. (1960). Average response to clicks in man recorded by scalp electrodes. *M.I.T. Technical Report, 380*, 1-158.

Green, G. G. R., & Kay, R. H. (1973). The adequate stimuli for channels in the human auditory pathways concerned with the modulation present in frequency-modulated tones. *Journal of Physiology, 234*, 50-52.

Green, G. G. R., & Kay, R. H. (1974). Channels in the human auditory system concerned with the waveform of the modulation present in amplitude- and frequency-modulated tones. *Journal of Physiology, 241*, 29-30.

Green, G. G. R., Kay, R. H., & Rees, A. (1979). Responses evoked by frequency-modulated sounds recorded from the human scalp. *Journal of Physiology, 296*, 21-22.

Hillyard, S. A., Picton, T. W., & Regan, D. (1978). Sensation, perception and attention: Analysis using ERPs. In E. Callaway, P. Teuting, & S. H. Koslow (Eds.), *Event related brain potentials in man* (pp. 223-341). New York: Academic Press.

Kay, R. H., & Matthews, D. R. (1972). On the existence in human auditory pathways of channels selectively tuned to the modulation present in frequency-modulated tones. *Journal of Physiology, 225*, 657-677.

Kuwada, S., Batra, R., & Maher, V. L. (1986). Scalp potentials or normal hearing and hearing impaired subjects in response to sinusoidally amplitude-modulated tones. *Hearing Research, 21*, 179-192.

Linden, R. D., Campbell, K. B., Hamel, G., & Picton, T. W. (1985). Human auditory steady-state evoked potentials during sleep. *Ear and Hearing, 6*(3), 167-174.

Namerow, N. S., Sclabassi, R. J., & Enns, N. F. (1974). Somatosensory responses to stimulus trains: Normative data. *Electroencephalography and Clinical Neurophysiology, 37*, 11-21.

Picton, W. W., Hillyard, S. A., Krause, H. I., & Galambos, R. (1974). Human auditory evoked potentials: I. Evaluation of components. *Electroencephalography and Clinical Neurophysiology, 36*, 179-190.

Rance, G., Rickards, F. W., Cohen, L. T., Di Vidi, S., & Clark, G. M. (1995). *The automated prediction of hearing thresholds in sleeping subjects using auditory steady-state evoked potentials, 16*, 499-507.

Rees, A., Green, G. G. R., & Kay, R. H. (1986). Steady-state evoked responses to sinusoidally amplitude-modulated sounds recorded in man. *Hearing Research, 23*, 123-133.

Regan, D. (1966). Some characteristics of average steady-state and transient responses evoked by modulated light. *Electroencephalography and Clinical Neurophysiology, 20*, 238-248.

Regan, D. (1968). A high frequency mechanism that underlies visual evoked potentials. *Electroencephalography and Clinical Neurophysiology, 25*, 231-257.

Regan, D. (1972). *Evoked potentials in psychology, sensory physiology and clinical medicine.* London: Chapman & Hall.

Regan, D. (1977). Steady-state evoked potentials. *Journal of the Optical Society of America, 67*, 1475-1489.

Regan, D. (1989). *Human brain electrophysiology: Evoked potentials and evoked magnetic field in science and medicine.* Amsterdam: Elsevier.

Rickards, F. W. (1983). *Auditory steady-state evoked potentials in humans to continuous amplitude-modulated tones.* Unpublished PhD thesis, University of Melbourne, Melbourne.

Rickards, F. W., & Clark, G. M. (1972). Field potentials in cat auditory nuclei in response to frequency and amplitude modulated sound. *Proceedings of the Australian Physiological and Pharmacological Society, 3,* 201.

Rickards, F. W., & Clark, G. M. (1984). Steady-state evoked potentials to amplitude-modulated tones. In R. H. Noda & C. Barber (Eds.), *Evoked potentials II* (pp. 163–168). Boston: Butterworth.

Rickards, F. W., Tan, L. E., Cohen, L. T., Wilson, O. J., Drew, J. H., & Clark, G. M. (1994). Auditory steady-state evoked potentials in newborns. *British Journal of Audiology, 28,* 327–337.

Spekreisje, H. (1966). *Analysis of EEG responses in man.* Unpublished PhD thesis, University of Amsterdam, The Hague.

Stapells, D. R., Galambos, R., Costello, J. A., & Makeig, S. (1988). Inconsistency of auditory middle latency and steady-state responses in infants. *Electorencephalography and Clinical Neurophysiology, 71,* 289–295.

Stapells, D. R., Linden, D., Suffield, J. B., Hamel, G., & Picton, T. W. (1984). Human auditory steady state potentials. *Ear and Hearing, 5*(2), 105–113.

Suzuki, T., & Kobayashi, K. (1984). An evaluation of 40-Hz event-related potentials in young children. *Audiology, 23,* 599–604.

CHAPTER 2

Introduction to Technical Principles of Auditory Steady-State Response Testing

M. SASHA JOHN
DAVID W. PURCELL

This chapter is dedicated to enthusiastic audiologists who have helped to push the field of auditory steady-state response testing forward.

Introduction

Auditory steady-state response (ASSR) techniques approximate the goals of objective evoked-response audiometry: No subjective responses are required on the part of the person being tested, and the detection of the evoked responses occurs automatically using statistical methods implemented by the computer.

Within such a testing paradigm, what is the role of the well-informed audiologist? Although automation provides the objective detection of ASSRs themselves, audiologists must be responsible for adjusting the protocol as the test progresses and for ensuring that the results make sense. Clinical audiology is, as we know, a mixture of science, art, and experience, and this will likely always be true regardless of the tool being used.

When performing ASSR testing, the audiologist is immediately faced with a number of questions related to technique, results, and their interpretation. Although answers have been obtained for some of these questions, several issues are still outstanding in this relatively new and constantly evolving field of steady-state evoked response testing. Furthermore, it is likely that the answer to a particular question may depend on the testing situation, and rules of thumb must be implemented using common sense and experience.

This chapter reviews the fundamental technical concepts that underlie stimulus generation, response detection, and threshold estimation. Several candidate "solutions" to a number of commonly encountered technical problems are presented as well. Some equations are provided to show how certain principles are functionally implemented, but the underlying math is largely sidestepped. Armed with this information, audiologists should feel more comfortable about interpreting the "objective" results that are provided by ASSR software packages and should be able to use the time available for testing in a more efficient and effective manner.

Overview of Auditory Steady-State Response Testing Techniques

This section provides an overview of what occurs during ASSR testing, as illustrated in Figure 2–1, and introduces some key terms and concepts, which are then reviewed in more detail throughout the chapter. The top of the figure depicts the creation of a stimulus, its presentation to a patient's left ear, the processing of the sound in the cochlea and the brain, and the recording of the resulting brain electrical activity as reflected in the electroencephalogram (EEG). The second row depicts the automatic processing of data and statistical evaluation of the response as accomplished by the ASSR software.

In order to obtain frequency-specific estimates of hearing, the ASSR stimuli can be presented sequentially or simultaneously. When multiple tones are tested simultaneously, this may be known as the *multiple auditory steady-state response* (MASTER) technique. Other names for this technique, such as *multiple-frequency ASSR* and *multiple-ASSR*, also are in use. Multiple carrier frequencies (Fc), each having a unique modulation frequency (Fm), can be added together to form a *compound stimulus* for use in testing (labeled "Sound" in the figure). During ASSR testing, this stimulus is converted from its digital representation within the computer's memory (known as the stimulus buffer) into an analog voltage signal, which is then provided to an acoustic transducer and presented as sound to the patient. Converting the stimulus from a digital set of numbers into an actual voltage signal of the sound is known as *digital-to-analog conversion*, whereas recording the EEG and storing it as a series of numbers in the computer's data buffer is termed *analog-to-digital conversion*. When both ears are tested, two stimulus buffers can be used to store the stimuli that will be delivered to the left and right ears.

Owing to the tonotopic representation of the cochlea, each of the one or more modulated carriers will be processed by relatively independent regions of the cochlea (see "Cochlea" in the figure). In each cochlear region, the response will be initiated at the modulation rate of each carrier. From the cochlea, the signals will travel more centrally (see "Brain" in the figure) through the primary auditory nerve (1) to the brainstem (2) and then, when the modulation rate

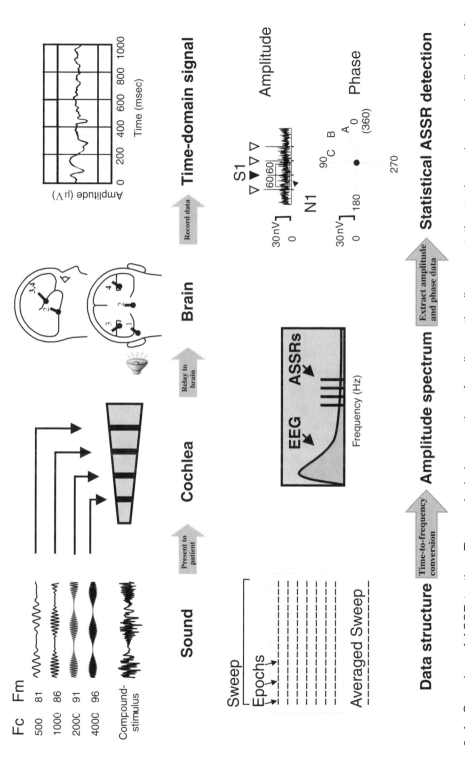

Figure 2–1. Overview of ASSR testing. *Top row* includes creation of auditory stimuli, presentation to the patient, and collection of epochs of EEG (including evoked-response) data. *Bottom row* includes organization of epochs into sweeps residing in a data structure, averaging of the data structure, time-to-frequency conversion of the averaged sweep, and statistical analysis of the resulting amplitude spectra using either amplitude-based or phase-based methods. For additional details, see text.

is slow enough (e.g., less than 70 Hz), the signal is bilaterally relayed to the ipsilateral and contralateral primary auditory cortex (3 and 4). Because the sources of the ASSR (and the corresponding locations and orientations of the recorded dipoles) can vary as a function of the age of the patient and the modulation rate being used, the optimal locations for placement of electrodes to record the evoked potentials also may vary (Herdman et al., 2002; John et al., 2000; Van der Reijden, Mens, & Snik, 2005).

Using scalp electrodes, the EEG signal can be recorded and then amplified (e.g., increased by a factor of 50,000) as well as filtered (e.g., using a high-pass filter of 10 Hz to remove low-frequency energy and a low-pass filter of 300 Hz to deter aliasing, as will be described), before undergoing analog-to-digital conversion. Once the EEG signal has been digitized into a series of numbers, it can be displayed on a computer screen as a time-series voltage-signal (labeled "Time-domain signal" in the figure). The recorded EEG signal will contain the brain activity evoked by the stimuli (known as *signal*—the ASSR), as well as ongoing brainwave activity that is unrelated to the processing of the sound stimuli (known as *noise*).

The material presented in the remainder of this section gets a little more complicated. It may be beneficial to simply skim it and get a general understanding of the concepts and terms. After reading the remainder of the chapter and returning to this section, this overview should be much easier to digest.

The EEG signal collected during the ASSR testing is stored in the computer's memory in segments known as *epochs*. These epochs can be of any length but normally are about 1 or 2 s in duration. As the recording continues and more epochs are collected into the data structure, these may be linked into larger segments known as *sweeps*. This maneuver serves to increase the length of the data segments that are submitted to the fast Fourier transform (FFT) algorithm, thereby increasing the frequency resolution of the amplitude spectra used to evaluate the ASSR (as described further later in the chapter). Sweeps may last any amount of time, but in Figure 2–1, these last 16 s and form rows of our dataset. Accordingly, a test record that lasts about 2 minutes will result in a dataset (labeled "Data structure" in the figure) with 8 rows; where each row is a 16-s sweep (8×16 s = 128 s), and the columns are the individual 1-s epochs. In order to increase the size of the signal (i.e., ASSRs) relative to the size of the noise (i.e., the unrelated EEG activity), known as the *signal-to-noise ratio* (SNR), the sweeps can be added together in order to obtain an "average" sweep. This is the same logic that underlies collecting a large number of transient responses to click stimuli: Components such as wave V are time-locked to the click-stimulus; unrelated background activity is not, so the latter type of energy averages toward zero as more responses are collected.

The averaged sweep can then be converted from the time domain into the frequency domain to produce a *spectrum* (often only the "amplitude spectrum" is shown), which provides an estimate of all of the different frequencies present in the averaged sweep. The ASSRs will show up as peaks in the amplitude spectrum at the frequencies at which the auditory steady-state stimuli were modulated (see "Amplitude spectrum" in the figure).

The final portion of Figure 2–1 illustrates that ASSRs can be detected using statistics that evaluate either the amplitude or the phase of the ASSRs. Amplitude-based statistics, such as the F-test, will evaluate if the energy of a particular ASSR (labeled S1 in the figure) is statistically of greater amplitude than that of a background noise estimate (calculated as the average energy within the box labeled N1). The amplitudes of the signal and noise are compared as a ratio, known as the *F-ratio*, which is evaluated using 2 (numerator) and $2n$ (denominator) degrees of freedom, where n is the number of noise frequencies that were used to create the noise estimate (i.e., the width of the box N1). With use of 120 frequencies as the noise estimate (60 above, and 60 below, the ASSR frequency), the F-ratio that must be exceeded to detect a signal at the $p < .05$ level is 1.75 (i.e., the amplitude of the signal must be 1.75 times as big as the amplitude of the noise to be statistically detected).[1] Generally, as more frequencies are used to create the noise estimate, the estimate becomes more stable, and therefore the criterion that must be met for the F-ratio to reach significance is decreased.[2]

Phase-based statistics are used to detect ASSRs by evaluating the "phases" of the responses to see if these are nonrandomly distributed. As shown later on, ASSR phases are related to the time interval between when a portion of the modulated stimulus was presented and when that same portion was processed by the brain (as evidenced by an evoked response). The assumption is that if the auditory system is "locking" to the modulations of the auditory stimulus, then the sets of evoked responses will occur at similar times (i.e., the phases will be similar).

ASSR data often are displayed in polar plots (see Figure 2–1, bottom row, right). A *polar plot* is a two-dimensional coordinate system in which each ASSR can be plotted as a point determined according to its phase and amplitude. The two axes define all angles between 0 and 360 degrees (i.e., throughout a full circle), and as one moves counterclockwise, the phase values increase from 0 to 90 to 180 to 270 to 360 degrees. ASSRs are plotted so that their amplitude is reflected as the length of a line that starts at the center of the graph (filled circle in Figure 2–1) and extends outward as a function of its size. The polar plot in the figure shows three ASSRs in the upper right

---

[1]The enterprising reader may note the use of the square root of values reported in statistical tables showing critical values of the F-distribution. The square root of these values is used because the F-ratio estimates of signal and noise are reported in terms of amplitude, rather than power. Also, 2 and $2n$ degrees of freedom, rather than 1 and n, are used because the amplitudes of the signal and noise are estimated from measures computed using both amplitude and phase (for detailed discussion, see Lins et al., 1995).

[2]With use of 16 frequencies (i.e., 8 above and 8 below the frequency of ASSR), the F-ratio criterion increases to 1.82 (for 0.05, at 2 and 32 degrees of freedom), because this estimate will be more noisy than one obtained by averaging the values of 120 frequencies together. Although the F-ratio has been increased, this test is not more conservative. The F-ratio criterion is merely increased to compensate for less bins being used in the noise estimate. The only way to make the F-ratio more conservative is to increase the statistical criterion for a given degrees of freedom (require $p < .01$ instead of $p < .05$). This has been a source of some confusion. Studies have shown that changing the number of frequencies that contribute to the noise estimate does not lead to differences in detection efficacy when the significance level is held constant (e.g., Valdes et al., 1997).

corner, wherein response 'A' represents an ASSR with a phase of 15 degrees and an amplitude of 50 nanovolts (nV); response B represents an ASSR with a phase of 45 degrees and an amplitude of 60 nV; and response C represents an ASSR for which the reader is now encouraged to provide an estimated value.[3] The ASSRs seem to be clustered in the upper right quadrant, rather than residing in all four quadrants, and a phase statistic may be used to formally determine if this intuitively nonrandom distribution is statistically improbable at a specified probability level, such as $p < .05$. As in the case of the amplitude statistic, as the number of phase values that are assessed increases (i.e., degrees of freedom increases), the value of the statistical test criterion may become smaller, although the p value needed to reach significance will remain at a set probability level (e.g., $p < .05$).

Stimulus Considerations

Creation of Auditory Steady-State Stimuli

A large number of stimuli have been used for evoking ASSRs. Figure 2–2 shows six examples of such stimuli, each having different advantages and disadvantages. The first stimulus is a sinusoidally amplitude-modulated (AM) 1000-Hz tone for which the frequency of modulation (Fm) is 80 Hz. The amplitude spectrum shows that this stimulus has energy at the 1000-Hz carrier frequency (Fc), and at two sidebands located at the Fc ± Fm. When the modulation depth is 100%, which causes the amplitude envelope to decrease to zero every cycle of the modulator, the sidebands are only 50% of the amplitude of the carrier. The second stimulus is a mixed-modulation (MM) stimulus in which both amplitude and frequency modulation occur at 80 Hz. The amplitude modulation depth commonly is set at 100%. Frequency modulation depth often is set at about 20%, which means that the stimulus roves ±10% from the center carrier frequency (Cohen, Rickards, & Clark, 1991; John, Dimitrijevic, & Picton, 2003). Because adjusting the maximum frequency (of the FM glide) to coincide with the maximum amplitude (of the AM envelope) generally evokes the largest ASSR, the spectral power of the stimulus is shifted by about 100 Hz to be slightly higher than the 1000-Hz center frequency (arrow labeled "Shift" in Figure 2–2). Although it is possible to compensate for this shift by defining the center frequency to be slightly lower than 1000 Hz, this usually is not done. The MM stimulus still is fairly frequency-specific, because the amplitudes of the extended sidebands drop off rapidly from the central frequency. The MM stimulus tends to elicit larger responses (in adults for 500, 1000, and 2000 Hz stimuli, and in infants for 1000 and 2000 Hz) than those occurring with use of amplitude modulation (the ASSRs are about 20% larger than when using simple AM stimuli) or frequency modulation alone (John, Brown, Muir, & Picton, 2004). The third type of stimulus is an exponential AM stimulus, in which the sine wave envelope has been raised to a power of 2 (i.e., squared). Exponential AM stimuli are similar to conventional AM stimuli except that their rising and falling slopes are steeper, causing a slight decrease in its acoustic spectral specificity. Exponential stimuli have been shown to produce

---

[3]The ASSR for C has a phase of 80 degrees and amplitude of 40 nV.

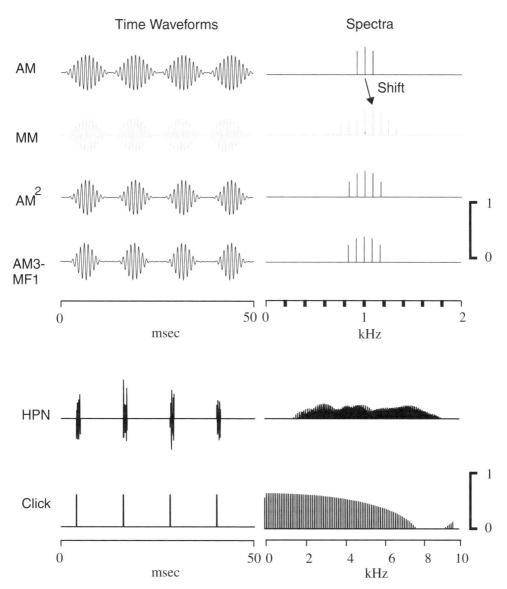

Figure 2–2. Time waveforms and associated amplitude spectra for several types of auditory steady-state stimuli. The *top* four stimuli show different manners of modulating a 1000-Hz carrier at 80 Hz. The *bottom* two rows show modulated high-pass noise (HPN) stimuli (2 to 8 kHz) and clicks as examples of "transient" stimuli that may be presented at 80 Hz to rapidly evoke ASSRs. The HPN stimulus was created by multiplying a rectangular window with high-pass noise. For greater frequency specificity, this stimulus could have been filtered, or alternatively, a different AM envelope, such as an exponential envelope, could have been used. Scale is logarithmic.

larger responses at lower (e.g., 500 Hz) and higher (e.g., 4000 Hz) carrier frequencies in both adults and infants (John, Dimitrijevic, & Picton, 2002a; John et al., 2004). Because the MM and exponential stimuli enhance responses to different carrier frequencies, protocols may become more efficient by using both of these types of stimuli, or by using MM stimuli with exponential envelopes. The fourth stimulus is an extended sideband (ES) stimulus, which can be defined with multiple (e.g., 4) rather than 2 sidebands (Sturtzebecher, Cebulla, & Pschirrer, 2001). In this stimulus each sideband is separated from the central carrier by a distance that is a multiple of the modulation rate—for example, Fc ± 80 Hz for the first set of sidebands, Fc ± 160 Hz for the second set of sidebands, and so on. There is a high degree of similarity between the amplitude spectrum of an ES stimulus and that of the exponential stimulus, and expectedly both of these have been found to provide increases in ASSR amplitudes of about 20%, mostly for the low- and high-frequency carriers.[4] The ES stimulus is interesting because it is created by combining multiple (in this case, three) AM carriers, and can be easily customized with additional spectral peaks having well-defined amplitudes. For example, rather than using three AM carriers, four, five, or even six carriers (which may each be adjusted to have different amplitudes) can be used to form the ES stimulus. Although these latter types of stimuli may not be optimal for high-intensity ASSR testing (owing to the decreased acoustic spectral specificity of the stimuli), their cochlear place specificity may be adequate at lower intensities (e.g., 35 dB), for which spectral spread of energy within the cochlea is decreased.

There is always a tradeoff in evoked potential testing between frequency speci-ficity and response definition or amplitude, whereby less frequency-specific stimuli tend to elicit larger responses. If the audiologist is willing to forgo some specificity, the ASSRs can grow considerably in size. The fifth stimulus is an AM high-pass noise (HPN) (i.e., 2 to 8 kHz) stimulus. The sixth type of stimulus is a click stimulus. These last two types of stimuli (as well as various types of chirp stimuli) have been shown to evoke ASSRs that are large enough to rapidly (e.g., within 1 to 2 minutes) be detected in both adults and infants when presented at 30 to 35 dB nHL, and have been proposed as a screening tool (Cebulla, Sturzebecher, Elberling, & Wafaa, 2007; Hekimoglu, Ozdamar, & Delgado, 2001; John et al., 2003). What is common to all of these stimuli is that the ASSR is elicited at the modulation frequency (or repetition rate in the case of clicks).

Figure 2–3 portrays how a simple AM stimulus is created through either sine wave multiplication or sine wave addition. On the left side of the figure, the top row shows three cycles of an 80-Hz sine wave. By adding 1 to this signal, all negative values are removed, and by dividing this signal by 2, the values will range between 0 and 1. This is the *modulation envelope* of an AM stimulus. The modulation envelope is then multiplied by a carrier signal in order to obtain the amplitude-modulated carrier. The amplitude spectrum, at the bottom of the figure, shows that the AM stimulus contains energy at the Fc (1000 Hz), as well as at two sidebands with half the amplitude of the Fc (because the modulation depth is

---

[4]It should again be noted that the improvements in ASSR amplitude offered by different stimulus types may be somewhat age-specific and frequency-specific. For example, ES stimuli may be better than MM stimuli in adults at 500 Hz, whereas in infants, the opposite may be found (Van der Reijden, 2007).

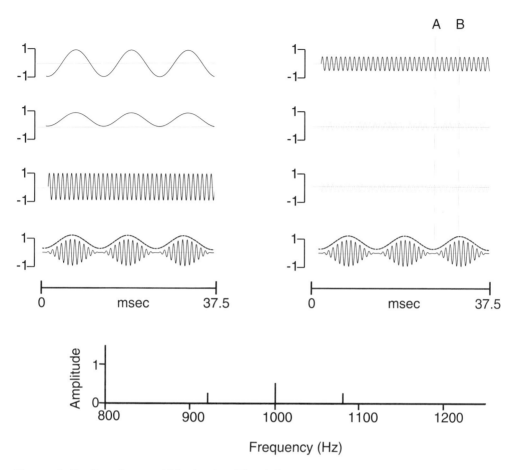

Figure 2–3. Creating an AM stimulus. The *left column* shows the waveforms that are used during AM creation using sine wave multiplication. The *dotted line* above the AM stimulus of row 4 is not part of the actual stimulus and is merely provided to highlight the stimulus envelope. The *right column* shows how sine wave summation can be used to produce the same AM waveform. *Vertical line* A shows a time point at which the peaks of the carrier add "destructively" with the peaks of the sideband waveforms to produce a value of 0 (i.e. −0.5 + (+0.25) + (+0.25), and *vertical line* B shows a time point at which the peaks add "constructively" to produce a value of 1 (i.e., +0.5 + 0.25 + 0.25). The *bottom* of the figure shows the amplitude spectrum obtained by submitting the AM waveform of row 4 to an FFT algorithm. The spectrum shows that the carrier tone has an amplitude of 0.5 (arbitrary units) and the sideband tones are half as large. An unmodulated carrier would have an amplitude of 1, rather than 0.5.

100%). These sidebands appear at the frequencies Fc − Fm (920 Hz) and Fc + Fm (1080 Hz). Because the amplitude spectrum reflects all the frequencies present in the AM signal, it follows that by adding together these 3 sinusoids then we can create an AM signal. The right side of Figure 2–3 shows that if a 1000-Hz tone is added with a 920-Hz tone and a 1080-Hz tone (which are adjusted to be 50% as large), then the same AM stimulus is obtained. This occurs because the positive peaks of the carrier signal become aligned with either the positive or negative peaks of the 2 sideband signals (which have different phases than the central carrier). Investigators may use either sine-wave multiplication or addition in order to create the AM stimuli used for ASSR recordings, but these are two sides of the same coin and arrive at identical AM stimuli.

Independent of the stimuli used (continuous or transient), or methods of stimulus creation, two rules must be followed to permit the ASSRs to remain time-locked to the stimuli and subsequently enable accurate response evaluation in the frequency domain.

- *Rule 1*: Auditory steady-state stimuli must be created so that the modulation envelope (or repetition rate in the case of transient stimuli) fits exactly into the stimulus buffer without truncation of a cycle. The stimulus buffer is a segment of computer memory that holds the values representing the stimulus. These values are converted to an analog waveform and presented as an acoustic stimulus by the acoustic transducer.

- *Rule 2*: The stimulus buffer must be exactly the same duration as that of the data buffer into which the ASSR data are stored.

For reasons which will be explained, the data buffer into which the ASSR responses are stored (i.e., a "data epoch") often lasts 1024 ms, rather than 1000 ms. Likewise, according to Rule 2, the stimulus buffer also must last 1024 ms. Consequently, in order to adhere to these two rules, auditory steady-state stimuli will

often be defined with peculiar modulation rates (e.g., 83.0078 Hz, rather than 85 Hz). By setting the modulation rate at 83.0078, exactly 85 cycles of the recorded ASSR will fit into the data epoch.

Figure 2–4 graphically demonstrates this issue using 3-Hz amplitude modulation of a 38-Hz carrier stimulus (these relatively slow integer frequencies are selected for illustration purposes and normally would not be used in ASSR testing). The top row stimulus shows what occurs when the stimulus buffer used during collection of the first data epoch lasts exactly 1000 ms. In this case, a 3-Hz modulation envelope and a 38-Hz carrier frequency fit exactly into the first epoch. A second epoch, with an identical stimulus, could then be played as soon as the stimulus for the first epoch ends. The transition between the first and second epoch would occur smoothly without any abrupt changes (these "discontinuities" are more formally termed *transients* in the literature) in either the stimulus envelope or the carrier signal.

The second row of the figure shows that when the stimulus buffer epoch (and hence the data buffer) is extended from 1000 ms to 1024 ms (a more favorable duration, as explained in the next section of this chapter), both the modulation envelope and the modulated carrier signal depart from zero and begin the next cycle of the modulated stimulus (see the stimulus waveform between times A and B). As a result, when the stimulus for the second epoch begins, there is a mismatch between the end of the first stimulus and the beginning of the second stimulus. This is a problem for two reasons. First, this will produce a "click" once every 1.024 s, which will decrease frequency specificity by activating many regions of the cochlea. Second,

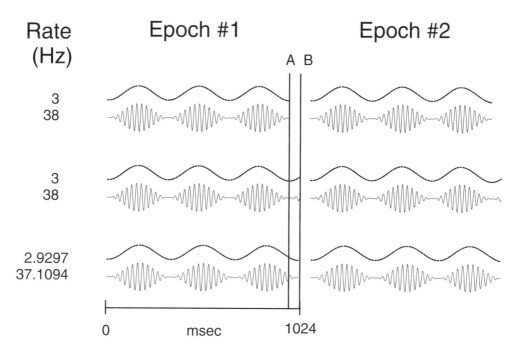

Figure 2–4. Adjusting stimulus characteristics as a function of epoch duration. The *top row* shows that a 3-Hz envelope and a 38-Hz AM carrier frequency fit exactly into a stimulus buffer of 1000 points (which ends after 1 s at *vertical bar* A). The *second row* shows that when the stimulus buffer is increased to 1024 points (which ends after 1.024 s at *vertical bar* B) that slightly more than 3 cycles (and 38 cycles of the carrier) fit into the buffer. The *third row* shows that decreasing the modulation and carrier frequencies slightly again allows an integer number of cycles to fit exactly into the stimulus buffer.

the recorded response also will not fit evenly into the data epoch, which will lead to problems such as spectral leakage, as described later on.

The third row shows that by decreasing the modulation frequency to 2.9297 Hz (i.e., 3 * [1000/1024]) and the carrier frequency to 37.1094 Hz (i.e., 38 * [1000/1024]), an integer number of cycles of the modulation waveform, as well as the carrier waveform, will fit into the stimulus buffer (and the elicited ASSRs that it evokes will similarly fit into the data epoch). The stimulus can be played continuously, and transitions between stimulus buffers will not be heard. Accordingly,

in the literature, these "unique" frequencies commonly are used in order to adhere to the principles of ASSR recording.

Calibration of Auditory Steady-State Stimuli

Multiple-modulated carriers can be used to simultaneously test several ranges of frequency-specific hearing, so long as each is modulated at a unique modulation frequency (Lins & Picton, 1995). When multiple-modulated carriers are used, each of these is individually calibrated before these are combined into a compound stimulus, which is presented to at least one ear during testing. The addition of four individual stimuli normally causes about 5 to 6 dB increase in RMS intensity. Therefore, an auditory steady-state stimulus having carriers of 500, 1000, 2000, and 4000 Hz that were calibrated individually at 50 dB SPL will actually be experienced as 55 dB SPL by the listener. We suggest that no compensation need be made to reduce the intensity of the stimulus by 5 to 6 dB, the logic being that each of the four carrier signals will be processed in a different region of the cochlea. In other words, from the standpoint of the cochlea, the frequency-specific sound energies in the compound stimulus are processed relatively independently.

Time-to-Frequency Conversion

ASSRs are contained in the EEG data that are collected. These data represent a series of voltages that are measured from scalp electrodes in consecutive moments in time (i.e., a time series). Conventionally, these data are converted into the frequency domain in order to evaluate the ASSRs. This is known as *time-to-frequency conversion*, or *spectral analysis*. Toward this end, an algorithm called the Fourier transform often is used that decomposes any time waveform into a series of sinusoidal signals, as illustrated in Figure 2–5. On the left side of the figure, rows 1 and 2 show 5-Hz and 20-Hz sine waves, having amplitudes of 2 and 1,

respectively. Row 3 shows a signal that was created by adding the 5-Hz and 20-Hz signals together. The fourth row shows the amplitude spectrum which was obtained by submitting the signal of row 3 to a Fourier transform. As expected, there are spectral components at 5 Hz and 20 Hz, with amplitudes of 2 and 1, as occurred in the original waveform components. This also occurs on the right side of the figure. Are there any differences between the signals shown in the left and right columns?

In Figure 2–5, the summed waveforms on the left side of row 1 are upside down relative to those on the right, and in terms of phase these differ by 180 degrees. The stimulus on the left starts at zero and moves toward positive 2; the stimulus on the right starts at zero and moves toward negative 2. As a result, although the "amplitude spectra" of the complex waveforms on row 3 are identical, the "phase spectra" shown in row 5, are different: the left column phase spectral components have values of only zero (see arrows) and the right column phase spectrum reflects the 180-degree phase of the 5-Hz sinusoid. From this example, it should be clear that so long as both the amplitude and phase data are available, any time series waveform can be accurately represented in the frequency domain. All ASSRs, therefore, will always have both amplitude and phase values, although both of these may not be formally derived, and subsequently used, in the detection of the evoked responses.[5]

Now that the general principles of Fourier analysis have been introduced, some discussion is merited about the

---

[5]By way of clarification, it should be noted that in other texts, or in ASSR software packages, the Fourier transform algorithms may define phase relative to cosine; therefore, the phases in the examples of Figure 2–5 would actually be −90, −90 and +90, −90. For simplicity, the discussion

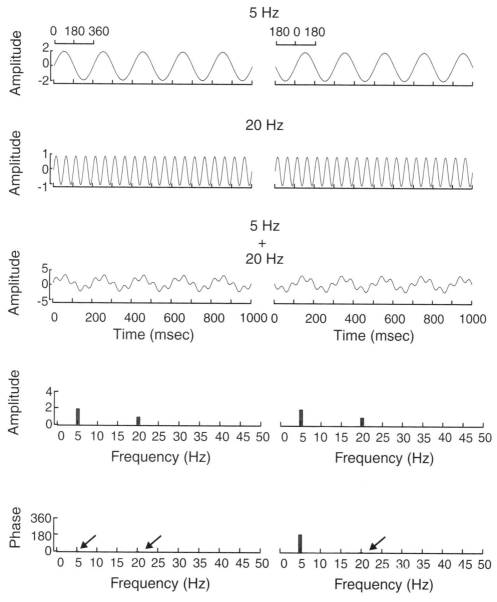

Figure 2–5. Basic principles of time-to-frequency conversion. A 5-Hz and a 20-Hz signal are combined to produce a time series waveform having both of these frequencies. An FFT algorithm can decompose any time series waveform into a series of sinusoids, in which each spectral component will be defined with an amplitude and phase value. The signals of the *left column* all have a phase of zero degrees (*arrows*), whereas the 5-Hz signal in the *right column* has a phase of 180 degrees.

of FFTs and phase within this chapter consistently uses sine phase. Additionally, FFT algorithms would return many non-zero phases for bins that have near-zero amplitudes. The phase plots of Figure 2–5 are deceptively clean (as these should be for teaching purposes).

complications that can occur during its use with real-world ASSR data. A particular type of Fourier transform, called the *fast Fourier transform* (FFT), is widely used owing to its computational speed. The FFT achieves its efficiency by requiring that the number of data points that are submitted to it be set at a positive integer power of 2 (i.e., 2 ^ N). For example, 16 (2 ^ 4) or 1024 (2 ^ 10) data samples may be used. In the collection of neurophysiological data (e.g., of the EEG), the analog signal from the electrodes and amplifier must be converted into a digital signal at a particular rate. Often, the hardware used to perform this analog-to-digital conversion is designed to convert data at integer submultiples of 1 s. For example, sampling data every 1 ms constitutes an acquisition rate of 1000 Hz. A problem occurs because the FFT is designed to operate on data containing, for example, $2^{10} = 1024$ points, and the hardware provides 1000 points per second. This is why data are collected for epochs lasting for 1.024 s, rather than simply for 1 s. As described in the previous section, this requires some adjustment of the stimulus so that the evoked ASSRs will fit correctly (seamlessly) into the data buffer that lasts 1.024 s (1024 points collected at 1000 Hz).

Although the FFT will create a digital representation of any time series waveform, as with any digital representation of real-world information, the final result will have a degree of accuracy that is related to the conversion process: The conversion will never be perfect. This is well known in applications that fall in the spatial domain. For example, an 8 megapixel camera will produce a sharper picture than a 1-megapixel camera. As the "spatial resolution" increases, so does the fidelity of the digital repre-

sentation. In the case of the FFT, the frequency representation improves as a function of two factors:

1. *Duration*: Spectral resolution increases as the duration of data submitted to it increases (the relationship being resolution = 1/time, where resolution is in Hz and time is in seconds). Spectral resolution defines the width of the spectral "bins" of the amplitude spectrum. Each bin can be thought of as a container that holds the sum of the signal energies that exist within a frequency range across which the bin is defined. If 1 s of data is submitted to the FFT, then a 1-Hz (1/1 s) resolution is obtained for each bin. Increasing the duration of data to 2 s will provide a 0.5-Hz (1/2-s) resolution, whereas 10 s yields 0.1-Hz (1/10-s) resolution.

2. *Sampling rate*: Spectral range also increases as the sampling rate increases. The FFT will calculate energy at all frequencies that exist below half the sampling rate—known as the *Nyquist frequency*. If the data are sampled at 1000 Hz, then the FFT algorithm will calculate energy at discrete frequencies between 0 and 500 Hz, because 500 Hz is the Nyquist frequency. Increasing the sampling rate to 2000 Hz will allow the FFT to calculate energy at frequencies up to 1000 Hz.

As illustrated in Figure 2–6, these two characteristics of the FFT algorithm have several implications for measurement of ASSRs. The figure shows a hypothetical case in which an auditory steady-state stimulus, modulated at 83 Hz, was used

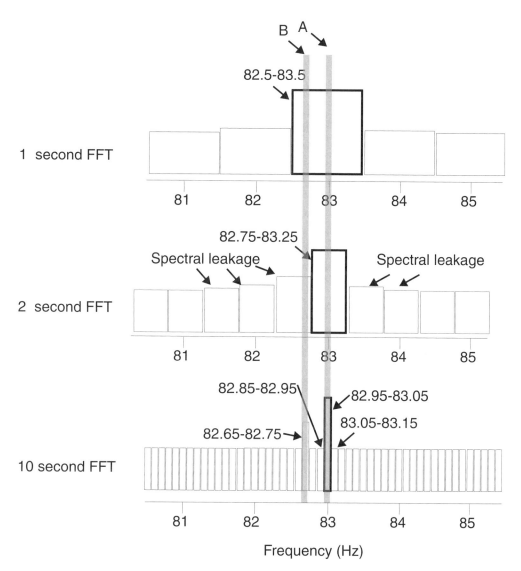

Figure 2–6. Influence of spectral resolution on estimating ASSR energy. The amplitude spectra for simulated ASSR data sweeps lasting 1, 2, and 10 s yield spectral estimates with resolutions of 1.0, 0.5, and 0.1 Hz, respectively. Both ASSR energy at 83 Hz and a noise peak at 82.7 Hz are well resolved in the *bottom* spectra but affect the measurement of the ASSR in the two *top* spectra. The two *faded vertical bars* show where the 82.7-Hz and 83.0-Hz energy fit within the bins of the three different amplitude spectra.

to evoke an 83-Hz ASSR. In the following discussion, an attempt is made to estimate the ASSR after time-to-frequency conversion of averaged evoked-response data ("average sweeps") that are defined to have three different durations. In this example, the modeled signal consists of the ASSR signal at 83 Hz, as well as some broad-band noise energy that serves to approximate background EEG energy.

This energy is about equal at all of its frequencies (i.e., white noise), except that the noise signal also has a randomly occurring peak at 82.7 Hz.

In the top row of Figure 2–6, the simulated average sweep contains a single 1-second epoch and results in an amplitude spectrum having bins that are 1 Hz wide. The 83-Hz ASSR is represented nicely by the 83-Hz spectral bin because it contains energy centered at 83 Hz and spanning 1 Hz (i.e., ±0.5 Hz). However, the 82.7-Hz noise energy also is present in this bin and is indistinguishable from the energy of the ASSR. In rows 2 and 3, the duration of the simulated average sweep has been increased to 2 and 10 s, resulting in amplitude spectra with 0.5-Hz bins and 0.1-Hz bins, respectively. In the amplitude spectrum of the 10-s data sample, the frequency resolution is fine enough to accurately detect the "noise" energy at 82.7 Hz. In the 1-s FFT and 2-s FFT, the frequency resolution is not fine enough to detect the noise energy, so this energy is evaluated in the 83-Hz bin as part of the ASSR signal. In the 1-Hz spectrum, the 82.7-Hz energy falls directly within that bin and therefore is measured with the rest of the energy that falls within that bin. In the 0.5-Hz spectrum, because the 82.7-Hz noise energy falls off-center of a neighboring bin, the bin doesn't receive the energy well, and it spills into or "leaks" into neighboring spectral bins. Because the 82.7-Hz noise is not centered in the middle of a bin (for either the 1- or 2-Hz spectra), its energy 'leaks' across a number of neighboring spectral bins, causing the bins on the left and right of the ASSR bin to become slightly elevated. This leakage will be higher within the FFT bins that flank the left side of the ASSR bin, because 82.7-Hz energy is skewed more to the left side of

the 83-Hz bin (in the case of the 1-Hz spectrum), than to the right. A sharp reader will notice that 1-, 2-, and 10-s datasets are used for this example, rather than 1.024, 2.048, and 10.24 s, as would be likely to occur in measuring real ASSR data.

Response Detection

Sources of Energy at the Modulation Frequency

An attractive feature of many auditory steady-state stimuli is that these do not contain energy at the modulation frequency. Instead, the spectral profile contains energy at the carrier and at Fc ± Fm. For example, a 1000-Hz carrier tone that is modulated at 80 Hz will have energy at 920 Hz (Fc − Fm), 1000 Hz (Fc), and 1080 (Fc + Fm), but will not have any energy at 80 Hz itself. It is only because the auditory system transforms the acoustic energy by nonlinear processes such as rectification (e.g., the hair cells fire more when pushed in one direction) and compression (e.g., the hair cells fire less, per unit increase, at higher intensity levels) that it is possible to measure the activity in the EEG at 80 Hz. At least five sources of energy, however, may contribute to the energy that is held in the 80-Hz FFT bin where the evoked response is measured, rather than simply energy related to the ASSR:

1. True ASSR energy that has been evoked within the brain by the acoustic steady-state stimulus.

2. Physiologically based noise energy that exists in the brain as background EEG, or that is tonically present in the electromyogram

(EMG), which occurs over a range of frequencies including the same frequency at which the ASSR occurs.

3. Physiologically based evoked energy that is not generated in the brain. Several sources of physiological activity can be evoked by the sound, at the frequency of modulation, which do not necessarily indicate that the stimulus evoked an ASSR from the central auditory nervous system.

   a. Three types of muscle responses are the postauricular muscle response (PAMR), the sternocleidomastoid response (recorded from the lateral neck), and the posterior neck muscles (recorded from the inion electrode). These are increasingly likely to be elicited by sound energy over 70 dB SPL and under 1000 Hz but are mainly mediated through the vestibular system and are not necessarily related to processing of sound with respect to hearing. Unfortunately, there is no easy manner to disentangle neural responses from other physiological responses that are evoked by the stimulus. With some work, it is possible to identify a vestibular response by comparing different intensities or electrode montages. A PAMR type of response may not show the changes in latency, with changes of intensity, as would occur with the ASSR and may be larger with use of a mastoid-to-Cz, rather than an inion-to-Cz, configuration.

   b. Another source is the cochlear microphonic. Similarly, cochlear

microphonic can be distinguished from ASSR by testing at several intensities, because microphonic shows little if any latency change with intensity.

4. Instrumentation or "electromagnetic" energy that is created during the transduction of the stimulus. This type of energy may be created at the level of the acoustic transducer and may be due to a nonsymmetrical speaker that rectifies or compresses the stimulus. This energy also may be created within the instrumentation itself, for example, if the audio-amplifiers are positioned sufficiently close to the EEG amplifier to permit energy induction. Because many audiologists rely on low-power ear inserts (e.g., EAR-3A) for presentation of the stimulus, this is not usually an issue. However, with use of higher-intensity stimuli, even with the EAR-3A, or with use of bone conduction transducers, energy emitted from the transducer may be recorded as an ASSR.

5. Aliased energy that is spuriously detected at lower frequencies, although it actually exists at higher frequencies. This type of energy can be created when stimulus-related energy is not sufficiently attenuated by the filtering and sampling rate settings defined within the data acquisition protocol. Although a low-pass filter can be used before the analog-to-digital conversion of the EEG signal in order to attenuate stimulus energy, this reduction may not sufficiently remove all of this energy to prevent aliasing.

There also are other sources of energy that can enter into the frequency bin where the ASSR is measured. For example, energy from lower frequencies, which does not fit exactly into a bin, can "leak" into higher-frequency bins. Noise energy from the EEG amplifiers also may contribute to the noise floor across the entire spectrum. These types of energy likely contribute very little to the energy measured as the ASSR and, although noted here, are not discussed further, because they normally are of little functional importance.

Although ASSRs are small, the hope is that what is being evaluated is energy of type 1, and normally this is the case. Energy of type 2 may cause trouble in the first minute or two of a recording period because sometimes a random spike of energy can occur at the frequency of the ASSR that looks like a clear and rapidly significant response (e.g., appearing in the first 30 seconds) that subsequently disappears as recording progresses. By recording long enough that the background EEG activity is sampled sufficiently, this type of energy should converge toward zero. Energy of types 3, 4 and 5 often is not an issue and can largely be ignored in many situations, but it is important to understand the conditions under which these phenomena may occur, how to tell if these are occurring, and possible solutions. The two most likely situations in which artifact will produce spurious ASSRs are those in which high-intensity air conduction stimuli and bone conduction stimuli are used. These sources of artifact are considered elsewhere in this book and are briefly addressed in the last section of this chapter.

Measuring Energy at the Modulation Frequency

An amplitude spectrum of ASSR sweep data has three types of signals. As shown in Figure 2–7, these comprise the actual ASSR energy (S1), noise energy that occurs at the same frequency as for the ASSR (N1), and noise energy at other frequencies (N2). The top portion of Figure 2–7 shows that the energy present in the spectral bin where the ASSR is measured may be estimated with an amplitude equal to A1 if only the ASSR signal (S1) is present. If a secondary type of energy also is present that is at the same frequency as for the ASSR but is not related to the response, then this noise energy (N1) will cause the amplitude of the ASSR that is measured to be either A2 (overestimation of actual size of ASSR) or A3 (underestimation of actual size of ASSR), depending on whether this noise energy is "in phase" or "out of phase," respectively, with the true energy of the ASSR. The bottom portion of Figure 2–7 shows that the energy normally considered to be simply the ASSR may either be increased or decreased, depending on the relative phases of the non-ASSR and true ASSR energy (the vector sum of the energy). The polar plots graphically show geometrically how the estimate of the ASSR (A2 or A3) can vary with the magnitude and phase of the noise (N1) that contaminates the estimate of the true ASSR signal (S1). The measured ASSR (A2 or A3) is the vector sum of these two residents of the response's frequency bin: signal S1 and noise N1. On the left polar plot, where the noise (N1) is approximately in phase, the measured ASSR (A2) is slightly overestimated, whereas on the right polar plot, where the noise (N1) is

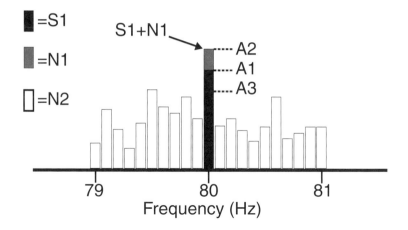

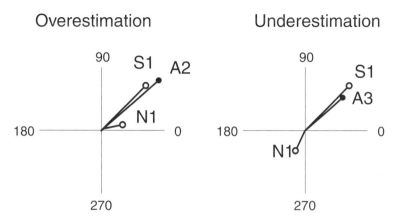

Figure 2–7. What's in the ASSR frequency bin? The *top* of the figure illustrates that noise energy (N1) present at the same frequency as that of the ASSR signal (S1) may cause either overestimation (A2) or underestimation (A3) of ASSR amplitude relative to the true amplitude (A1). Noise energy at adjacent frequencies (N2) can be used to estimate how much noise energy (N1) may be present in the ASSR estimate. The *bottom* of the figure shows polar plots illustrating how the vector sum of the signal energy (S1) and noise energy (N1) lead to over- or underestimation of the ASSR amplitude that is measured.

approximately out of phase, the measured ASSR (A3) is underestimated.

Early in an ASSR recording using lower-intensity stimuli, before the averaged sweep contains a large amount of data, or when large artifact-related energy randomly occurs, the noise (N1) can be considerably larger than the actual ASSR (S1). This noise energy can be incorrectly detected as an ASSR, which then "disappears" as the test progresses, because the noise energy will not have a constant amplitude or phase. It is assumed that the true ASSR (S1) is relatively constant in amplitude and phase, for given stimulus and patient variables, which is why it is detected as averaging progresses. Because the energy in all neighboring spectral bins (N2) is simply "noise" and does not contain any ASSR energy, these bins can be used to estimate how much noise may be in the Fm bin itself. Noise estimates based on background noise energy (N2) also can be used to objectively detect an ASSR, by comparing the amplitude in the bin corresponding to the Fm (our best estimate of S1) with this background noise energy. The F-test permits this comparison to occur at a specified level of statistical significance.

Measuring Responses at Harmonics of the Modulation Frequency

An amplitude-modulated tone often will evoke an ASSR that is detected primarily at the modulation frequency, especially when presented at intensities below 60 dB SPL. When ASSRs are evoked by stimuli at higher intensity levels, by transient stimuli such as clicks or tone-bursts, or by AM stimuli that are not sinusoidally modulated (e.g., rows 3 and 4 of Figure 2–2), then the ASSR responses also may be measured at the higher harmonics of the modulation rate. As the energy of the stimulus moves to more broadly spaced side-bands, an increase in harmonic energy of the evoked ASSRs also occurs (Cebulla, Sturzebecher, & Elberling, 2006; John et al., 2002a). This is not necessarily because the auditory system is responding two or three times for each cycle of the stimulus, but rather because the stimulus envelope (and hence the evoked

response which follows it) cannot be represented by a simple sine wave. When a sine wave departs from its prototypical shape, for example, having steeper rise times or plateau regions near the maximum or minimum values, then these deformations are represented in the FFT as higher harmonics of the fundamental frequency. Infant ASSRs may sometimes show more harmonics than are found in adult ASSRs, but this is not uniformly true across the population. At least in adults, using more than the fundamental harmonic in statistical assessment of the ASSR response may provide better performance (e.g., faster and greater detection rates) over detection algorithms that rely only on the first harmonic especially with stimuli that are designed to evoke responses at these higher harmonics. (e.g., Cebulla et al., 2006)

Amplitude- versus Phase-Based Statistical Methods of Auditory Steady-State Response Detection

A common question is whether it is better to use amplitude- or phase-based techniques in the detection of ASSRs. A number of "amplitude-only" measures (e.g., F-ratio) and "phase-only" measures (e.g., phase coherence), as well as measures that combine amplitude and phase (e.g., Hotelling's T^2 and magnitude-squared coherence), have been compared using adult ASSR data, and these seem to provide approximately similar detection sensitivity and specificity (Dobie & Wilson, 1996; Picton, 2001; Valdes et al, 1997). In reality, both amplitude and phase contribute to the characteristics of the ASSR that is measured, regardless of what measure is relied on to detect the response.

In amplitude-based statistical techniques, which evaluate the amplitude of an ASSR and often compare this to the size of a noise estimate, both amplitudes and phases of the individual ASSR sweeps contribute to the size of the average ASSR that is statistically assessed. The top left side of Figure 2–8 shows a vector-averaged response (filled circle) that is calculated as the mean of 5 simulated subaverage

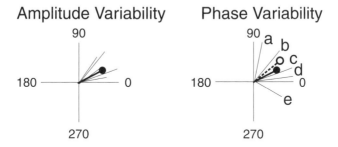

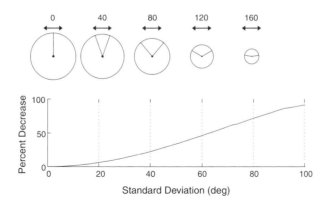

Figure 2–8. Functional overlap of amplitude-based and phase-based statistics. The *top panel* contains two polar plots showing individual ASSRs (or ASSR subaverages) and the vector-averaged mean ASSR that is calculated. In the plot on the *left*, there is little phase variability, and so amplitude variability mostly influences the mean phase value. In the plot on the *right*, there is more phase variability, which is further increased by a small-amplitude ASSR with a divergent phase. The two resulting mean ASSRs (*filled circle*) are identical. Without response e, the resulting mean amplitude would have been larger (*open circle*). The *bottom panel* illustrates how the amplitude of the mean ASSR decreases as phase variability increases. The sizes of the circular phase graphs (above the amplitude variability graph) have been adjusted to be spatially proportionate to the reduced ASSR amplitude that results with selected values of phase variability.

ASSRs. Because there is little phase variance, the average ASSR is mostly a function of amplitude variability. As may occur with real ASSRs, the larger ASSRs tend to be closer to the phase of the mean response, whereas the smaller ASSRs show relatively more divergence. Generally, as the size of an ASSR decreases (e.g., as may occur with lower-intensity stimuli), the variance of the phases of the ASSRs will increase. Both true attenuation of response amplitude and an increase in the phase variance of the individual subaverages will cause the averaged ASSR that is measured to be smaller. Hence, when only amplitude of the ASSR is assessed, both amplitude and phase variance implicitly contribute to the size of the ASSR. Even though the F-test compares amplitude of the averaged ASSR to the amplitude of noise bins, the averaged ASSRs are a result of both amplitudes and phases of the individual ASSRs.

On the top right side of Figure 2–8, the amplitudes are equivalent for the ASSRs labeled *a* through *d*. Response *e*, which is slightly smaller than the other ASSRs, has a different phase; consequently, the averaged response (filled circle) is smaller in amplitude than would be calculated if response *e* had not occurred. The average ASSR that would have been obtained without response *e* is shown by the open circle. Again, both phase and amplitude have altered the size of the averaged ASSR that is measured. In "phase-based" statistical detection of ASSRs, amplitude of the responses also contributes in an implicit fashion. From a physiological standpoint, phase stability will increase with larger responses because these larger signals are somewhat the result of tighter synchrony in the physiological response. From a signal processing standpoint, the increased signal-to-noise ratio (SNR) of larger ASSRs will serve to reduce the relative contribution of noise energy that is at the same frequency as the ASSR, but which may have a different phase.

The divergent response in *e* would have altered statistical estimates based upon either response amplitude or phase coherence. Either increased phase variance or decreased response amplitude in the elicited signal may lead to a similar result in the ASSR measured, regardless of whether amplitude or phase is assessed. It also should be noted that even though the individual ASSRs in the righthand polar plot are larger than those on the left, the increased phase variance produces an ASSR of the same size.

How does this interaction between amplitude and phase play out in actual practice? The bottom portion of Figure 2–8 models the relationship between the standard deviation of the phases from a sample of simulated sweeps, and the percent by which the resulting averaged ASSR will be attenuated compared to the situation in which all the phases were identical. The results were obtained by generating a set of 200 sine waves of equal amplitude, but with phases that were randomly and uniformly distributed across a specified range. The circular plots above the chart show how the size of the ASSR will decrease as a function of phase variability.[6] For example,

---

[6]The term *variability*, rather than *variance*, is used because the phase values were uniformly rather than normally distributed in this simulation. The amplitude decrease corresponding to a particular standard deviation value was almost identical for both normal and uniform distributions, but phase distributions for very small signals may be closer to uniform, so the latter was chosen.

when the standard deviation is 20 (e.g.., about 3 out of 4, of the phases fall within a 40 degree range) the size of the vector-averaged ASSR will be decreased by about 5%, whereas a standard deviation of 40, will cause a decrease of about 23%. It is reasonable to propose that ASSRs that reach significance in the averaged data for 30- to 50-dB stimuli, and which are mainly distributed within 90 degrees of the mean phase value, are probably decreased by about 10 to 15% compared with what these would be if there was no phase variability. This estimate would likely become larger for lower intensities and smaller for higher intensities. It may be helpful for the audiologist to consider the range of phases that are graphically depicted while conducting ASSR testing of patients. By comparing the single-sweep amplitudes and phase variability of the current recording to that of higher intensity recordings from the patient, the audiologist can roughly predict the final size the ASSRs of the current recording. When only the phase of the cumulative average is shown (as occurs using ASSR packages such as MASTER software), it is important to remember that the phase variability will decrease as the recording continues, because each subsequent sweep represents a smaller percentage of the total data.

Strategies of Response Detection

The audiologist may choose from among a number of methods for assessing whether or not a response is present. Three strategies are most commonly used.

1. *Strategies with preset duration criterion* may be employed in which each stimulus intensity is evaluated for a fixed duration. For example, a period of 10 minutes may be used to collect responses at each intensity level. Because the amplitudes of ASSRs at lower intensities (e.g., 30 dB SPL) are relatively small, these will need more time to reach significance than those collected at higher intensities. In order to increase the efficiency and sensitivity of the test protocol, the times used for the lower intensities may be increased relative to those used at higher intensities. For example, although a period of 5 minutes may be used to collect responses at 60 dB SPL, it is likely that about 20 minutes will be needed to collect responses at 30 dB SPL and lower (assuming that normal adult thresholds are available for at least some frequencies). Population-normative data can be used to set these times.

2. *Strategies using preset noise-level criterion* may be used in which target noise levels must be reached before responses are evaluated for each stimulus intensity. One can simply require that the noise estimate meet a fixed criterion such as 10 nV (where this value is defined as the 95% confidence interval and would be associated with about 6 nV RMS). Because the amplitudes of ASSRs at lower intensities (e.g., 30 dB SPL) are smaller, the noise levels for these intensities should be lower than for those collected at higher intensities to achieve a favorable SNR. Population-normative data can be used in order to set these noise level criteria (95% confidence

intervals) for adults and infants where the noise level is set by dividing the lower amplitude ASSRs of the population by 1.75 (assuming that 120 bins of noise are used in the noise estimate, because the F-test relies on this ratio of signal amplitude to noise amplitude in order to obtain a significance level of $p < .05$). The noise level of a recording will decrease with the square root of the number of sweeps in the average, assuming that the noise for each sweep remains more or less the same. The data that are collected early in the current recording can be used to estimate how long it may take to reach a specific noise level using the following equation[7]:

$$T = S (B/N) \wedge 2 \qquad \text{(Equation 1)}$$

where T is the time required to reach the criterion noise level, S is the time for each sweep, B is the single-sweep noise amplitude level, and N is the target amplitude noise level that has been defined for the test (John, Purcell, Dimitrijevic, & Picton, 2002b).

If the audiologist waits until after the first four sweeps are collected in order to assess the ASSR noise level in a potentially more representative fashion (because the first sweep often is the noisiest), the equation can be modified with a simple adjustment. The equation becomes

$$T = S ((B' * Sw \wedge (1/2)) /N) \wedge 2$$
$$\text{(Equation 2)}$$

where B' is the noise level of the averaged sweep as assessed at the current sweep, Sw is the current sweep number, and $\wedge$ (1/2) denotes the calculation of the square root (see text of Table 7 in John et al., 2004). Additionally, when an estimate of the amplitude of an ASSR is available (from either self- or population-normative data), it is possible to estimate the noise level that will be needed for that response to reach significance at the $p < .05$ level by dividing this amplitude by 1.75.

It is likely more sensible to use a protocol with a noise level criterion, rather than preset times. The recording duration is somewhat irrelevant because a "low noise" patient can sometimes provide significant ASSRs, even at 30 dB SPL, within a few minutes. Conversely, if a patient's EEG record is characterized by a relatively larger amount of background noise, then a much longer testing period will be required for the ASSRs to be recognized, or there may be too much noise for the ASSRs to be detected even if the recording was lengthened indefinitely. Due to this latter situation, when noise level criteria are relied on, these should be used in conjunction with a maximum time limit, because it is not possible to record indefinitely. In higher-noise patients, simply stopping the test because a time limit has been reached does not ensure that an adequate SNR has been achieved. If the noise levels of the ASSR test data are not sufficiently attenuated

---

[7]These equations use Excel-friendly conventions and can be cut and pasted directly into that program. The use of $\wedge$ 2 indicates a squaring of that term; $\wedge$ (1/2) is the square root.

because the patient is not relaxed, then the test results may not be valid and the test will have to be redone. When testing high-noise infants, sometimes performing the test in one ear rather than both ears will enable the infant to become more relaxed. Although this may take longer, it will require less time than redoing the entire examination.

3. *Strategies using multiple comparisons.* Rather than, or in addition to, using either a maximum time limit or target noise level, the test procedure at each intensity level may continue until the response reaches significance. This type of multiple-comparison strategy is not as straightforward as one might like and has been a point of some controversy. The problem here is that when an ASSR is statistically detected, this occurs using a specified degree of statistical confidence. Using a $p < .05$ criterion means that there is a 1 in 20 (5%) risk that this result occurred simply by chance, and a 19 in 20 (95%) likelihood that this result is real. However, if the same ASSRs are sequentially evaluated as each new sweep of data is added to the average sweep, then the likelihood increases that one of these statistical tests will reach significance simply by chance. This likelihood can be computed as $1 - (1 - p) \wedge N$, where N is the number of tests that were carried out and $p = .05$, or other initial probability level at which the test was assessed (Sankoh, Huque, & Dubey, 1997).

A standard technique for addressing this issue is to apply a *Bonferroni correc-* *tion*, which simply divides the level of significance by the number of comparisons that are done. In the case of an ASSR test, this strategy may quickly become impractical. For example, if an audiologist simply relies on a rule that as soon as the response is significant, it will be considered present, then the statistical test will be adjusted to $p < .05$ divided by the number of sweeps collected. If each sweep lasts 16 s, then already by the 10th sweep (160 s into a test that may last 20 minutes!) the statistical test now will require significance at the $p < .005$ (0.05/10) level, instead of the 0.05 level. Rather than requiring the ASSR-to-noise ratio to reach a value of 1.75 (needed for $p < .05$ with typical degrees of freedom for the noise estimate), this is increased to 2.35 (needed for $p < .005$). In some instances, such as when testing at lower intensity levels, this may be physiologically impossible to achieve. Luts, Van Dun, Alaerts, and Wouters (2007) recently reported that changing the level of significance from $p < .05$ to $p < .01$ caused the number of detected responses to decrease from 74% to 59%, using 32-sweep (16.384 s/sweep) recordings from adults and infants. Although the Bonferroni technique has protected against detection of an ASSR when it is actually noise (avoiding type II false-negative errors—hearing loss missed), it inadvertently did this at the cost of deterring the detection of real ASSRs (thereby increasing type I false positive errors—normal hearing identified as hearing loss).

Studies using both modeled and real ASSR data have shown that the Bonferroni correction is too conservative for use with multiple-comparison ASSR testing (Sturzebecher, Cebulla, & Elberling, 2005). Because the ASSR data are combined into a cumulative average, the consecutive estimates are highly correlated, making repeated testing much less of an issue except at the early part of the recording. Sankoh et al (1997) offer an adjusted Bonferroni equation that reduces the adjustment in relation to the strength of correlation of the data. It probably is fair to assume that after 5 to 10 minutes of testing, consecutive estimates of the amplitude or phase of the signal and background noise, are correlated at about the 0.75 level (where 1 is a perfect correlation), although in reality the correlation often is likely to be higher. After assessment of the data at 10 different times, rather than using a Bonferroni-corrected criterion of $p < .005$, the criterion can be set at $p < .028$. From a physiological perspective, this is a more feasible compromise. An equation for computing this adjusted significance level is

$$Pa = 1 - (1 - p) \wedge (1/(N \wedge (1 - r)))$$
(Equation 3)

where Pa is the adjusted p value, p is the desired p value to be maintained during multiple comparisons (e.g., 0.05), N is the number of comparisons that will be made (e.g., 10), and r is the correlation coefficient of the data computed between the prior and current iterations being evaluated (e.g., 0.75). An online calculator for obtaining these adjusted p values is available at www.quantitativeskills.com/sisa/calculations/bonfer.htm.

By using some (common) sense, a number of additional strategies may be employed to mitigate statistical concerns. For example, rather than assessing ASSRs after every sweep, these can be assessed after pre-set intervals have elapsed. If ASSRs are collected at 30 dB, it is unlikely that these will reach significance within the first 5 to 10 minutes, especially for 500- and 4000-Hz stimuli that evoke

smaller responses. The ASSRs may first be assessed after 8 minutes and then every 5 minutes thereafter. For a 28-minute test, if the responses are evaluated after 8, 13, 18, 23, and 28 minutes, then this will cause an adjustment of the required significance level from 0.05 to 0.01 (if the Bonferroni correction is used, or 0.033 if equation 3 is used). Similarly, the first statistical assessment of the data can be delayed until a selected noise level criterion is reached.

In an alternative multiple-comparison strategy, rather than decreasing the statistical probability level that is used to detect the presence of a response, the number of significant estimates that are required to occur sequentially can be increased above 1 in order for a response to be detected. Luts et al (2007) presented MM stimuli to infants at 40 dB SPL and found that an error rate of 5% could be maintained, while testing sequentially over time, by requiring that an ASSR be identified as significant (at the $p < .05$ level) across eight consecutive sweeps. As expected, decreasing the number of consecutive sweeps required for an ASSR to be considered significant led to increased spurious detection rates. This mirrors findings from our laboratory (unpublished data) in which ASSRs were evoked in infants using broadband AM noise stimuli (presented at 30 dB SPL). We found that 7 consecutive sweeps led to an error rate of 5% (*note*: Luts et al. tested 2, 4, 6, and 8 sweeps but not 7). It is likely that seven is not a "magic number." Using a 7-sweep criterion led to the 5% error rate by reducing the impact of the random occurrence of a noise energy spike, as a function of averaging, so that the noise energy in the bins of the spurious responses was reduced to less than 1.75 times the amplitudes of the adjacent noise bins (the criterion used by the F-test in these examples). In the population of infants tested within these two studies, the heterogeneity of the noise across adjacent frequencies (the noise structure) of the EEG probably was similar. If an individual patient is not relaxed (or sedated) and relatively larger spikes of noise energy randomly occur in the patient's EEG, then this "rule" may not hold (it also may not hold for testing in adults, in whom the structure of the noise may be different). Audiologists who are uncomfortable with this approach should simply rely on a rule wherein the ASSR is not evaluated until the noise amplitude has met a given criterion. Still, this type of approach is intriguing and bears further investigation.

Several additional considerations are warranted on this topic. The issue of sequential comparisons is complicated and relates primarily to testing low-intensity stimuli. In assessment of large ASSRs evoked in adults with moderate-intensity stimuli, the responses often will be unambiguously clear, because they are many times larger than the background noise floor and have stable phases: Multiple comparisons are not an issue. In the case of ASSRs evoked by lower-level-intensity stimuli, often the SNR will not be high enough until more than about 10 minutes has passed. Issues of repeated testing will be more relevant early in the recording period. In the case in which individual sweeps of 16.384 s are cumulatively combined with an average sweep, then in 10 minutes, 37 sweeps will have been collected before the most recent sweep. Early in the measurement, after, for example, 5 sweeps have been recorded, the average ASSR amplitude estimate may be 50 nV. If the sixth sweep contains an ASSR with an amplitude of 70 nV (due

to noise, as well as some actual fluctuation in ASSR amplitude and/or phase), then this will increase the average ASSR amplitude estimate to 53.33, or (5 * 50 + 70)/6. Later in the recording, for example, after 37 sweeps, the average ASSR amplitude estimate would be affected much less by the sweep containing the 70 nV ASSR. In this case, the average ASSR amplitude would increase to only 50.53, or (37 * 50 + 70)/38, an effect that is one-sixth as large. What are the functional implications of these considerations?

When performing ASSR testing at lower intensities, if an ASSR measurement is repeatedly oscillating between being detected significantly and not meeting the statistical criterion, then the ultimate outcome of these oscillations may not be important in deriving the final test result (present versus not present). If an ASSR is significant after 20 minutes, nonsignificant after 21 minutes, and then significant at 22 minutes, these fluctuations are more likely to be due to fluctuations in the background noise, rather than to changes in the size of the ASSR itself, which is assumed to be approximately constant at frequencies above 70 Hz. What this fluctuation probably indicates is the existence of a weak response that is close to the noise floor. Rather than worrying about statistical issues of repeated testing, it may be more helpful to assess whether the phase value of the ASSR is "normal" and then to consider whether the noise level has met a criterion that is low enough that a small ASSR would be detected.

If time permits, then the testing protocol may be increased by 5 dB, and more data can be recorded. If this latter data record produces a significant ASSR, then the size of the significant response can be used to determine whether the

ASSR at the slightly lower intensity was a true "almost" positive. If this latter record is not significant, then these data can be combined with the prior record to evaluate whether the ASSR then becomes significant. If significance is obtained in this amalgamated recording, then threshold can be estimated, for example, at the intensity of the slightly higher recording (i.e., 5 dB higher than the original recording). Alternatively, testing can continue until the maximum time limit is reached or ASSR remains significant for a specified number of sweeps (e.g., 7 sweeps). In this type of situation, the ability to independently and dynamically control the stimulus intensity, or at least to test multiple carrier frequencies that are set at different intensity levels (which remain fixed over the testing period), would be of great assistance. These features are just now beginning to be offered in clinical systems.

Switching Between Single and Multiple Auditory Steady-State Stimuli

The presentation of a number (n) of multiple-modulated carriers to each ear often is seen as advantageous because the simultaneous presentation of stimuli allows the data to be captured in a single recording session of m minutes, rather than n recording sessions each lasting m minutes. Although it is certain that one will record m times more data than if a single modulated stimulus was presented to each ear, the testing protocol is not made n times faster (John et al, 2002b). This is because the different modulated carriers produce ASSRs of different sizes and often the recording at a given intensity will last until the smallest of the ASSRs reaches significance. Additionally, multiple carrier stimuli are useful for reasons aside from providing the possibility of more efficient ASSR testing. First, in the real world, sounds usually do not occur in isolation, although this is what is tested in pure-tone audiometry. Speech is composed of complex mixtures of sounds, and the speaker (the sound's "signal") typically is experienced in a background of unrelated sound (the "noise"). Testing with multiple-frequency stimuli therefore provides a more similar picture of what may occur outside of the clinic in real-world hearing.[8] Second, because multiple regions of the tonotopically organized auditory system each are activated by their own stimulus, this deters adjacent regions from responding to "off-frequency" energy that is of high enough intensity to enter the filter bandwidth of this adjacent region. In other words, when presented at similar intensity levels, multiple carriers act to provide a level of functional masking.

Single-ASSR testing provides its own benefits. Above 60 dB, the interactions between adjacent regions of the cochlea may produce unpredictable results, one of which is that the ASSRs will be smaller for multiple- than for single-modulated carriers. In cases of hearing loss, no response to certain components of the multiple-ASSR stimulus may be obtained (Picton et al., 1998), whereas single-ASSR testing may rapidly lead to a significant response (although this may occur from

---

[8]It should also be noted that testing with single stimuli can sometimes produce thresholds which are closer to those obtained with pure-tone audiometry, which may be seen as an advantage, and an argument for using single stimuli.

an "off-frequency" place if masking is not used, especially when stimuli above 60 dB are presented).[9] Both single- and multiple-ASSR testing thus provide unique benefits and complementary types of information. For both low- and high-intensity stimuli, it may be useful to switch between the two paradigms in assessing thresholds.

With use of lower-intensity stimuli (e.g., less than 40 dB SPL), either the 500- or the 4000-Hz response may be considerably smaller than the 1000- and 2000-Hz responses. These latter two responses may become significant relatively quickly, but the audiologist may need to sit and wait for one of the other responses to be detected. In this case, the audiologist may perform more efficient testing by establishing threshold of the three larger responses and then testing the "rogue" response by itself, if there is sufficient time. Another alternative is to reduce the intensity of the stimuli which have reached significance while continuing to test the not-yet-detected stimulus at the same intensity (or increasing this intensity), if this option is available on the ASSR software. We have shown that it is possible to use interstimulus intensity differences of 20 dB, in normal-hearing subjects, without causing interstimulus interactions when adjacent carriers are separated by at least one octave (John et al, 2002b).

When using high-intensity stimuli above 70 dB, it can be a good idea to switch from multiple to single stimuli (or to decrease from four to two modulated carriers per ear) for a number of reasons. Above 60 dB, interactions between multiple stimuli (separated by one octave) will begin to make the multiple stimuli less efficient than using single stimuli.

With strongly sloping hearing loss, the use of multiple stimuli becomes less efficient, because some thresholds will be very high and others very low, causing responses to become significant at very different times. Furthermore, the multiple stimuli have an intensity that is 5 to 6 dB higher than the single stimulus, making it perceptually louder than the test level; such stimuli may cause some discomfort at higher intensity levels, or when the patient has low thresholds for some of the carriers. When recording ASSRs to stimuli above 80 dB, it is a good idea to consider the clinical circumstances in terms of both patient comfort and potential damage from continuous presentation of stimuli at this intensity (this will not be a major consideration if the test lasts for only 90 seconds but can become a problem if the test continues for 10 to 15 minutes without any breaks). Although some commercial systems automatically limit the duration of testing at these higher intensities, others may not, and it is up to the audiologist to use judgment in these instances.

Calculations of Phase, Phase Delay, and Latency

The fast Fourier transform will always provide estimates of both amplitude and phase for ASSRs. Although the amplitude measure of the ASSR is somewhat straightforward, phase measures and their underlying concepts are much less so.

Figure 2–9 shows the envelope of an 80-Hz AM stimulus as well as three hypothetical ASSRs evoked in response to this

---

[9]The single-ASSR is again more similar to audiometric testing, in which pure tones usually are not presented in notched noise to produce a standard behavioural audiogram.

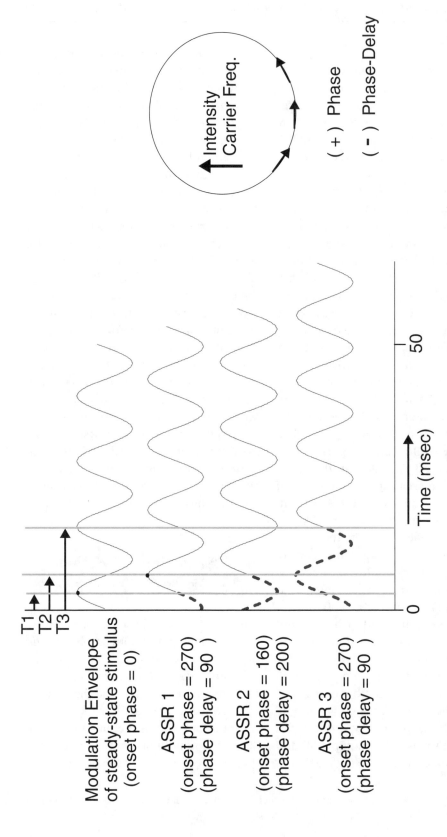

Figure 2–9. Concepts of phase, phase delay, and latency. *Left panel:* The *top* sine wave shows four cycles of an 80-Hz envelope (for an AM stimulus) so that four cycles (12.5 ms each) occur within a 50-ms time span. The *bottom* three waveforms are hypothetical ASSRs that are elicited by the corresponding segment of the stimulus waveform. Because the start of the ASSRs are delayed relative to the start of the stimulus waveform, these also end later. *Right panel:* A graphical mnemonic for remembering how phase, latency, and phase delay change as a function of increases in intensity and carrier frequency.

stimulus. The ASSR will be delayed by some duration relative to the auditory steady-state stimulus. This delay is a function of several smaller delays, such as the time it takes for the stimulus to arrive at the eardrum (e.g., when the sounds are presented through ear inserts, the sound requires about 0.9 ms to travel through the tube from the speaker to the ear); the traveling wave time as the sound energy is transmitted to and processed by the "biological filter" of the appropriate tonotopic area of the cochlea; and the synaptic and conduction delays along the auditory fibers and within the structures of the brainstem. In the case of cortical responses, which can be increasingly elicited by stimuli modulated below 70 Hz, additional delays may result as the evoked signals are relayed to the cortex. The EEG amplifier also will add delays such as those caused by its filtering circuitry (for a detailed review of all sources of delay, see John & Picton, 2000).

In a majority of studies in the ASSR literature, authors will report the phase values of ASSRs or may report the phase variance when referring to the stability of a response. Generally, phase variance increases as the intensities of the stimuli decrease, and is higher for the 500-Hz responses, probably as a result of less synchronized population activity, especially at the lower intensity levels. A small number of studies have attempted to make sense of ASSR phase values by converting these values into latencies. These studies refer not only to phase but also to a measure termed *phase delay*. The concepts of phase delay and ASSR latency are somewhat complex. However, latency measurements of transient ABRs are common, and accordingly some effort should be made to clarify how latency is calculated in the case of ASSRs.

The relationship between phase and phase delay is straightforward. Phase delay is calculated simply by subtracting a phase value of the response from 360 degrees, which is the phase value of the standard stimulus (actually, the phase of the stimulus is 0 degrees, which is the same as 360, because a circle starts and ends at the same point). For example, a phase value of 90 degrees has a phase delay of 270 degrees. What is the purpose of this transformation?

ASSR #1 in Figure 2–9 is delayed, relative to the modulation envelope, by a duration (T1), which for this example extends a quarter-cycle (i.e., 90 degrees) into the stimulus envelope waveform. In the case of ASSR #2, the response is delayed by a duration (T2) which spans about 200 degrees of the stimulus waveform. If the ASSRs are measured using an FFT, phase values of 270 and 160 degrees would be obtained, rather than 90 (360 − 270) and 200 (360 − 160) degrees. This is a problem because although the onset of ASSR #2 is delayed relative to ASSR #1, the measured phases decrease, rather than increase. This result is the opposite of what one would expect. It occurs because the FFT calculates the phase values of the ASSRs at $t = 0$ (the start of the analysis window), rather than the difference in phase between the stimulus envelope and the evoked response. By subtracting the phase value from 360, phase is redefined relative to the stimulus envelope: If the interval between the start of the stimulus and start of the response increases, so will phase delay.

A more "physical" example may elucidate the issue further. Imagine that the stimulus and evoked-response waveforms are a series of virtual hills and valleys. If an ant starts at a location defined by 0 degrees (where time T = 0) and crawls along the stimulus envelope to the first peak, then this is the location defined by 90 degrees (where time is now T1). If a second ant starts crawling at the same time (T = 0) and crawls along the ASSR #1 waveform to the first peak, it will have to start at a location of the ASSR waveform defined by 270 degrees and then crawl to the top of the first hill by approximately the time defined by T2. Although the phase value that the FFT provides will tell us at what "location" of the ASSR waveform the second ant started (i.e., the initial phase), what we really want to know is how much later this ant arrives at the top of her hill (i.e., 90 degrees) compared with the time when the first ant arrived at the top of *her* hill. The delay between the arrival of the second ant relative to that of the first is the phase delay.

How are phase delays converted into measures of latency? ASSR #1 is delayed (relative to the start of stimulus envelope) by the time designated T1, which here spans about 90 degrees of the stimulus envelope. For a modulation envelope of an 80-Hz AM stimulus, a full cycle is calculated as 1000 ms/80 which yields a result of 12.5 ms. Each full cycle or "wavelength," therefore, lasts 12.5 ms. Because ASSR #1 is delayed by 90 degrees, the equivalent time can be calculated as 90/360 * 12.5 ms, or 3.125 ms. Although 3.125 ms is too fast to be an actual delay recorded using real 80-Hz ASSRs (normally in the range of 12 to 20 ms), this value can be used for purposes of this demonstration.

In the case of the second ASSR, the response is delayed by the time designated by the arrow T2, which here spans about 200 degrees or slightly more than half a cycle (i.e., 180 degrees) of the

modulation envelope. Because ASSR #2 is delayed by 200 degrees, we can calculate an equivalent time as 200/360 * 12.5, or 6.94 ms.

In the case of the third ASSR, the response is delayed by the time designated by the arrow T3, which here spans about 450 degrees or about 90 degrees plus one full cycle of the modulation envelope. Although ASSR 3 is delayed by 450 degrees, values of phase usually are reported between 0 and 360 degrees, so the FFT will return a result of 270 degrees. This ambiguity of phase is sometimes referred to as *phase circularity* or *phase ambiguity* (and also by less pleasant names which you, yourself, may be thinking of now). As just discussed, a phase delay value of 90 degrees yields an equivalent time of 90/360 * 12.5 ms, which equals 3.125 ms. If a full cycle of the stimulus is assumed to have occurred prior to the phase value being measured, then this leads to (360 + 90)/360 * 12.5 ms which is a 15.625-ms delay. If it is assumed that two full cycles have occurred, or (2 * 360 + 90)/360 * 12.5 ms, then the latency estimate is 28.125 ms. In the case of ASSRs evoked by stimuli in the 80-Hz range, a reasonable assumption is that one full cycle of the stimulus has occurred before this measurement was made, because from a physiological standpoint, 3 ms is too fast and 28 ms is too slow. A constant value of 12.5 ms was added to the calculations of the latency based on these and other considerations during analysis of measured phase delays. This method is part of what has been termed the *preceding cycle technique* (John et al., 2000). Another method of calculating delays is called *apparent latency* (Regan, 1966, 1989) and is discussed in Chapter 3. The preceding cycle technique provides latency estimations that are in fair agreement with early estimations of latency provided using apparent latency (e.g., Cohen et al., 1991). The two methods are mathematically similar, although they use different strategies to approach their results. Calculation of ASSR latency is a controversial topic in which a number of assumptions must be made that are not necessarily valid (Bijl & Veringa, 1985; Hari, Hamalainen, & Joutsiniemi, 1989). Laten-

cies reported in the literature should be seen as well-educated estimations to be discussed using some caution.

The right side of Figure 2–9 shows a picture that embodies this discussion of phase, phase delay, and latency. As stimulus intensity and carrier frequency are increased, phase delay (and hence latency) *decreases*, while "onset phase" of the ASSR *increases* (this is shown with empirical data in Figure 2–10).[10]

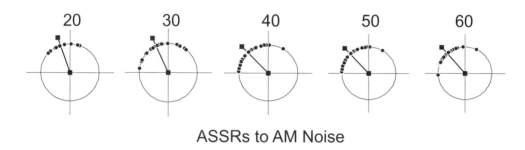

ASSRs to AM Noise

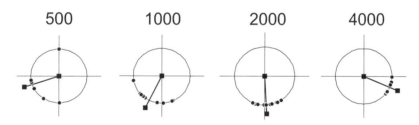

ASSRs to exponential SAM tones

Figure 2–10. Phase distributions of infant ASSRs are stable and predictable. The figures show ASSR phase delay values evoked by AM noise presented at 20 to 60 dB SPL (*top*), and exponentially modulated AM tones (*bottom*) using an exponential set to 2. Counterclockwise rotation follows a decrease in phase delay.

---

[10]As modulation rate increases over small ranges (e.g., from 80 to 95 Hz), phase delay increases, whereas increasing from 80 to 180 Hz will cause phase delay to decrease, ostensibly because the generators for these responses occur earlier in the auditory system (see John & Picton, 2000, for a detailed discussion).

The Use of Phase for Increasing Detection Efficiency in Auditory Steady-State Response Testing

The use of phase in detection of the response is accomplished formally using statistical tests that assess whether a set of phase values is random or coherent. Phase also may be used to bias both amplitude-based and phase-based tests. The idea implemented in this latter type of test is that if the phase of an ASSR is similar to an expected phase, then the statistical test can be positively biased (rewarded) so that the ASSR is more likely to reach significance. If the phase of an ASSR is not similar to a phase that is expected, then the statistical test can be negatively biased (punished) so that the ASSR is less likely to reach significance. In this manner, ASSRs that have the correct phase reach significance more quickly (and with greater sensitivity), and spurious responses are rejected more quickly (Dobie & Wilson, 1994; Picton et al., 2001; Zar, 1999).

Commercial ASSR systems have not yet implemented phase-biasing techniques, probably because of the issue of choosing expected phases. This may not always be an easy task. The expected phase values can vary with the types of stimuli, intensities, and transducers which are used, as well as with pathologic conditions of the auditory system (e.g., the degree of hearing loss) and the age of the patient. These factors complicate the use of population-based normative data as a basis for selecting phase values since the experimental variables used for the collection of normative data must match those used for ASSR testing of a particular patient. Furthermore, phase values derived from normative data collected on different commercial systems would likely not be the same as a result of differences in stimuli, filter settings, or other signal processing factors. As an alternative to population-normative data, self-normative data collected for a patient at higher intensities, or at other frequencies that are tested simultaneously, may be used. Because phase will change somewhat regularly as a function of intensity, carrier frequency, and modulation rate, the audiologist may use knowledge of phase to distinguish between real and spurious candidate ASSRs, and this can be used intelligently to adjust the test protocol. Although this implicitly works against the goal of an independent, objective hearing measure, an important point is that the ASSR techniques are still relatively young, so some time may be required for these types of strategies to be formally implemented within commercial ASSR systems. Comparing phases of ASSRs evoked at different intensities is similar to what audiologists sometimes do with identification of wave V in both tone-ABR and click-ABR tests, in which increases in latency of wave V, which accompany decreases in intensity, are used to determine spurious peaks in the ABR waveform.

The top row of Figure 2–10 shows ASSR phase delay values to amplitude-modulated noise presented from 60 to 20 dB SPL in a group of newborn infants. The thick line shows the mean phase delay, which decreases (counterclockwise) with increasing intensity. Only results of significant ASSRs are shown (n = 37, 41, 40, 34, 12 for 60 to 20 dB SPL, respectively, although visually fewer data appear owing to overlap of the circles). Except for a few cases, values fall within 90 degrees for all intensities. For clinical efficacy, a formal implementation of phase-biasing within the test statistic is effective when the observed distribution is primarily within 90 degrees of the expected phase (Picton et al., 2001). The single data point for the ASSRs in the upper right quadrant (the outliers), at 60, 50, and 40 dB, is from the same patient. Setting the expected phase value based on self-normative, rather than population-normative, data could have worked better in this case, as discussed later on.

The data show that in normal-hearing young infants, the phase values across the population are fairly reliable at different intensities of a stimulus. An audiologist who is testing an infant may use this type of population-normative data to guide the testing procedure. For example, at 30 dB, all of the responses of the population fall between 0 and 180 degrees. If an ASSR being assessed seemed like it was not going to reach significance, the audiologist could check to see if the phase value fell within this 0- to 180-degree range. If it did not, then the likelihood is increased that the ASSR would not be detected at that intensity even with further testing. In cases in which an infant awoke before the end of a testing period (e.g., before background noise levels reached a selected criterion), an assessment of the phase values may give the audiologist a manner of deciding whether a response might have occurred if testing had continued. In some instances (e.g., with an impaired auditory system), an infant's ASSR phase values may diverge from that expected using population norms. Using a self-norm, rather than population norm, may assist in this type

of case, where a phase value obtained at a higher intensity (e.g., 60 dB) can be used to derive an expected phase for a lower intensity before initiation of the test (e.g., 30 dB). For example, a constant value such as 10 degrees can be subtracted from the phase value obtained at 60 dB in order to estimate the phase that is expected at 50 dB, and an additional 10 degrees for every 10 dB step thereafter.

The lower row of Figure 2–10 shows values from 12 newborn infants (aged 3 to 15 weeks; only significant responses are shown). There are clear differences between the phase-delay values in the upper row and those in the lower row of the figure that are due to several differences between the stimuli used. In the upper row the stimulus was AM noise modulated at the same rate and presented at different intensity levels, whereas in the bottom row, exponential sinusoidally amplitude-modulated (SAM) tones were presented at 55 dB SPL, each tone being modulated at a different rate. The large shifts in phase values between the upper and lower rows are related to the different modulation envelopes used in the two test protocols (as well as the use of tones rather than noise).

The regularity of the changes with intensity (top row in Figure 2–10) and carrier and modulation frequency (bottom row) suggests that deriving expected phase from either population norms or self-norms will work well. The expected phases may be used either in formal phase-biasing techniques or in an informal method that enables audiologists to anticipate whether a small ASSR may reach significance at lower intensity levels, and for detecting spurious responses that may occur as a result of infiltration of the ASSR frequency bin by noise energy.

Issues of Artifact

Because issues related to performing ASSR testing with bone conduction (or high intensity air-conducted stimuli) are reviewed in Chapter 11 by Small and Stapells, as well as within several articles in the literature (e.g., Gorga et al., 2004; Picton & John, 2004; Small & Stapells, 2004), the technical aspects of how to avoid artifact are not reviewed here. Instead a description of how non-ASSR electromagnetic energy can enter the ASSR bin and create spurious detection of ASSRs is provided.

On the top left of Figure 2–11, a 1000 Hz carrier is shown that is modulated at 80 Hz. It is converted from a digital to an analog signal at a rate of 32 kHz, which typically is the minimum rate used for generation of steady-state stimuli. This is so fast that individual time points in the figure are not distinguishable, and the waveform appears as a continuous line. The black dots represent samples of a concurrent analog-to-digital conversion at 500 Hz. This is the minimum sample rate that would normally be used for obtaining the EEG during ASSR measurements. The right panel shows the resampled waveform, which results from using the 500-Hz analog-to-digital rate. The 500-Hz sampling rate is not fast enough to accurately represent the original waveform. Rather than an AM 1000-Hz stimulus, which has no energy at the modulation frequency, the undersampled waveform contains energy *only* at the modulation rate (this energy is positively biased above zero volts, which is known as a "DC offset," but the offset does not affect our ASSR estimate).

This energy at the modulation rate can be mistaken for an ASSR when two unde-

sirable conditions happen together. First, electromagnetic energy from the stimulus must somehow contaminate the EEG electrodes or EEG amplifier before the analog-to-digital conversion circuitry. Second, the analog low-pass filters of the EEG amplifier must have too shallow a roll-off slope, or attenuation factor, to completely attenuate the high-frequency energy of the stimulus. Once the signal has been digitized, subsequent digital filtering will not be able to remove this contamination because the energy from higher frequencies has already been aliased into the lower-frequency region, where it cannot be distinguished from the true energy related to the physiological responses and other noise.

The middle portion of Figure 2–11 shows the energy that exists in an auditory steady-state stimulus having four AM carriers. Also shown is how 6 dB/octave and 12 dB/octave low-pass, anti-aliasing filters will attenuate the stimulus energy to prevent it from entering the ASSR bin (the filters have been staggered in the drawing for clarity, but they are meant to have similar cutoff frequencies; the vertical amplitude axis is different for the ASSR stimulus and for the filters). Filter A would fail to eliminate electromagnetic energy from the 500-Hz carrier that was induced on the "input" signal that is recorded (e.g., by the electrodes picking up signals generated from the acoustic transducers).

The bottom portion of Figure 2–11 shows how stimulus energy can be aliased or "folded" back into the spectral range within which the ASSR is measured (i.e., 70 to 120 Hz), when either a 1000-Hz or 1250-Hz sampling rate is used to collect data. When 1000-Hz sampling is used (left column), the FFT will provide estimates of the EEG signal energy from 0 to

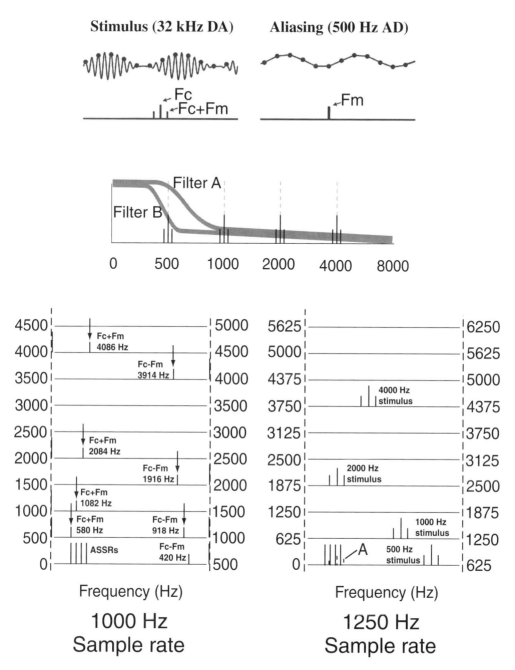

Figure 2–11. Issues of aliasing. Aliased energy from the stimulus can show up as spurious ASSRs. The *left top panel* shows a 1000-Hz tone amplitude modulated at 80 Hz, and that same tone sampled at 500 Hz (*black dots*). The *right top panel* shows the waveform produced by the 500-Hz sampling rate. Although the original waveform contains energy at Fc ± Fm, the undersampled waveform contains energy at Fm, which is the frequency at which the ASSR will be evoked. The *middle portion* of the figure shows two filters, A and B, in relation to the stimulus energy. The *bottom portion* of the figure shows where the aliased energy will show up in the resulting amplitude spectra. Using a 1000-Hz or 1250-Hz sampling rate will cause the aliased energy to show up as ASSR energy or noise energy, respectively.

the Nyquist frequency of 500 Hz. In other words, the 1000-Hz sampling rate, which is what might be used in actual ASSR testing, provides only the bottom row shown in the left column spanning from 0 to 500 Hz. This is a truncated version of the true EEG spectrum. If sampling at 10,000 or 100,000 Hz, rather than 1000 Hz, was relied upon, then aliasing would not be an issue, and a better representation of the true energy in the EEG would be obtained. Sampling at such high rates, however, puts a large burden on the computer's memory and resources, so this normally is not done.

Ten rows in Figure 2–11 show spectral segments of the true EEG spectrum. In the left column, the spectral ranges of each segment sequentially increase in 500-Hz steps and altogether show the range 0 to 5000 Hz. For example, the bottom row illustrates the lowest-frequency range, 0 to 500 Hz, and the row above that is the next-highest range, 500 to 1000 Hz. The four large spikes in the bottom row represent the signals estimated at the ASSR frequencies. The modulation rates are 80, 82, 84, and 86 Hz for the carriers 500, 1000, 2000, and 4000 Hz, respectively. The rows above this cannot be captured accurately with a sampling rate of 1000 Hz. Unfortunately, without adequate low-pass filtering, the energy contained in these higher-frequency rows will be aliased to the 0- to 500-Hz range and can show up as spurious energy at the frequencies at which the ASSRs occur. What energy exists in the high-frequency spectral ranges shown in the upper rows of the left column? The carrier sidebands at Fc + Fm and Fc − Fm (marked by downward-pointing arrows) will alias *exactly* into the spectral bins where the ASSRs are measured. The carrier frequencies themselves alias to 0 Hz and do not affect the ASSR estimates.

By using a sampling rate of 1250 Hz, the stimulus energy aliases into the noise bins, rather than into the ASSR bins. This noise artifact is shown by the dotted lines labeled as A on the bottom row of the right column which is the aliased spectral energy of the stimulus. Of note, although using a sampling rate of 1250 Hz will prevent spurious ASSR detection, the energy that aliases into the noise bins will serve to increase the noise energy estimate against which the ASSR signal may be compared. If a measure such as the F-120 is used, which evaluates 60 bins on each side of the ASSR bin for the noise estimate, this additional energy may average out to become of little consequence; however, a statistic that relies upon only 10 bins per side (i.e., an F-20), may not fare as well.

These issues of aliased artifact can be avoided entirely by using low-pass filters with sufficiently steep slopes before digitization, or by using higher analog-to-digital conversion rates. The sampling rate must be high enough that the Nyquist frequency is above the highest frequency in the stimulus. For example, a 4-kHz carrier (and its sideband energy at Fc ± Fm) could be accurately represented by a sampling rate of 10 kHz with a Nyquist frequency of 5 kHz.

It is possible to test for electromagnetic signal–related artifacts by playing sounds above a set intensity level (e.g., 80 dB SPL) while simultaneously recording from electrodes that have been placed in a glass of saline. This is a very stringent test because no biological noise is present, so this test can easily result in false ASSR detection (e.g., with energy levels that are much lower than normal, such as 0.04 nV, because the noise floor can be 0.01 nV or lower). A more useful test may be to record from a patient who has very-low-noise EEG signal and to occlude the transducer (or, more stringently, put it into a Zwislocki coupler so that the acoustic impedance is similar to what occurs in the ear) so that there is no way that the patient can hear the sounds (this is easy to do with ear-insert speakers). It also is possible to identify aliasing-related artifact by changing the filter setting of the ASSR equipment, or the sampling rates used to collect EEG data, and investigate the changes in ASSR amplitude that occur when the electrodes are in saline.

Three common methods of decreasing the risks and effects of artifact are to use insert earphones, rather than headphones; to braid the EEG electrode wires; and to use non-mastoid references for bone conduction stimuli. An additional method is to use stimuli that are designed to alternate within each epoch, or to alternate stimulus polarity across different epochs, so that on average, any aliased energy will cancel itself out (Picton & John, 2004; Small & Stapells, 2004). As noted earlier, when filtering and sampling rates are not sufficient to completely attenate aliased energy, it is possible to decrease the effects of aliasing-related artifact by selecting analog-to-digital conversion rates as a function of the energy profile of the stimulus, so that the stimulus energy will not alias back into the ASSR bins.

Auditory Steady-State Response Testing with Different Audiometric Configurations

In performing ASSR testing in patients, the degree of hearing loss can alter the testing procedure. In cases of mild hearing loss, ASSRs evoked by stimuli at 60 dB SPL are relatively large and can become significant within 2 to 5 minutes. However, for certain types of disorders, or when thresholds are greatly elevated, the responses at 60 dB may be small (i.e., 60 dB SPL may only be 5 to 10 dB SL). In such instances, the background noise must be reduced sufficiently by collecting additional sweeps of data. Because the amplitude of the noise is decreased by the square root of the number of sweeps collected at a given intensity level (i.e., the duration of the test), this may take some time. In infants, in order to detect small signals of about 10 to 15 nV evoked by steady-state stimuli that are modulated at rates of 80 to 100 Hz, and presented at moderate intensity levels, the noise must be reduced to levels of about 5 to 9 nV (root-mean-square). This noise level also may be required when hearing loss is present, even with testing at higher levels. Additionally, if the recording time is arbitrarily set too short, then small responses will not be recognized, and the estimated thresholds (even using regression) will be elevated (Luts & Wouters, 2004; Picton, John, Dimitrijevic, & Purcell, 2003). As a result of physiological recruitment, the size of ASSRs may grow rapidly with testing at 5 dB above threshold in cases of hearing loss above, for example, 60 dB, and 90 seconds may be sufficient to obtain useful threshold information. If, however, the ASSRs from normal patients are assessed after only 90 seconds of recording, thresholds will be about 20 dB higher than if recordings are allowed to go as long as 12 to 18 minutes at near-threshold levels. The material presented elsewhere in this chapter must be contemplated within the context of these issues.

Summary

This chapter reviewed some basic technical concepts of ASSR testing. The emphasis has been on clarification of particular issues that seem to repeatedly reemerge both in the clinic and in the literature, as a result of a misunderstanding of these principles. It also has provided some insight into the nature of the energy that is measured both as the ASSR and background noise. This material has been presented to elucidate a number of phenomena that emerge during ASSR testing: If an ASSR is immediately significant and then stops being significant after 4 or 5 sweeps, the audiologist may now not become concerned that an ASSR strangely "vanished," but will realize that the initial "ASSR" could have been due to noise energy in the same bin as the ASSR. Furthermore, rather than conceptualizing ASSR testing as an automated method, and simply waiting for an ASSR to reach significance, audiologists can use other available strategies, such as examining the phase of the ASSR, evaluating the current level of EEG noise with respect to a noise criterion, retesting the ASSR using a single modulated carrier, and using sequential testing with appropriate statistical considerations.

A public forum that is not specifically related to any specific commercial system is currently available to the community of ASSR users and is located at http://www.mastersystem.ca.

Key Points

- There are two factors that determine the characteristics of the frequency bins of amplitude spectra: The first is the length of the dataset that is submitted to the FFT algorithm, and the second is the rate at which the data were sampled. The length of the dataset determines the frequency resolution so that for every doubling of the data set duration (i.e., sweep length), the frequency resolution is also doubled. For example, a 1-s data set will produce a frequency resolution of 1 Hz, and a 2-s data set will produce a frequency resolution of 0.5 Hz. The sampling rate will determine the maximum frequency which can be represented by the FFT. This maximum frequency (the Nyquist frequency) is half the sampling rate.

- It is important to ensure that the modulation rates of the auditory steady-state stimuli fit exactly into the stimulus buffer. This will enable the stimulus to be played continuously without discontinuities between the end of one stimulus buffer and the beginning of the next. Using modulation rates that exactly fit into the stimulus buffer also ensures that an integer number of evoked ASSRs will fit exactly into the data buffer, causing the ASSRs to fit exactly into the frequency bins of the FFT without producing "spectral leakage."

- A Bonferroni correction, achieved by dividing the statistical criterion (e.g., $p < .05$) by the number of statistical tests carried out, is too conservative for use in ASSR testing because the ASSR estimates during the later parts of the testing session may be highly correlated. It also is too conservative because it may be physiologically impossible to produce an ASSR large enough to meet the statistical adjustment, especially at lower intensities.

■ Different types of energy can reside in the frequency bin in which an ASSR is measured: (1) true ASSR energy; (2) background EEG; (3) the electromyogram (EMG); (4) non-brain-evoked activity including postauricular muscle response (PAMR), sternocleidomastoid response (recorded from the lateral neck), and the posterior neck muscles (recorded from the inion electrode); (5) the cochlear microphonic; (6) instrumentation or "electromagnetic" energy at the frequency of the ASSR; (7) general noise energy from the EEG amplifiers; (8) aliased energy; and (9) energy from lower frequencies, which does not fit into a bin exactly, that "leaks" into higher-frequency bins that are used to assess ASSRs.

Acknowledgments. The authors wish to thank Terry Picton, Hedvig Soderlund, Patricia van Roon, Heleen Luts, and Gary Rance for reviewing the manuscript. Funding from CIHR enabled collection of the infant data presented in Figure 2–10.

References

Bijl, G. K., & Veringa, F. (1985). Neural conduction time and steady-state evoked potentials. *Electroencephalography and Clinical Neurophysiology, 62*, 465–467.

Cebulla, M., Sturzebecher, E., Elberling, C., & Wafaa, S. D. (2007). *New chirp stimuli for hearing screening.* International Evoked Response Audiometry Study Group (IERASG) XX IERASG Meeting, Bled, Slovenia.

Cebulla, M., Sturzebecher, E., & Elberling, C. (2006). Objective detection of auditory steady-state responses: Comparison of one-sample and q-sample tests. *Journal of the American Academy of Audiology, 17*(2), 93–103.

Cohen, L. T, Rickards, F. W, & Clark, G. M. (1991). A comparison of steady-state evoked potentials to modulated tones in awake and sleeping humans. *Journal of the Acoustical Society of America, 90*, 2467–2479.

Dobie, R. A., & Wilson, M. J. (1996). A comparison of t test, F test, and coherence methods of detecting steady-state auditory-evoked potentials, distortion-product otoacoustic emissions, or other sinusoids. *Journal of the Acoustical Society of America, 100*, 2236–2246.

Dobie, R. A., & Wilson, M. J. (1994). Phase weighting: A method to improve objective detection of steady-state evoked potentials. *Hearing Research, 79*(1–2), 94–98.

Gorga, M. P., Neely, S. T., Hoover, B. M., Dierking, D. M., Beauchaine, K. L., & Manning, C. (2004). Determining the upper limits of stimulation for auditory steady-state response measurements. *Ear and Hearing, 25*(3), 302–307.

Hari, R., Hamalainen, M., & Joutsiniemi, S. L. (1989). Neuromagnetic steady state responses to auditory stimuli. *Journal of the Acoustical Society of America, 86*, 1033–1039.

Herdman, A. T., Lins, O., Van Roon, P., Stapells, D. R., Scherg, M., & Picton, T. W. (2002). Intracerebral sources of human auditory steady-state responses. *Brain Topography, 15*(2), 69–86.

Hekimoglu, Y., Ozdamar, O., & Delgado, R. (2001). *Chirp and click evoked auditory steady state responses.* Institute of Electrical and Electronics Engineers Engineering in Medicine and Biology Society IEEE EMBS 23rd Annual International Conference, Istanbul, Turkey.

John, M. S., Brown, D. K., Muir, P. J., & Picton, T. W. (2004). Recording auditory steady-state responses in young infants. *Ear and Hearing*, 25(6), 539-553.

John, M. S., Dimitrijevic, A., & Picton, T. W. (2003). Efficient stimuli for evoking auditory steady-state responses. *Ear and Hearing*, *24*(5), 406-423.

John, M. S., Dimitrijevic, A., & Picton, T. W. (2002a). Auditory steady-state responses to exponential modulation envelopes. *Ear and Hearing*, *23*, 106-117.

John, M. S., Purcell, D. W., Dimitrijevic, A., & Picton, T. W. (2002b). Advantages and caveats when recording steady-state responses to multiple simultaneous stimuli. *Journal of the American Academy of Audiology*, *13*(5), 246-259.

John, M. S., & Picton, T. W. (2000). Human auditory steady-state responses to amplitude-modulated tones: phase and latency measurements. *Hearing Research*, *141*(1-2), 57-79.

Lins, O. G., & Picton, T. W. (1995). Auditory steady-state responses to multiple simultaneous stimuli. *Electroencephalography and Clinical Neurophysiology*, *96*, 420-432.

Lins, O. G., Picton, T. W., Boucher, B. L., Durieux-Smith, A., Champagne, S. C., Moran, L. M., et al. (1996). Frequency-specific audiometry using steady-state responses. *Ear and Hearing*, *17*(2), 81-96.

Luts, H., Van Dun, B., Alaerts, J., & Wouters, J. (2007). *Objective detection of ASSR: Do's and don'ts.* International Evoked Response Audiometry Study Group (IERASG) XX Meeting, Bled, Slovenia.

Luts, H., & Wouters, J. (2004). Hearing assessment by recording multiple auditory steady-state responses: the influence of test duration. *International Journal of Audiology*, *43*(8), 471-478.

Picton, T. W., & John, M. S. (2004). Avoiding electromagnetic artifacts when recording auditory steady-state responses. *Journal of the American Academy of Audiology*, *15*(8), 541-554.

Picton, T. W., John, M. S., Dimitrijevic, A., & Purcell, D. (2003). Human auditory steady-state responses. *International Journal of Audiology*, *42*(4), 177-219.

Picton, T. W., Dimitrijevic, A., John, M. S., & van Roon, P. (2001). The use of phase in the detection of auditory steady-state responses. *Clinical Neurophysiology*, *112*, 1692-1711.

Picton, T. W., Durieux-Smith, A., Champagne, S. C., Whittingham, J., Moran, L. M., Giguere, C., et al (1998). Objective evaluation of aided thresholds using auditory steady-state responses. *Journal of the American Academy of Audiology*, *9*(5), 315-331.

Regan, D. (1989). *Human brain electrophysiology: Evoked potentials and evoked magnetic fields in science and medicine.* Amsterdam: Elsevier.

Regan, D. (1966). Some characteristics of average steady-state and transient responses evoked by modulated light. *Electroencephalography and Clinical Neurophysiology*, *20*, 238-248.

Sankoh, A. J., Huque, M. F., & Dubey, S. D. (1997). Some comments on frequently used multiple endpoint adjustment methods in clinical trials. *Statistics in Medicine*, *16*(22), 2529-2542.

Small, S. A., & Stapells, D. R. (2004). Artifactual responses when recording auditory steady-state responses. *Ear and Hearing*, *25*(6), 611-623.

Sturzebecher, E., Cebulla, M., & Elberling, C. (2005). Automated auditory response detection: Statistical problems with repeated testing. *International Journal of Audiology*, *44*(2), 110-117.

Sturzebecher, E., Cebulla, M., & Pschirrer, U. (2001). Efficient stimuli for recording of the amplitude modulation following response. *Audiology*, *40*, 63-68.

Valdes, J. L., Perez-Abalo, M. C., Martin, V., et al. (1997). Comparison of statistical indicators for the automatic detection of 80 Hz auditory steady state responses. *Ear and Hearing*, *18*, 420-429.

Van der Reijden, C. S., Mens, L. H., & Snik, A. F. (2007). Improving recording and stimulus conditions of ASSRs in infants and adults. International Evoked Response Audiometry Study Group (IERASG) XX Meeting, Bled, Slovenia.

Van der Reijden, C. S., Mens, L. H., & Snik, A. F. (2005). EEG derivations providing auditory steady-state responses with high signal-to-noise ratios in infants. *Ear and Hearing, 26*(3), 299–309.

Zar, J. H (1999). *Biostatistical analysis* (4th ed., pp. 618–624). Upper Saddle River, NJ: Prentice Hall.

CHAPTER 3

The Stimulus-Response Relationship in Auditory Steady-State Response Testing

DAVID W. PURCELL
HILMI R. DAJANI

This chapter explores how the auditory steady-state response (ASSR) changes with the stimulus that is used to elicit it. In the previous chapter, a variety of stimuli were described, such as amplitude-modulated (AM) tones, tone pairs, repeated clicks and tone bursts, and more complex waveforms that include a combination of amplitude and frequency modulation. The effects of these different stimulus types are discussed next, but it is important to recognize that in general, the stimuli used to elicit ASSRs share three defining parameters that play important roles in the response. These

three stimulus parameters in common are rate, intensity, and carrier frequency.

The *rate* is the frequency at which the stimulus varies in amplitude, frequency, or both. For AM or frequency-modulated (FM) stimuli, rate refers to the modulation frequency. For tone pairs that cause beating, rate refers to the rate of the beat, or fluctuation in amplitude envelope, which is the difference in frequency between the two carrier tones. Finally, for click or tone burst stimuli, rate is the frequency of stimulus repetition. Rate is particularly important because it is the frequency at which the response is evaluated in the spectrum of the averaged electroencephalogram (EEG) sweeps. Because many common stimuli include explicit amplitude modulation, this chapter generally refers to rate as the *modulation frequency*.

The most familiar of the three common stimulus parameters is *intensity*, which, as it normally does, refers to the root-mean-square (RMS) level of the presented stimulus specified with a decibel scale such as dB SPL (sound pressure level), dB HL (hearing level), or dB SL (sensation level). Finally, the *carrier frequency* is the frequency of the sinusoid to which modulation is applied. By specifying the carrier frequency, the response can be initiated from a desired characteristic region in the tonotopic cochlea. Sometimes broad-band noise is used instead of a tone, in which case there is no carrier frequency, but rather a noise carrier. This chapter describes the effects of these parameters in detail.

Many clinical instruments use ASSRs elicited by stimuli whose modulation rates are unique to each ear. Analysis of the average EEG spectrum then typically treats responses from the two ears as independent. However, the ASSR also can be elicited using identical modulation rates in each ear simultaneously. This allows these binaural measurements to be compared with monaural measurements elicited by the same stimulus. Alternatively, dichotic unmodulated stimuli can be presented to each ear. The response then relies on interactions in the auditory nervous system to produce modulation through binaural beating. These methods allow binaural interactions to be studied. This chapter discusses the binaural techniques that have been developed and their potential value for future clinical use.

Modulation Rate

In humans, the effect of modulation rate on the ASSR has been investigated over a broad frequency range: from about 2 Hz up to about 600 Hz (e.g., Campbell, Atkinson, Francis, & Green, 1977; Cohen, Rickards, & Clark, 1991; Galambos, Makeig, & Talmachoff, 1981; Geisler, 1960; Rickards & Clark, 1984; Rees, Green, & Kay, 1986; Stapells, Linden, Suffield, Hamel, & Picton, 1984). When all other stimulus parameters are held constant, the amplitude and phase of the ASSR varies with modulation rate. Figure 3–1, reproduced here from a report by Picton, John, Dimitrijevic, and Purcell (2003; their Figure 10), plots data from many studies that looked at different ranges of modulation. These studies did not use uniform carrier frequencies or stimulus levels, but the plots show the general effect of modulation rate on the amplitude of the response. It can be seen that at very low frequencies (below 10 Hz), and in the region of 40 Hz, the response is at its largest. Another, smaller amplitude peak is evident in the range 80 to 100 Hz, after which the response decreases towards both zero and the noise floor at higher modulation rates.

Most investigations of modulation rate have used sequential measurements wherein the modulation rate (as well as all other stimulus parameters) is fixed during a given measurement and then changed in between measurements. This is because the Fourier transform typically used in the analysis requires there to be no changes in stimulus or response for optimal performance. Using other analysis techniques, however, does make it possible to change a stimulus parameter, such as modulation, within a given measurement. By ramping or sweeping

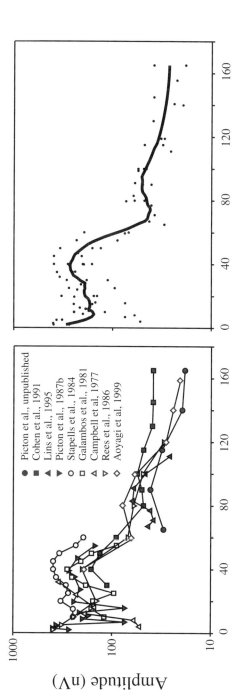

Rate or Modulation Frequency (Hz)

Figure 3–1. Effects of stimulus rate or modulation frequency. The *left graph* shows data from nine different studies in which the rate of stimulation or the modulation frequency was manipulated. The stimuli were all AM tones, except for the Galambos study, which used clicks, and the Stapells study, which used tone bursts. Stimulus intensity varied between 55 and 70 dB HL. The data were made comparable using the following procedures: Peak-to-peak amplitudes have beer halved to make them equivalent to baseline-to-peak measurements. The amplitudes of the responses to binaural stimuli also have been halved. The binaural effect varies with different stimulus rates, with binaural responses being about 200% of the monaural responses at rapid rates (Lins et al., 1995) and 150% at slow rates (Rees et al., 1986). Responses measured by visual analysis in the time domain usually are larger than measured by computer analys s in the frequency domain, because the peaks in the time domain are enhanced by superimposed activity at other frequencies. Responses measured in the time domain were therefore multiplied by 0.75 to make them equivalent to those recorded in the frequency domain. Most of the results at frequencies less than 60 Hz are for awake participants. If the participants were asleep, these amplitudes probably would be reduced by a factor of 2 or 3 (Cohen et al., 1991). The actual stimuli in each of the experiments were as follows: Picton et al. (unpublished studies): AM tones at 60 dB SPL (measurements combined over multiple carrier frequencies); Cohen et al. (1991): 55 dB HL tones, AM, binaural; Lins et al. (1995): 1000-Hz AM tone at 60 dB SPL; Picton et al. (1987b): 70 dB nHL AM 1000-Hz tones; Campbell et al. (1977): 500-Hz AM tone; Stapells et al. (1984): 60 dB nHL tone bursts of 500 Hz; Galambos et al. (1981): clicks of unspecified intensity; Rees et al. (1986): 60 dB SL AM 1000-Hz tones; Aoyagi et al. (1999): 50 dB HL AM 1000-Hz tones. The *right graph* plots the general trend of the various datasets plotted on the left. Each point on the *smooth curve* was fitted using a window of 22 points, with the points weighted using a bisquare function of the distance from the point being smoothed, and with the lines between the smoothed points interpolated using a second-degree polynomial. (Reprinted with permission from Picton, T. W., John, M. S., Dimitrijevic, A., & Purcell, D. W., *International Journal of Audiology, 42*(4), 177–219, 2003 [Figure 10, p. 191]; see http://www.informaworld.com)

modulation frequency, the effect of rate can be observed more continuously over a desired range (Linden, Campbell, Hamel, & Picton, 1985; Regan, 1973, 1989; Sapsford, Pickworth, & Jones, 1996). Figure 3–2, adapted from a report by Purcell, John, Schneider, and Picton (2004; their Figure 2), shows the average ASSR from five awake participants to an AM 1-kHz tone that was swept in modulation rate from 35 to 100 Hz over 15.36 s. The largest response is at a rate just above 40 Hz, and a smaller, local maximum is evident just above 90 Hz.

As mentioned previously, when the modulation rate of a tone increases beyond 100 Hz, the response decreases in amplitude and ultimately cannot be distinguished from background noise. The amplitude of the ASSR can be increased by using a noise carrier instead of a tone (John, Lins, Boucher, & Picton, 1998; Rees et al., 1986). This may allow the effect of higher modulation frequencies to be observed before the response dis-

appears into the noise. Figure 3–3, also adapted from a report by Purcell et al. (2004; their Figure 5), shows the average ASSR amplitude and phase responses from 14 sleeping young adults at two different ranges of modulation of a noise carrier. Panel a) shows rates from 20 to 100 Hz and a maximum in the response amplitude can again be seen just above 40 Hz. A second, albeit smaller peak is evident in the region of 90 Hz. Panel c) plots data for rates from 100 to 600 Hz. Although some fine structure can be seen in the amplitude versus rate function, the ASSR decreases in amplitude until it is no longer distinguishable from noise at about 485 Hz. The depth of modulation used to obtain the data in Figure 3–3 was only 25%. As discussed later, a modulation depth of 100% would have evoked a larger response and may have permitted the response to be detected at even higher modulation rates. The low modulation depth and sleep are responsible for the smaller amplitudes in Figure 3–3

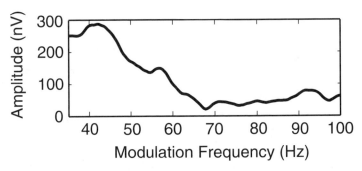

Figure 3–2. Grand average of responses from five awake participants. Response amplitude is shown as the rate was swept from 35 to 100 Hz for 100% amplitude modulation of a 1-kHz pure-tone carrier presented at 60 dB SPL. (Adapted with permission from Purcell, D. W., John, M. S., Schneider, B. A., & Picton, T. W., *Journal of the Acoustical Society of America*, *116*(6), 3581–3593, 2004 [Figure 2, p. 3585]. Copyright 2004, Acoustical Society of America.)

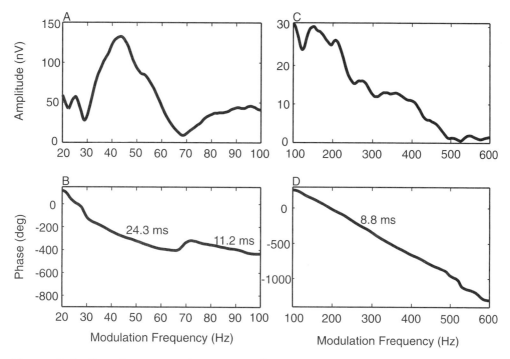

Figure 3–3. Grand average of responses from 14 young sleeping adults. Panels A (amplitude) and B (phase) show the responses to 25% amplitude-modulated white noise presented at 60 dB SPL in the range 20 to 100 Hz. Similarly, panels C (amplitude) and D (phase) show the responses for the range 100 to 600 Hz. (Adapted with permission from Purcell, D. W., John, M. S., Schneider, B. A., & Picton, T. W., *Journal of the Acoustical Society of America, 116*(6), 3581–3593, 2004 [Figure 5, p. 3588]. Copyright 2004, Acoustical Society of America.)

compared with those in Figure 3-2, in which participants were awake and the depth was 100%.

The focus thus far has been the effect of modulation rate on the ASSR, but detection and estimation also are dependent on the level of the background EEG noise in the spectrum. This background noise is not "white" (equal or flat across frequency) but rather decreases with increasing frequency. To estimate the amplitude and phase of an ASSR, the relative level of the noise in the frequency region where the response is expected must be taken into consideration. As dis-

cussed earlier, this is determined by the modulation rate of the stimulus. In ASSR measurements, the background noise usually is estimated from the Fourier transform for a set of frequency bins that bracket the response frequency. A commonly used noise estimate employs the average of 60 bins on either side of the ASSR that span a range of about 7.32 Hz (sweep length is 16.384 s). Figure 3-4, reproduced from the published report by Picton and associates (2003; their Figure 7), shows the average EEG noise spectra from 2 to 200 Hz for 20 sleeping or drowsy participants, along with the

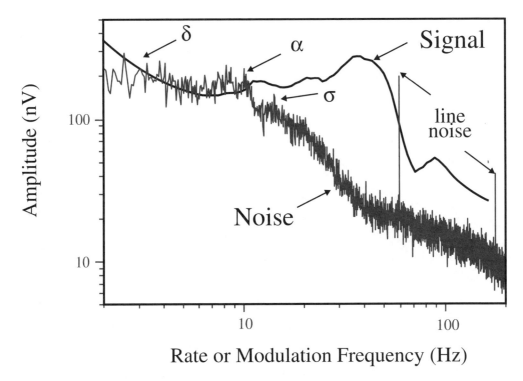

Rate or Modulation Frequency (Hz)

Figure 3–4. Measurements of signal and noise at different frequencies. The noise data were obtained from the spectra recorded when no stimuli were presented (Picton et al., 2001). For each of 20 subjects, 24 sweeps of 16.4 s were combined using weighted averaging. The plotted data represent the average (phase disregarded) of the amplitude spectra across the 20 participants. The two *vertical lines* represent the activities at the frequency of line noise and its third harmonic (60 and 180 Hz). The subjects were drowsy or asleep, and the background EEG noise shows slow delta activity (δ) with small peaks at the frequency of the alpha (α) rhythm (10 Hz) and spindle (σ) activity (14 to 16 Hz). The *smooth line* superimposed on the noise data plots the general amplitudes of the steady-state responses from Figure 3–1 using log-log coordinates, rather than the semilog coordinates used in that figure. (Reprinted with permission from Picton, T. W., John, M. S., Dimitrijevic, A., & Purcell, D. W., *International Journal of Audiology, 42*(4), 177–219, 2003 [Figure 7, p. 187]; see http://www.informa world.com.)

average ASSR response from Figure 3–1. Below 10 Hz, the noise is largest, thus making it more difficult to detect responses. Between 10 and 40 Hz, the noise drops quickly; it then decreases more slowly above 40 Hz.

In any given frequency range, the level of the ASSR (the signal of interest) relative to the level of the noise determines whether the response will be detectable. It also determines how accurately its amplitude and phase can be estimated. This is quantified with the *signal-to-noise ratio* (SNR), which is the ratio of the power of the signal to the power of the noise. Often it is represented in dB, so an SNR of 3 dB indicates that the power of the ASSR signal is approximately twice that of the noise. The *F-ratio*, commonly used to statistically evaluate whether a response is likely present, also compares the power of the signal estimate to the power of the noise estimate. The statistical significance of the response varies in part with the degrees of freedom of the noise estimate. However, for a noise estimate obtained using a reasonable number of Fourier transform bins, an SNR of 6 dB will indicate that the likelihood of the signal actually being noise is lower than $p < .05$ (*aside*: an SNR of 6 dB tells us the RMS amplitude of the ASSR is twice that of the noise). To obtain optimal estimates of ASSR amplitude and phase, it is desirable to have an SNR as large as possible.

As explained previously, the noise estimate can be obtained from frequencies neighboring the ASSR. If a statistical test indicates that the spike at the ASSR frequency is unlikely to be just noise, the amplitude of this spike often is treated as if it were the true ASSR amplitude. However, this estimate of ASSR amplitude also is contaminated by noise. The Fourier transform bin at the ASSR frequency contains both the true ASSR and noise (see Elberling & Don, 2007, pp. 104–105; Picton, Dimitrijevic, Perez-Abalo, & Van Roon, 2005, Appendix on p. 156). The level of this noise probably is similar to that of the noise estimate obtained at nearby frequencies. In practice, if the SNR is very good (e.g., greater than 10 dB), then the impact of the noise contamination will be small. This fact is pointed out here simply to raise awareness that as measurement conditions become poor, the numerical estimate of SNR will approach a ratio of 1, or 0 dB. This is because the signal estimate from the ASSR frequency bin becomes essentially only noise. If access to the true ASSR amplitude were

possible, then the ratio would approach 0, or a large negative value in dB, for extremely noisy conditions or a very small response.

At a given modulation rate, SNR can be maximized by increasing the ASSR amplitude, or by decreasing the background noise. Ways to increase ASSR amplitude include increasing stimulus intensity and also depth of modulation, as discussed further later on. Some studies also have suggested combining multiple recording channels (van der Reijden, Mens, & Snik, 2004) and the use of different channel sets for adults and infants (van der Reijden, Mens, & Snik, 2005). The noise can be decreased through an appropriate use of noise rejection and weighted averaging (John, Dimitrijevic, & Picton, 2001a), but the most important factor is recording time (Luts & Wouters, 2004; Picton et al., 2005). A longer recording time allows more sweeps in the average, which theoretically decreases the amplitude of the noise by $\sqrt{N}$ (noise power decreases by N), where N is the number of sweeps (e.g., Elberling & Don, 2007 [see pp. 106–109]; John, Dimitrijevic, & Picton, 2002a). In practical terms, however, the clinician is of course limited to how much time is available for any given measurement.

In review, ASSR amplitude (and hence power) varies with modulation frequency. The background EEG noise also varies with frequency. Therefore, SNR, the important relationship between signal and noise, will vary with frequency. The EEG noise and ASSR data from Figure 3–4 can be used to roughly demonstrate how SNR might change across frequency. In Figure 3–5, it is clear that some frequency bands are better than others for obtaining the ASSR, given a finite time available for collecting data. Here, the

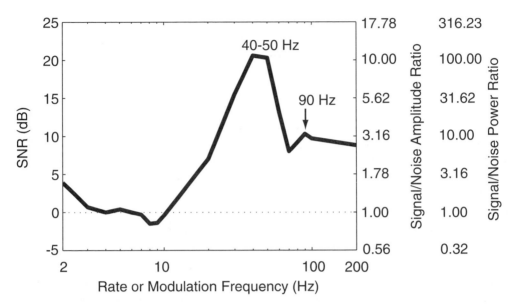

Figure 3–5. Signal and noise data from Figure 3–4 are replotted as signal-to-noise ratio (SNR) using a decibel scale on the *left vertical axis*. The *right vertical axis* shows the SNR values as a ratio of amplitudes and a ratio of powers. The best SNR occurs between 40 and 50 Hz, with a second, smaller peak at 90 Hz.

noise estimate is the average of 20 participants from whom 24 sweeps of 16.4 s were processed with weighted averaging. Both the background noise and (low-frequency) ASSR amplitude can be significantly affected by subject state, as discussed in Chapter 5 on subject-related variables. Of note, whereas the noise curve in Figure 3–4 was from sleeping participants, the ASSR curve was from awake individuals for frequencies less than 60 Hz. As a result, the curve in Figure 3–5 is instructive of only the general relationship between signal and noise. The background EEG noise would be expected to be higher for awake individuals (Cohen et al., 1991 [see their Figure 2]; Dobie & Wilson, 1998).

It can be seen in Figures 3–1 through 3–3 that the ASSR from the 40-Hz region is larger than at higher modulation rates. Despite the higher noise floor relative to higher frequencies, the SNR is relatively favorable in the region of 40 Hz. Therefore, measurements from this frequency band can be done reasonably quickly in waking adults, provided that muscle noise is controlled with proper head and neck support. The second region with a favorable SNR is between 80 and 100 Hz. The 40-Hz region typically is two to five times larger in amplitude than the 90-Hz region in waking adults (Picton, 2007), but this factor is smaller in sleep. Because infants have reduced responses in the 40-Hz range compared with adults (Levi, Folsom, & Dobie, 1995; van der Reijden et al., 2005) (see also Chapter 5) and it is desirable to test them while they sleep to reduce muscle artifacts, measuring ASSRs with modulation rates between 80 and 100 Hz can minimize recording time and maximize detection efficiency. Owing to their favorable SNR, these two frequency regions (40 to 50 Hz and 80 to 100 Hz) have been identified as efficient modulation rates for measuring ASSRs (Cohen et al., 1991 [see their Figure 9 and Table III]; Levi, Folsom, & Dobie, 1993; Dobie & Wilson, 1998). There is also evidence that the SNR in the 108- to 125-Hz range is similar to that in the 90-Hz range (Picton et al., 2005), making it useful as well for estimating audiometric thresholds. Of note, however, some modulation rates may elicit a smaller ASSR, such as near 70 Hz in Figure 3–5. If a particularly unfavorable rate is used, it could potentially lead to a poor SNR and subsequent overestimation of the behavioural hearing threshold at the carrier frequency associated with that modulation rate (e.g., Brennan & Stevens, 2007). Purcell and colleagues (2004) suggest that these dips in the ASSR amplitude versus modulation rate function could be due to destructive (out-of-phase) summation of responses from cortical and brainstem sources.

In addition to ASSR amplitude, modulation rate also affects the latency of the response (Rickards & Clark, 1984). Latency is a more easily understood measurement for transient-evoked potentials like the auditory brainstem response (ABR). For the ABR, the stimulus has a short duration (e.g., click) and the delay between the stimulus and the onset of the response (e.g., wave I) can be easily measured. The ASSR is an ongoing steady-state response that is elicited by a stimulus that lasts for many minutes at a time. There are therefore no obvious points in time to measure a delay between stimulus and response. The latency of the ASSR can, however, be estimated by calculating a delay value called *apparent latency* (Regan, 1966, 1989) or group delay (Goldstein, Baer, & Kiang, 1971; O Mahoney & Kemp, 1995).

Apparent latency makes use of the change in ASSR phase over a range in modulation frequency. It often is calculated by fitting a line to phase measurements made at several discrete modulation frequencies, or by using a swept modulation rate as described earlier. The equation for apparent latency makes sense if it is interpreted in terms of the units involved:

$$\text{Apparent latency (ms)} = 1000 \times (-\Delta\theta / 360°) / \Delta f$$

where

$\Delta\theta$ is the difference in ASSR phase (in degrees) between the highest modulation rate and the lowest modulation rate in the measurement range

Δf is the difference (in Hz) between the highest and lowest modulation rates in the measurement range

Dividing $\Delta\theta$ by 360 degrees per cycle gives the number of cycles elapsed over the measurement range. Dividing this by Δf in Hz, or cycles per second, leaves the units of seconds. Multiplying by 1000 milliseconds per second converts to milliseconds (ms), which is an appropriate unit for the physiological delays involved. The negative sign reconciles the fact that response onset phase decreases with increasing modulation rate (leading to a negative $\Delta\theta$), whereas latency must be a positive number. Said another way, the slope of the ASSR onset phase versus modulation frequency line is negative. In practice, the measured response onset phase is corrected using the onset phase of the acoustic stimulus measured in the ear canal. Instead of onset phase, response phase can be represented as phase lag, which is the difference between stimulus onset phase and response onset phase. It has a positive slope, so the negative sign in the foregoing equation is not required.

For apparent latency to be meaningful, the phase versus rate function must be linear and the measurement dominated by a single neural generator for the range of interest. This implicitly suggests that the measurement has very good SNR, but single-channel measurements cannot inform us about the possible presence of multiple sources of similar magnitude. To be dominant, a given generator's signal at the electrodes would require a magnitude much larger than the signals from any other generators (e.g., more than 20 dB larger).

In addition to amplitude, Figure 3–3 shows ASSR phase as a function of modulation rate. In panel B it can be seen that the slope of the phase response is different between the 40- and 90-Hz regions. The slope was steeper and the apparent latency (24.3 ms) was longer when calculated for the range 35 to 55 Hz. For the range 75 to 90 Hz with a shallower slope, the apparent latency was much shorter at only 11.2 ms. Panel D illustrates a further small decrease in apparent latency to 8.8 ms for the range 110 to 450 Hz.

Herdman and coworkers (2002a) determined the intracerebral sources of the ASSR at modulation rates of 12, 39, and 88 Hz. At both lower modulation rates, the measured ASSR represented the sum of sources in the brainstem and auditory cortex. However, at 88 Hz, the measurement was dominated by short latency brainstem activity. The measured phase data in the 40-Hz region of Figure 3–3 probably are due to the sum of a short latency brainstem source and longer latency cortical sources. The calculated value of 24.3 ms, therefore, probably underestimates the true latency of the cortical sources. For example, using magnetoencephalography (MEG) (albeit with different sinusoidal AM tone stimuli), Ross, Borgmann, Draganova, Roberts, and Pantev (2000) reported an apparent latency of 48 ms for cortical sources at a modulation rate of 40 Hz. At higher modulation rates, the apparent latencies near 10 ms are more likely to represent an accurate estimate of latency from brainstem sources. Purcell and colleagues (2004) modeled this change of source contributions from low to high modulation rates and found good correspondence with the measured data. Neural generators are discussed in detail in Chapter 4. See Table 1 in the published report by Picton and associates (2003) for a review of other latencies published in the literature.

Stimulus Intensity

Increasing stimulus intensity causes growth of ASSR amplitude and a decrease in latency (Galambos et al., 1981; Lins, Picton, Picton, Champagne, & Durieux-Smith, 1995; Picton, Skinner, Champagne, Kellett, & Maiste, 1987b; Picton et al., 2003; Rodriguez, Picton, Linden, Hamel, & Laframboise, 1986; Stapells et al., 1984; Vander Werff & Brown, 2005). Great individual variability, however, is observed in the absolute value of the amplitude for any given stimulus. Figure 3–6 shows some example average amplitudes at a rate of 80 Hz and level of 64 dB SPL that will be discussed in detail in the following section on stimulus type. As presented in the previous section, the 40-Hz response can be two to five times larger

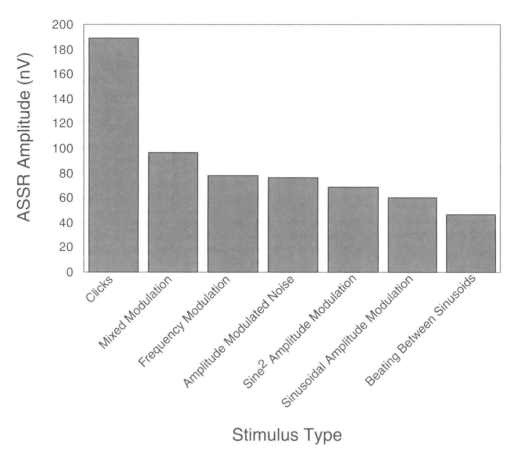

Figure 3–6. Average ASSR amplitudes from five participants in response to different stimuli with envelope or repetition rates of 80 Hz (numerical data are reported by Picton [2007, p. 445]). The intensities of the sounds were matched at 64 dB SPL.

than in the 80-Hz range, depending on subject factors. The growth in response amplitude is linear when the stimulus pressure change is, as usual, represented with a decibel scale (Galambos et al., 1981; Rees et al., 1986; Ross et al., 2000; Stapells et al., 1984). Recent data show that ASSR growth may be steeper above 60 dB SPL (Picton, Van Roon, & John, 2007 [see their Figure 7]). Response amplitude does, however, saturate at high stimulus levels (90 dB HL) (Picton et al., 2003). The response amplitude versus stimulus intensity slope varies

with stimulus type, rate, and carrier frequency (Rodriguez et al., 1986). Hearing loss increases this slope, which may be a physiological measure of recruitment (Picton et al., 2005). Picton and colleagues (2005) show average and individual amplitude changes with stimulus intensity for young, elderly, and hearing-impaired persons (see the Picton report's Figures 3, 5, 6, and in particular 9, with ±1 standard deviation ranges). Vander Werff and Brown (2005) also show individual and average examples of amplitude and phase changes for normal hearing and different hearing loss configurations as stimulus intensity is varied (see their Figures 5 through 7).

Changes in ASSR amplitude with increasing stimulus level begin in the cochlea. The higher intensity stimulus spreads basally on the basilar membrane and involves more sensory hair cells. This broadening of the response region will activate more afferent nerve fibers, which in turn increase the input to the ASSR generators in the brainstem and auditory cortex. Owing to traveling wave delays, not all of these fibers will fire in phase, but the net effect is an increase in synchronous neural activity. The effect on ASSR latency also begins with the changes in the basilar membrane response. Cochlear filter buildup time is shorter at higher intensities, and the peak of the response is closer to the middle ear. Above the level of the cochlea, synaptic delays will be smaller due to more contributing presynaptic inputs at each junction (Picton et al., 2003).

Stimulus Type

As discussed in Chapter 2 on recording ASSRs, a variety of stimulus types can be used to elicit ASSRs. The acoustic spectra of some are less frequency-specific than others (e.g., clicks and AM noise) but may still have applications in screening and research. Figure 3–6 shows average ASSR amplitudes from five participants in response to some of these stimuli with envelope or repetition rates of 80 Hz (numerical data are reported by Picton [2007, p. 445]). The intensities of the sounds were matched at 64 dB SPL (i.e., RMS). However, psychophysical detec-

tion is a function of duration and spectral content, which varies for the different stimuli. For any stimulus, the average detection threshold of normal-hearing persons is defined as 0 dB nHL (normal hearing level). Because sound pressure level (dB SPL) was fixed, the presentation level above normal-hearing threshold would be expected to vary for the different stimuli. This may have contributed to the relative ASSR amplitudes, because they were not matched in dB nHL. For clicks and AM noise, 64 dB SPL is only 46 dB nHL (46 dB above the threshold of normal-hearing persons). The more tonal stimuli were higher above threshold, with a level of 56 dB nHL. If the clicks and AM noise were matched in normal hearing level by raising their intensity 10 dB, their ASSR amplitudes would be larger (Picton, 2007).

It is clear that clicks elicit a relatively large response compared with other stimulus types, and although not shown, tone pip responses also are relatively large (John, Dimitrijevic, & Picton, 2003; Stürzebecher, Cebulla, & Neumann, 2003). However, the click is a broad-band stimulus, containing energy across a wide-frequency spectrum. It is therefore not useful for obtaining frequency-specific estimates of audiometric thresholds (at least without using masking noise to obtain derived bands). Beating between two sinusoids produces the smallest response—normally about 70% of the response to sinusoidal amplitude modulation (Picton et al., 2005)—and has not been favored in clinical ASSR instruments.

In Figure 3–6, the second-largest ASSR was elicited by a mixed-modulation (MM) stimulus. This stimulus contains both amplitude and frequency modulation at the same rate. The two types of modulation appear to be processed relatively independently by the auditory system. The response is therefore similar to the sum of the responses to AM and FM stimuli presented independently (Cohen et al., 1991; John, Dimitrijevic, van Roon, & Picton, 2001b). The possibility of multiple pathways is supported by the shorter apparent latency of responses to frequency modulation compared with those from amplitude modulation (John et al., 2001b; Picton et al., 1987b). The caveat of mixed modulation is that the AM and FM responses must add in phase (constructively) to achieve a large ASSR, and this is difficult to guarantee owing to individual variability and carrier frequency effects. Independent AM and FM (IAFM) stimuli differ from mixed modulation in that the rates used for amplitude and frequency modulation are different. The response at each rate is somewhat smaller than when the individual responses are measured in separate recordings (Dimitrijevic, John, Van Roon, & Picton, 2001; Picton et al., 2003).

The "add constructively" caveat for mixed modulation is sufficiently limiting that Picton and colleagues (e.g., Picton, 2007) now prefer to use amplitude modulation with an exponential sinusoidal envelope. A squared or cubed sinusoidal amplitude modulation ($\sin^2$ or $\sin^3$) produces both larger response amplitudes and longer latencies as the exponent is increased (John et al., 2002a). The effect is, however, largest for low and high carrier frequencies. The acoustic stimulus becomes less frequency-specific as the exponent increases, but this is not sufficient to limit cochlear place specificity in practice (Picton et al., 2003).

By optimizing SNR through choice of modulation frequency and stimulus type, we are able to most accurately estimate behavioural thresholds. For example, if the background noise is equal in two measurements at similar modulation rates, an exponentially modulated stimulus normally will elicit a larger ASSR than that to a sinusoidally modulated stimulus. This would improve the SNR, allowing the ASSR to be detected with a stimulus intensity closer to the true behavioural threshold. Accordingly, the accuracy of the threshold estimate improves. Research is ongoing to improve ASSR stimuli by maximizing the response amplitude. For example, Stürzebecher, Cebulla, Elberling, and Berger (2006) are investigating a chirp stimulus designed to better synchronize the response initiated in a narrow cochlear region by making use of modeled traveling wave delays (they also are using multiple harmonics of the modulation rate in the analysis).

Modulation Depth

ASSR amplitude increases as the depth of modulation is increased from low values to 100%. As is the case for stimulus intensity, this increase is linear when the depth of amplitude modulation is expressed using a logarithmic scale (Rees et al., 1986; Ross et al., 2000). Modulation depth commonly has been represented using decibels (20 log m, where m is the modulation depth from 0 to 1) in psychophysical work involving the behavioural detection of amplitude modulation (e.g., Viemeister, 1979).

For amplitude modulation, a higher modulation depth produces larger fluctuations in the envelope of the stimulus. At 100% amplitude modulation, the envelope goes to zero during each modulation cycle:

$$\text{Percent amplitude modulation} = 100(\text{max} - \text{min})/(\text{max} + \text{min})$$

where max and min are the maximum and minimum peak amplitudes of the modulated carrier. If the maximum amplitude of the envelope is fixed for different modulation depths, then a 100% AM signal will have a smaller RMS intensity than a signal with only 50% modulation depth. This is because where the envelope goes to zero for 100% amplitude modulation, there is no carrier signal contributing energy to the RMS value. The ASSR amplitude thus will reach its maximum at a depth of 50% if the stimulus is fixed in maximum envelope amplitude (Lins et al., 1995; Picton et al., 1987b). Adjusting the maximum envelope amplitude to maintain equal RMS intensity for different depths, however, produces the largest ASSR for 100% amplitude modulation (Dimitrijevic et al., 2001; John et al., 2001b). ASSR phase is unaffected by depth of amplitude modulation for values larger than 25% (Picton et al., 2003).

Frequency modulation also elicits a larger ASSR as the depth of modulation is increased. This has been measured up to depths of 50% for the 80-Hz modulation range (John et al. 2001b) and 50% (Picton, Dauman, & Aran, 1987a) or 90% (Picton et al., 1987b) for the 40-Hz modulation range. Response phase is unaffected by the depth of frequency modulation. Care is required in reading the literature to note how individual studies define the amount of frequency modulation (the aforementioned studies all use the same definition). Engineers use the modulation index, which varies with modulation frequency instead of percentage frequency modulation, and the ASSR literature has used more than one definition of percentage frequency modulation (see Picton et al., 2003, p. 193).

Carrier Frequency

The amplitude of the ASSR varies with carrier frequency, and this variation is itself a function of the modulation range. Most work has been done for carrier frequencies between 500 Hz and 4000 Hz, which typically are spaced at octave intervals. The most common stimulus frequencies are then 500, 1000, 2000, and 4000 Hz, but values such as 250 or 1500 Hz, or very high frequencies (e.g., 12,000 Hz, as described by Tlumak, Durrant, and Collet [2007]), also are reported. These common carrier frequencies are, of course, chosen to be most consistent with behavioural threshold testing and important speech frequencies.

In the 40-Hz modulation range, the largest ASSR response occurs for the lowest carrier frequencies. As the carrier frequency is increased, the amplitude of the response decreases (Galambos et al., 1981; Picton et al., 1987b; Rodriguez et al., 1986; Ross, Draganova, Picton, & Pantev, 2003). This is in contrast with responses in the 80-Hz modulation range. Of the common carrier frequencies, 500 Hz generally has the smallest amplitude and is the most difficult to detect near behavioural threshold. At higher intensities, however, the 500-Hz response may actually be larger than the response to higher frequencies. A literature meta-analysis by Herdman and Stapells (2003) found threshold estimates at 500 Hz to be the least accurate, which reflects the smaller amplitude and hence worse SNR of the response at this carrier frequency. Chapter 7 discusses behavioural threshold estimation with the ASSR in detail. The highest 80-Hz ASSR amplitudes are found for carriers in the 1000- to 2000-Hz range, with amplitudes falling at 4000 Hz (John, Dimitrijevic, van Roon, & Picton, 2002b; John et al., 2001b, 2002a). It might be hypothesized that this band-pass shape reflects the best sensitivity region of the human ear, but these results hold for stimuli presented at constant dB HL values across carrier frequency (Dimitrijevic et al., 2002). In other words, raising the stimulus intensity at extreme carrier frequencies to compensate for human sensitivity is insufficient to equalize ASSR amplitude across carriers.

The latency of the ASSR decreases with increasing carrier frequency, which is partly a reflection of the shorter stimulus traveling wave delay to the characteristic region of the carrier on the basilar membrane. Previously reported decreases in latency between carriers of 500 and 4000 Hz range from 4 to 18 ms, with a mean of 9.5 ms (for individual study values, see Table 1 in Picton et al., 2003).

Single and Multiple Stimuli

Two of the most galvanizing concepts in ASSR measurement are the use of multiple simultaneous carrier frequencies in a given ear (Regan & Regan, 1988), and of concurrent testing of both ears (Lins & Picton, 1995). The promise of simultaneously evaluating the integrity of both cochleae at multiple frequencies is very attractive for rapidly demonstrating integrity of the auditory system in screening applications, and for objectively estimat-

ing behavioural thresholds. The use of multiple frequencies allows different regions of the cochlea to be tested so that audiometric configuration is properly identified (Herdman, Picton, & Stapells, 2002b). This helps to avoid false negatives (i.e., persons with hearing loss are not identified), which can occur when broad-band stimuli are used in screening applications. For example, hearing losses limited to any particular-frequency region of the cochlea (low-, middle-, or even high-frequency) may not be detected using the click-evoked ABR as a screening tool because the unmasked stimulus can elicit a response from any functional region (reviewed by Stapells [2000; see p. 15]). Tone-burst ABRs are of course frequency-specific, but different frequencies and ears normally are tested sequentially. Some clinical ASSR instruments now apply the four carrier frequencies 500, 1000, 2000, and 4000 Hz simultaneously in both ears. This measurement could theoretically be accomplished eight times faster than sequential ASSR measurements at the same frequencies. If a suprathreshold screening application were carried out with the eight stimuli, the full eightfold savings in time could potentially be realized. During threshold estimation, however, when it is necessary to wait for all responses to be recognized, the multiple-stimulus measurement is only two to three times faster than sequential measurements (John et al., 2002b). This is partly because not all instruments can vary the carrier intensities independently (John et al., 2002b). If the current stimulus intensity is near threshold for one carrier, data may be collected for an extended period to allow the small ASSR attributed to that carrier to be detected (or not). Other carriers that are suprathreshold must wait their turn until the stimulus intensity is reduced. Independent adjustment of the carrier intensities can win back some of this time, but interactions may occur if some carriers are of substantially higher intensity than that of their neighbors (John et al., 2002b).

Research on the use of multiple stimuli at different carriers (at the same intensity) with modulation rates in the 80-Hz range has shown that interactions are minimal and acceptable if certain rules are followed. A maximum of four carrier frequencies may be used per ear (Lins & Picton, 1995). The separation of these carrier frequencies must be greater than half an octave, and the stimulus intensity must be 60 dB SPL or less (John et al., 1998). Multiple stimuli greater than 60 dB SPL can lead to a saturation of the response amplitudes (Picton et al., 2007). When higher intensities are needed because of hearing loss, a single carrier frequency and single ASSR measurement is required to avoid reduced ASSR amplitudes through interactions largely within the cochlea.

Despite the decrease in ASSR amplitude that may occur with multiple stimuli, the technique is still time-efficient so long as the amplitudes remain at least as large as $100/\sqrt{N}$ % of the single-stimulus values, with N being the number of simultaneous carriers in a given ear (John et al., 1998). For four carriers in one ear, the responses must remain at least 50% of their amplitude when elicited sequentially. Any reduction of ASSR amplitude requires a lengthened recording time to reduce the background noise sufficiently such that an acceptable SNR is achieved. This lengthened recording time in the multiple-stimulus case is still shorter than N sequential measurements—hence, the efficiency of the technique is maintained

(John et al., 1998, 2002b). Herdman and colleagues (Herdman & Stapells, 2001, 2003; Herdman et al., 2002b) have shown that thresholds are not different when estimated with multiple or single stimuli. Multiple-stimulus interactions may be greater in infants, but Hatton and Stapells (2007) determined that multiple stimuli are still more efficient than sequential single measurements.

Interactions of neural origin are larger for multiple stimuli with modulation rates in the range of 40 Hz (John et al., 1998; Ross et al., 2003). Despite these larger amplitude reductions, Van Maanen and Stapells (2005) found that the multiple-stimulus technique in the 40-Hz range is still preferred for rapidly obtaining accurate estimates of behavioural thresholds in adults.

Tests of Binaural Processing

Binaural processing plays a very important role in hearing, as it underlies the perception of static and moving sound sources within auditory space. Moreover, binaural processing plays an essential role in enhancing a target sound source, such as the voice of a particular speaker, relative to competing sounds in noisy environments (Hawley, Litovsky, & Culling, 2004). Unfortunately, the remarkable abilities of the intact binaural system often degrade with disorders of central auditory processing or with age. Decline in binaural processing may largely account for the difficulty many older people have in understanding speech involving competing speakers (Murphy, Daneman, & Schneider, 2006). As a consequence, electrophysiological measures of binaural processing may prove helpful in the assessment and treatment of some generally neglected aspects of hearing impairment. Before candidate tests are considered, however, a brief tour of the binaural system follows.

Nerve impulses that originate in the left and right cochleae meet in the superior olivary complex (SOC) of the lower brainstem, after traveling along the auditory nerve and across a relay stage in the cochlear nucleus. The SOC is the first stage in the auditory system at which a comparison between inputs from the two ears can be performed (e.g., Tollin & Yin, 2005). With pure tones, neurons in the SOC are sensitive to two types of interaural cues that are encoded in the patterns of nerve impulses arriving from the two ears: *interaural time differences* (ITDs) at low frequencies and *interaural level differences* (ILDs) at high frequencies (e.g., Riedel & Kollmeier, 2002). Sensitivity to ITDs has received special attention because it is an indicator of temporal processing in the auditory system, and because—in contrast with sensitivity to ILDs—it has been found to degrade with aging (Babkoff et al., 2002; Herman, Warren & Wagner, 1977). For low-frequency pure tones (below around 1000 Hz), auditory nerve fibers and relay neurons in the cochlear nucleus encode ITDs by firing only at a precise phase angle in the sinusoidal cycle (but not necessarily in every cycle) and are therefore said to be *phase-locked* to the tone (e.g., Joris, Carney, Smith, & Yin, 1994). In this case, ITDs can be considered equivalent to *interaural phase differences* (IPDs).

Beyond the SOC, ITDs and ILDs may be converted to location and movement information before being relayed to higher centers (Riedel & Kollmeier, 2002). Sensitivity to static and dynamic directional cues has been found in higher centers that include the nucleus of the lateral lemnicus (Kuwada, Fitzpatrick, Batra, & Ostapoff, 2006), the inferior colliculus (e.g., Rose, Gross, Geisler, & Hind, 1966; Spitzer & Semple, 1993), the primary auditory cortex (e.g., Sovijärvi & Hyvärinen, 1974), and specialized cortical areas outside the primary auditory cortex (Griffiths, Green, Rees, & Rees, 2000; Warren, Zielinski, Green, Rauschecker, & Griffiths, 2002). Although the exact nature of the physiological operations that are performed in the different neural stages is not well understood, conceptually an operation equivalent to the estimation of interaural correlation is thought to form a basis for a variety of binaural perceptual phenomena (e.g., Trahiotis, Bernstein, Stern, & Buell, 2005). Any degradation in auditory temporal processing, and in the timing of nerve firing specifically, should degrade the estimation of interaural correlation, thereby distorting binaural processing. To summarize, then, binaural processing is performed in multiple cortical and subcortical stations, and many of its functions probably depend on accurate phase-locking—particularly that occurring in the brainstem and in more peripheral pathways.

The complexity of the binaural system and the variety of binaural perceptual phenomena suggest that electrophysiological responses could be used to test binaural processing using any of a number of paradigms. Of the measures that have been proposed, the most thoroughly studied has been the *binaural interaction component* (BIC) (Dobie & Berlin, 1979; Dobie & Norton, 1980) in the brainstem and middle latency responses. The BIC, sometimes also called the binaural difference potential (e.g., Riedel & Kollmeier, 2002), is obtained by taking the difference between the sum of the responses to stimuli (usually clicks) presented monaurally and the response to the same stimuli presented binaurally. The brainstem BIC remains of limited clinical use because it is not always reliably detected, particularly in young children and neonates (Cone-Wesson, Ma, & Fowler, 1997; Stollman, Snik, Hombergen, Nieuwenhuys, & ten Koppel, 1996). Moreover, although the BIC is larger for the middle latency and long latency cortical responses (McPherson & Starr, 1993, 1995), it is not clear what this BIC represents in terms of binaural processing (Picton et al., 1985; Ross, Tremblay, & Picton, 2007). Other responses to transient binaural stimuli also have been investigated, including responses to sudden shifts in interaural correlation and in lateralization of broadband noise (Jones, Pitman, & Halliday, 1991; McEvoy et al., 1990).

ASSRs have been used to study the BIC at modulation rates in the range of 40 Hz (Picton et al., 1985) and 80 Hz (Lins et al., 1995). The main finding was that the binaural response was approximately equal to either monaural response at 40 Hz, but it was close to the sum of the monaural responses at 80 Hz. More recently, a number of other steady-state electrophysiological measures of binaural processing have been investigated in normal-hearing subjects. Wong and Stapells (2004) compared behavioural and electrophysiological binaural masking-level differences (BMLDs) using ASSR signals with a carrier frequency of 500 Hz, masked by 200-Hz-wide noise centered at 500 Hz. BMLDs are obtained by subtracting thresholds where either the signal or the noise is 180 degrees out of phase in the two ears (SπNo or SoNπ) from thresholds at which the signal and the noise are in phase binaurally (SoNo). These researchers found that "cortical" ASSRs (with a modulation frequency of 7 or 13 Hz), but not "brainstem" ASSRs

(with a modulation frequency of 80 Hz), demonstrated BMLDs that are similar to behavioural BMLDs, and only for the case of SπNo.

Another measure that has been investigated is the steady-state response to binaural beats (Draganova, Ross, Wollbrink, & Pantev, 2007; Karino et al., 2006; Schwarz & Taylor, 2005). When a pure tone is presented in each ear, and the two tones have different frequencies, a perceptually faint binaural beat is evoked. The binaural beat is due to neural interactions in central auditory pathways, probably starting in the SOC, and is thought to depend on neural activity that is phase-locked to the tones in the auditory periphery and to the beat frequency more centrally (Karino et al., 2006; Kuwada, Kin, & Wickesberg, 1979; Wernick & Starr, 1968). Schwarz and Taylor (2005) recorded a response to a beat frequency of 40 Hz using tones with a mean frequency of 400 Hz. However, they were not able to record a response with tones having a mean frequency of 3200 Hz, probably because this frequency exceeds the upper limit for phase-locking. Using whole-head MEG, and with two tones of 500 and 540 Hz generating a binaural beat at 40 Hz, Draganova and colleagues (2007) detected sources for the response in the primary auditory cortex. Karino and coworkers (2006) also used MEG recordings, but at the much lower beat frequencies of 4 and 6.66 Hz, and detected sources of the evoked response in parietal and frontal cortical areas in addition to the auditory cortex. The phase of the response showed great variability across subjects, which suggested that this response reflected higher-order cognitive processes that correspond to subjective fluctuations in the binaural beat.

Dajani and Picton (2006) tested the processing of interaural correlation directly, by measuring steady-state responses evoked by noise stimuli that alternated between two levels of interaural correlation ρ at a repetition frequency f_m (Figure 3–7A). Estimates of apparent latencies indicated that when the f_m was below around 8 Hz, the responses at f_m reflected cortical integration, while the responses at higher frequencies may have reflected the running cross-correlation in the high brainstem or primary auditory cortex. A particularly robust response was found at twice the repetition frequency when $f_m = 4$ Hz (i.e., at 8 Hz), which may have resulted from a superposition of late auditory responses. This response was most dependent on stimulus frequency content below 1000 Hz, suggesting a dependence on neural phase-locking. When ρ alternated between levels in the range of 0.2 to 1 and 0, the amplitude of this response in the grand-averaged signal varied linearly with ρ, and the physiological response threshold (ρ = 0.35) was close to the average behavioural threshold (ρ = 0.31) (Figure 3–7B). This linear variation in the response suggests that it may be a useful indicator of the estimation of interaural correlation by central neural circuits.

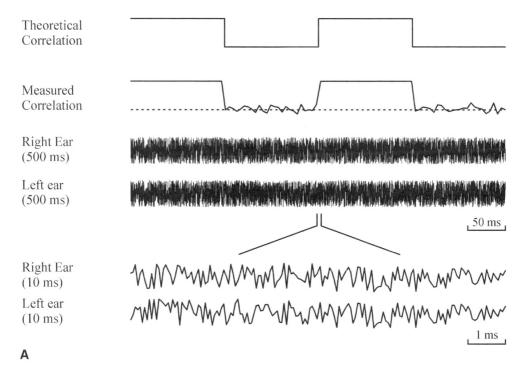

Figure 3–7. Steady-state responses to changes in interaural correlation. **A,** Stimulus. The *upper line* shows two cycles of interaural correlation, which alternates between the two levels of 1 and 0 at a rate of 4 Hz. The *second line* shows the correlation measured over 5-ms intervals. The *third* and *fourth lines* show the stimuli as presented to each ear. Note the lack of cycle-by-cycle amplitude variation. The *lower two lines* of the figure show a 10-ms epoch of the stimuli as it changes from the uncorrelated to the correlated section of the cycle. In the correlated section, identical stimuli occur in the two ears. *continues*

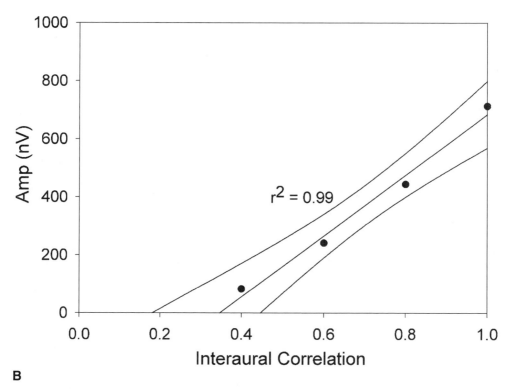

B

Figure 3–7. *continued* **B**, Effect of correlation. Interaural correlation alternated between 0 and ρ [ρ = 0.2, 0.4, 0.6, 0.8, 1] at a repetition frequency f_m = 4 Hz. Amplitudes of significant responses at the second harmonic of f_m (i.e., at 8 Hz) obtained with the grand-averaged signal are shown. A regression line with 95% confidence intervals also is shown. Response amplitudes are linearly related to ρ. (Adapted with permission from Dajani, H. R., & Picton, T. W., *Hearing Research, 219*, 85–100, 2006 [Figure 1, p. 86; Figure 8, p. 94]).

Although the three experimental approaches just described involve binaural steady-state responses, Ross, Fujioka, Tremblay, and Picton (2007) have proposed a novel approach that involves responses evoked by a change in the IPD within steady-state sinusoidal AM stimuli (Figure 3–8A). Although they recorded a brief cessation and reinstatement of the ASSR when the IPD changes, their main measurement was a transient auditory cortical response. These investigators found that, when the carrier frequency was 500 or 1000 Hz, significant transient responses could be detected in all subjects; however, when the carrier frequency was 1500 Hz, responses were absent in all subjects (Figure 3–8B). The threshold of the physiological response, determined at 1250 Hz for the group data, corresponded to the behavioural threshold at 1200 Hz. Therefore, they concluded that the physiological threshold probably reflected the upper limit of phase-locking in the brainstem. In a follow-up study with the same stimulus signal, Ross and associates (2007b) investigated the variation of the cortical responses with

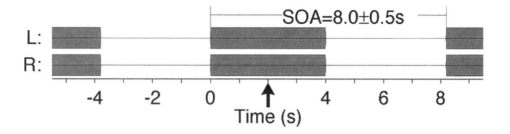

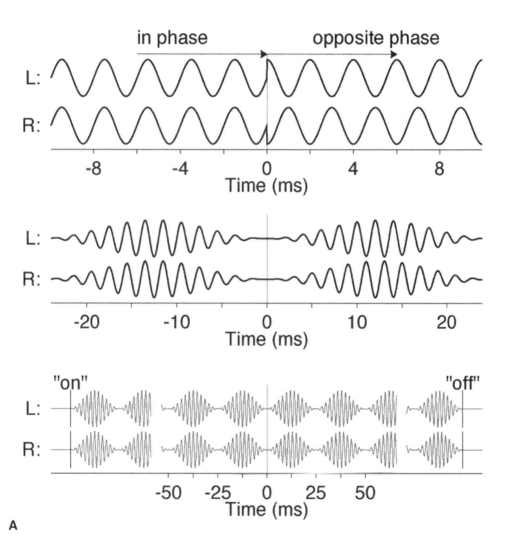

A

Figure 3–8. Responses to sudden changes in the interaural phase difference (IPD) within steady-state sinusoidal AM stimuli. **A**, Stimulus. *Top graph*: The stimulus sequence was composed of tone bursts (4 s in duration) presented dichotically with a stimulus-onset asynchrony (SOA) of 7.5 to 8.5 s. The *arrow* at 2 s after stimulus onset indicates the time point of the change in the IPD. *Second graph*: The 90-degree phase shifts, opposite in direction, result in a polarity reversal between left (L) and right (R) ears. *Third graph*: The phase shift occurs at the minimum point of the 40-Hz amplitude modulation. *Bottom graph*: The 40-Hz AM envelope defines the shape of stimulus onset, the phase shift, and the stimulus offset. *continues*

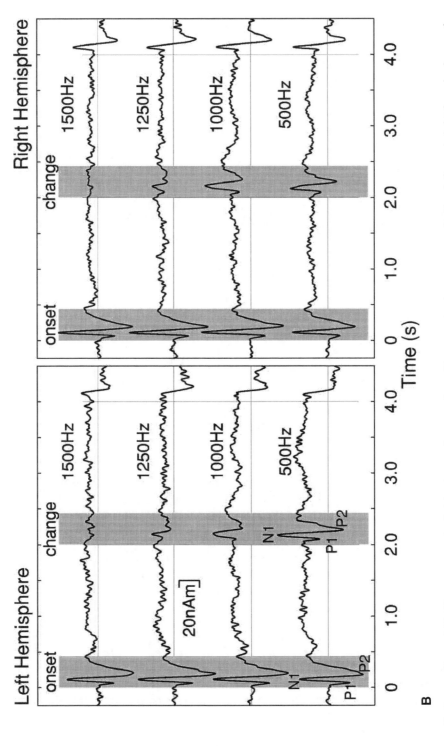

Figure 3–8. *continued* **B**, Responses. Individual waveforms of auditory evoked responses in the left and right hemispheres for each frequency tested. The response waveform at 500 Hz exhibits clear responses to the stimulus onset and IPD change (at 2.0 s). Whereas the onset responses are fairly consistent across all stimulus frequencies, the phase change response clearly diminishes with increasing stimulus frequencies and is absent at 1500 Hz. (Reprinted with permission from Ross, B., Tremblay, K. L., & Picton, T. W., *Journal of the Acoustical Society of America, 121*(2), 1017–1027, 2007 [Figure 1, p. 1018; Figure 4, p. 1021]. Copyright 2007, Acoustical Society of America.)

age. They detected responses for frequencies up to 1290 Hz in young subjects, but only up to 1130 Hz in middle-aged and 890 Hz in older adults. These results suggest that the proposed approach may provide a sensitive physiological indicator for the degradation of binaural processing with age.

Nevertheless, the development of clinically useful electrophysiological tests of binaural processing remains challenging for reasons including the following:

- Evoked responses in binaural tests sometimes are quite small and so may require excessive measurement time.

- Binaural perceptual phenomena are most salient at low frequencies. For example, the perception of auditory motion is limited to a few Hertz (Blauert, 1972). Responses at these frequencies may be susceptible to the effects of cognitive factors, such as attention, which would need to be controlled (e.g., Karino et al., 2006).

- An advantage of electrophysiological measures is that they often exhibit less variability across individual participants than do behavioural measures of binaural function (Ross et al., 2007a). Still needed, however, is demonstration of correlation between physiological and behavioural thresholds in individuals, which would require the study of a broad range of persons with different types and levels of hearing impairment.

Of the new experimental electrophysiological measures of binaural function that have been described, the one proposed by Ross and colleagues (2007a) currently is the most developed, because it has been shown to correlate with behavioural measures (in the group data) and to reflect the degradation of binaural processing with aging. However, because binaural processing is involved in a variety of perceptual phenomena (e.g., following moving sound sources, source localization, speech enhancement in noise, echo suppression), it is unlikely that a single measure is sufficient to assess the multiple subsystems of the auditory pathway that may be involved. Moreover, although the experimental measures described here probably depend on neural phase-locking and thus could be sensitive indicators of auditory temporal processing, there is a challenge to develop measures that distinguish between neural phase-locking—which is related to other auditory functions such as speech and musical pitch perception (e.g., Karino et al., 2006)—and processing that is specific to the binaural system.

This chapter has reviewed the ASSR stimulus-response relationship, as well as possibilities for tests of binaural processing. For further reading on these aspects of the ASSR, see the work of Picton (2007) and colleagues (Picton et al., 2003).

Acknowledgments. We sincerely thank Terence Picton for his advice as a reviewer of this chapter. Thanks also to Tracy Saunders and Blake Butler for their help in preparing this chapter.

References

Aoyagi, M., Suzuki, Y., Yokota, M., Furuse, H., Watanabe, T., & Ito, T. (1999). Reliability of 80-Hz amplitude-modulation-following response detected by phase coherence. *Audiology & Neuro-otology, 4*(1), 28–37.

Babkoff, H., Muchnik, C., Ben-David, N., Furst, M., Even-Zohar, S., & Hildesheimer,

M. (2002). Mapping lateralization of click trains in younger and older populations. *Hearing Research, 165*, 117–127.

Blauert, J. (1972). On the lag of lateralization caused by interaural time and intensity differences. *Audiology, 11*, 265–270.

Brennan, S., & Stevens, J. (2007). *How does the ASSR response amplitude vary with modulation rate for individual babies?* XX International Evoked Audiometry Study Group, Bled, Slovenia.

Campbell, F. W., Atkinson, J., Francis, M. R., & Green, D. M. (1977). Estimation of auditory thresholds using evoked potentials. A clinical screening test. *Progress in Clinical Neurophysiology, 2*, 68–78.

Cohen, L. T., Rickards, F. W., & Clark, G. M. (1991). A comparison of steady-state evoked potentials to modulated tones in awake and sleeping humans. *Journal of the Acoustical Society of America, 90*(5), 2467–2479.

Cone-Wesson, B., Ma, E., & Fowler, C. G. (1997). Effect of stimulus level and frequency on ABR and MLR binaural interaction in human neonates. *Hearing Research, 106*, 163–178.

Dajani, H. R., & Picton, T. W. (2006). Human auditory steady-state responses to changes in interaural correlation. *Hearing Research, 219*, 85–100.

Dimitrijevic, A., John, M. S., van Roon, P., & Picton, T. W. (2001). Human auditory steady-state responses to tones independently modulated in both frequency and amplitude. *Ear and Hearing, 22*(2), 100–111.

Dimitrijevic, A., John, M. S., van Roon, P., Purcell, D. W., Adamonis, J., Ostroff, J., Nedzelski, J. M., & Picton, T. W. (2002). Estimating the audiogram using multiple auditory steady-state responses. *Journal of the American Academy of Audiology, 13*(4), 205–224.

Dobie, R. A., & Berlin, C. I. (1979). Binaural interaction in brainstem-evoked responses. *Archives of Otolaryngology, 105*, 391–398.

Dobie, R. A., & Norton, S. J. (1980). Binaural interaction in human auditory evoked potentials. *Electroencephalography and Clinical Neurophysiology, 49*, 303–313.

Dobie, R. A., & Wilson, M. J. (1998). Low-level steady-state auditory evoked potentials: Effects of rate and sedation on detectability. *Journal of the Acoustical Society of America, 104*(6), 3482–3488.

Draganova, R., Ross, B., Wollbrink, A., & Pantev, C. (in press). Cortical steady-state responses to central and peripheral auditory beats. *Cerebral Cortex*.

Elberling, C., & Don, M. (2007). Detecting and assessing synchronous neural activity in the temporal domain (SNR, response detection). In R. F. Burkard, M. Don, & J. J. Eggermont (Eds.), *Auditory evoked potentials: Basic principles and clinical application* (pp. 102–123). Baltimore: Lippincott Williams & Wilkins.

Galambos, R., Makeig, S., & Talmachoff, P. J. (1981). A 40-Hz auditory potential recorded from the human scalp. *Proceedings of the National Academy of Sciences of the United States of America, 78*(4), 2643–2647.

Geisler, C. D. (1960). *Average responses to clicks in man recorded by scalp electrodes*. Technical Report No. 380. Cambridge, MA: MIT Research Laboratories of Electronics.

Goldstein, J. L., Baer, T., & Kiang, N. Y. S. (1971). A theoretical treatment of latency, group delay, and tuning characteristics for auditory-nerve responses to clicks and tones. In M. B. Sachs (Ed.), *Physiology of the auditory system; based on the proceedings of a workshop* (pp. 133–141). Baltimore: National Educational Consultants.

Griffiths, T. D., Green, G. G. R., Rees, A., & Rees, G. (2000). Human brain areas involved in the analysis of auditory movement. *Human Brain Mapping, 9*, 72–80.

Hatton, J. L., & Stapells, D. R. (2007). *Effects of single vs multiple-stimulus presentation on 80 Hz ASSR amplitudes and threshold: Results in young infants*. XX International Evoked Audiometry Study Group, Bled, Slovenia.

Hawley, M. L., Litovsky, R. Y., & Culling, J. F. (2004). The benefit of binaural hearing in a cocktail party: Effect of location and type of interferer. *Journal of the Acoustical Society of America, 115*, 833–843.

Herdman, A. T., Lins, O., van Roon, P., Stapells, D. R., Scherg, M., & Picton, T. W. (2002a). Intracerebral sources of human auditory steady-state responses. *Brain Topography, 15*(2), 69–86.

Herdman, A. T., Picton, T. W., & Stapells, D. R. (2002b). Place specificity of multiple auditory steady-state responses. *Journal of the Acoustical Society of America, 112*(4), 1569–1582.

Herdman, A. T., & Stapells, D. K. (2003). Auditory steady-state response thresholds of adults with sensorineural hearing impairments. *International Journal of Audiology, 42*(5), 237–248.

Herdman, A. T., & Stapells, D. R. (2001). Thresholds determined using the monotic and dichotic multiple auditory steady-state response technique in normal-hearing subjects. *Scandinavian Audiology, 30*(1), 41–49.

Herman, G., Warren, L., & Wagener, J. (1977). Auditory lateralization: Age differences in sensitivity to dichotic time and amplitude cues. *Journal of Gerontology, 32*, 187–191.

John, M. S., Dimitrijevic, A., & Picton, T. W. (2001a). Weighted averaging of steady-state responses. *Clinical Neurophysiology, 112*(3), 555–562.

John, M. S., Dimitrijevic, A., & Picton, T. W. (2002a). Auditory steady-state responses to exponential modulation envelopes. *Ear and Hearing, 23*(2), 106–117.

John, M. S., Dimitrijevic, A., & Picton, T. W. (2003). Efficient stimuli for evoking auditory steady-state responses. *Ear and Hearing, 24*(5), 406–423.

John, M. S., Dimitrijevic, A., van Roon, P., & Picton, T. W. (2001b). Multiple auditory steady-state responses to AM and FM stimuli. *Audiology & Neuro-otology, 6*(1), 12–27.

John, M. S., Lins, O. G., Boucher, B. L., & Picton, T. W. (1998). Multiple auditory steady-state responses (MASTER): Stimulus and recording parameters. *Audiology, 37*(2), 59–82.

John, M. S., Purcell, D. W., Dimitrijevic, A., & Picton, T. W. (2002b). Advantages and caveats when recording steady-state responses to multiple simultaneous stimuli. *Journal of the American Academy of Audiology, 13*(5), 246–259.

Jones, S. J., Pitman, J. R., & Halliday, A. M. (1991). Scalp potentials following sudden coherence and discoherence of binaural noise and change in the inter-aural time difference: A specific binaural evoked potential or a "mismatch" response? *Electroencephalography and Clinical Neurophysiology, 80*, 146–154.

Joris, P. X., Carney, L. H., Smith, P. H., & Yin, T. C. T. (1994). Enhancement of neural synchronization in the anteroventral cochlear nucleus. I. Responses to tones at the characteristic frequency. *Journal of Neurophysiology, 71*, 1022–1036.

Karino, S., Yumoto, M., Itoh, K., Uno, A., Yamakawa, K., Sekimoto, S., et al. (2006). Neuromagnetic responses to binaural beat in human cerebral cortex. *Journal of Neurophysiology, 96*, 1927–1938.

Kuwada, S., Fitzpatrick, D. C., Batra, R., & Ostapoff, E. (2006). Sensitivity to interaural time differences in the dorsal nucleus of the unanesthetized rabbit: Comparison with other structures. *Journal of Neurophysiology, 95*, 1309–1322.

Kuwada, S., Yin, T. C., & Wickesberg, R. E. (1979). Response of cat inferior colliculus neurons to binaural beat stimuli: Possible mechanisms for sound localization. *Science, 206*, 586–588.

Levi, E. C., Folsom, R. C., & Dobie, R. A. (1993). Amplitude-modulation following response (AMFR): Effects of modulation rate, carrier frequency, age, and state. *Hearing Research, 68*(1), 42–52.

Levi, E. C., Folsom, R. C., & Dobie, R. A. (1995). Coherence analysis of envelope-following responses (EFRs) and frequency-following responses (FFRs) in infants and adults. *Hearing Research, 89*(1-2), 21–27.

Linden, R. D., Campbell, K. B., Hamel, G., & Picton, T. W. (1985). Human auditory steady state evoked potentials during sleep. *Ear and Hearing, 6*(3), 167-174.

Lins, O. G., Picton, P. E., Picton, T. W., Champagne, S. C., & Durieux-Smith, A. (1995). Auditory steady-state responses to tones amplitude-modulated at 80-110 Hz. *Journal of the Acoustical Society of America, 97*(5 Pt 1), 3051-3063.

Lins, O. G., & Picton, T. W. (1995). Auditory steady-state responses to multiple simultaneous stimuli. *Electroencephalography and Clinical Neurophysiology, 96*(5), 420-432.

Luts, H., & Wouters, J. (2004). Hearing assessment by recording multiple auditory steady-state responses: The influence of test duration. *International Journal of Audiology, 43*(8), 471-478.

McEvoy, L. K., Picton, T. W., Champagne, S. C., Kellett, A. J. C. , & Kelly, J. B. (1990). Human evoked potentials to shifts in the lateralization of a noise. *Audiology, 29*, 163-180.

McPherson, D. L., & Starr, A. (1993). Binaural interaction in auditory evoked potentials: Brainstem, middle- and long-latency components. *Hearing Research, 66*, 91-98.

McPherson, D. L., & Starr, A. (1995). Auditory time-intensity cues in the binaural interaction component of the auditory evoked potentials. *Hearing Research, 89*, 162-171.

Murphy, D. R., Daneman, M., & Schneider, B. A. (2006). Why do older adults have difficulty following conversations? *Psychology and Aging, 21*, 49-61.

O Mahoney, C. F., & Kemp, D. T. (1995). Distortion product otoacoustic emission delay measurement in human ears. *Journal of the Acoustical Society of America, 97*(6), 3721-3735.

Picton, T. W. (2007). Audiometry using auditory steady-state responses. In R. F. Burkard, M. Don, & J. J. Eggermont (Eds.), *Auditory evoked potentials: Basic principles and clinical application* (pp. 441-462). Baltimore: Lippincott Williams & Wilkins.

Picton, T. W., Dauman, R., & Aran, J. M. (1987a). Responses evoked in "steady state" in man by means of a sinusoidal frequency modulation [Reponses evoquees en 'regime permanent' chez l'homme par la modulation sinusoidale de frequence]. *Journal of Otolaryngology, 16*(3), 140-145.

Picton, T. W., Dimitrijevic, A., Perez-Abalo, M. C., & Van Roon, P. (2005). Estimating audiometric thresholds using auditory steady-state responses. *Journal of the American Academy of Audiology, 16*(3), 140-156.

Picton, T. W., John, M. S., Dimitrijevic, A., & Purcell, D. (2003). Human auditory steady-state responses. *International Journal of Audiology, 42*(4), 177-219.

Picton, T. W., Rodriguez, R. T., Linden, R. D., & Maiste, A. C. (1985). The neurophysiology of human hearing. *Human Communication Canada, 9*, 127-136.

Picton, T. W., Skinner, C. R., Champagne, S. C., Kellett, A. J., & Maiste, A. C. (1987b). Potentials evoked by the sinusoidal modulation of the amplitude or frequency of a tone. *Journal of the Acoustical Society of America, 82*(1), 165-178.

Picton, T. W., van Roon, P., & John, M. S. (2007). Human auditory steady-state responses during sweeps of intensity. *Ear and Hearing, 28*(4), 542-557.

Purcell, D. W., John, S. M., Schneider, B. A., & Picton, T. W. (2004). Human temporal auditory acuity as assessed by envelope following responses. *Journal of the Acoustical Society of America, 116*(6), 3581-3593.

Rees, A., Green, G. G., & Kay, R. H. (1986). Steady-state evoked responses to sinusoidally amplitude-modulated sounds recorded in man. *Hearing Research, 23*(2), 123-133.

Regan, D. (1966). Some characteristics of average steady-state and transient responses evoked by modulated light. *Electroencephalography and Clinical Neurophysiology, 20*(3), 238-248.

Regan, D. (1973). Rapid objective refraction using evoked brain potentials. *Investigations in Ophthalmology, 12*(9), 669-679.

Regan, D. (1989). *Human brain electrophysiology: Evoked potentials and evoked magnetic fields in science and medicine.* New York: Elsevier Science.

Regan, M. P., & Regan, D. (1988). A frequency domain technique for characterizing non-linearities in biological systems. *Journal of Theoretical Biology, 133,* 293–317.

Rickards, F. W., & Clark, G. M. (1984). Steady-state evoked potentials to amplitude-modulated tones. In R. H. Nodar & C. Barber (Eds.), *Evoked potentials II* (pp. 163–168). Boston: Butterworth.

Riedel, H., & Kollmeier, B. (2002). Auditory brain stem responses evoked by lateralized clicks: Is lateralization extracted in the human brain stem? *Hearing Research, 163*(1–2), 12–26.

Rodriguez, R., Picton, T., Linden, D., Hamel, G., & Laframboise, G. (1986). Human auditory steady state responses: Effects of intensity and frequency. *Ear and Hearing, 7*(5), 300–313.

Rose, J. E., Gross, N. B., Geisler, C. D., & Hind, J. E. (1966). Some neural mechanisms in the inferior colliculus of the cat which may be relevant to localization of a sound source. *Journal of Neurophysiology, 29,* 288–314.

Ross, B., Borgmann, C., Draganova, R., Roberts, L. E., & Pantev, C. (2000). A high-precision magnetoencephalographic study of human auditory steady-state responses to amplitude-modulated tones. *Journal of the Acoustical Society of America, 108*(2), 679–691.

Ross, B., Draganova, R., Picton, T. W., & Pantev, C. (2003). Frequency specificity of 40-Hz auditory steady-state responses. *Hearing Research, 186*(1–2), 57–68.

Ross, B., Tremblay, K. L., & Picton, T. W. (2007a). Physiological detection of interaural phase differences. *Journal of the Acoustical Society of America, 121,* 1017–1027.

Ross, B., Fujioka, T., Tremblay, K. L., & Picton, T. W. (2007b). Aging in binaural hearing begins in mid-life: evidence from cortical auditory-evoked responses to changes in interaural phase. *Journal of Neuroscience, 27,* 11172–11178.

Sapsford, D. J., Pickworth, A. J., & Jones, J. G. (1996). A method for producing the co-herent frequency: A steady-state auditory evoked response in the electroencephalo-gram. *Anesthesia and Analgesia, 83*(6), 1273–1278.

Schwarz, D. W., & Taylor, P. (2005). Human auditory steady state responses to binaural and monaural beats. *Clinical Neurophysiology, 116*(3), 658–668.

Sovijärvi, A. R. A., & Hyvärinen, J. (1974). Auditory cortical neurons in the cat sensitive to the direction of sound source movement. *Brain Research, 73,* 455–471.

Spitzer, M. W., & Semple, M. N. (1993). Responses of inferior colliculus neurons to time-varying interaural phase disparity: Effects of shifting the locus of virtual motion. *Journal of Neurophysiology, 69,* 1245–1263.

Stapells, D. R. (2000). Frequency-specific evoked potential audiometry in infants. In R. C. Seewald (Ed.), *A sound foundation through early amplification* (pp. 13–31). Basel: Phonak AG.

Stapells, D. R., Linden, D., Suffield, J. B., Hamel, G., & Picton, T. W. (1984). Human auditory steady state potentials. *Ear and Hearing, 5*(2), 105–113.

Stollman, M., Snik, A., Hombergen, G., Nieuwenhuys, R., & ten Koppel, P. (1996). Detection of the binaural interaction component in the auditory brainstem response. *British Journal of Audiology, 30*(3), 227–232.

Stürzebecher, E., Cebulla, M., Elberling, C., & Berger, T. (2006). New efficient stimuli for evoking frequency-specific auditory steady-state responses. *Journal of the American Academy of Audiology, 17*(6), 448–461.

Stürzebecher, E., Cebulla, M., & Neumann, K. (2003). Click-evoked ABR at high stimulus repetition rates for neonatal hearing screening. *International Journal of Audiology, 42*(2), 59–70.

Tlumak, A. I., Durrant, J. D., & Collet, L. (2007). 80 Hz auditory steady-state responses (ASSR) at 250 Hz and 12,000 Hz. *International Journal of Audiology, 46*(1), 26–30.

Tollin, D. J., & Yin, T. C. T. (2005). Interaural phase and level difference sensitivity in low-frequency neurons in the lateral superior olive. *Journal of Neuroscience, 25,* 10648–10657.

Trahiotis, C., Bernstein, L. R., Stern, R. M., & Buell, T. N. (2005). Interaural correlation as the basis of a working model of binaural processing: An introduction. In A. N. Popper & R. R. Fay (Eds.), *Sound source localization*. New York: Springer.

van der Reijden, C. S., Mens, L. H., & Snik, A. F. (2004). Signal-to-noise ratios of the auditory steady-state response from fifty-five EEG derivations in adults. *Journal of the American Academy of Audiology, 15*(10), 692–701.

van der Reijden, C. S., Mens, L. H., & Snik, A. F. (2005). EEG derivations providing auditory steady-state responses with high signal-to-noise ratios in infants. *Ear and Hearing, 26*(3), 299–309.

Van Maanen, A., & Stapells, D. R. (2005). Comparison of multiple auditory steady-state responses (80 versus 40 Hz) and slow cortical potentials for threshold estimation in hearing-impaired adults. *International Journal of Audiology, 44*(11), 613–624.

Vander Werff, K. R., & Brown, C. J. (2005). Effect of audiometric configuration on threshold and suprathreshold auditory steady-state responses. *Ear and Hearing, 26*(3), 310–326.

Viemeister, N. F. (1979). Temporal modulation transfer functions based upon modulation thresholds. *Journal of the Acoustical Society of America, 66*(5), 1364–1380.

Warren, J. D., Zielinski, B. A., Green, G. G. R., Rauschecker, J. P., & Griffiths, T. D. (2002). Perception of sound-source motion by the human brain. *Neuron, 34*, 139–148.

Wernick, J. S., & Starr, A. (1968). Binaural interaction in the superior olivary complex of the cat: An analysis of field potentials evoked by binaural-beat stimuli. *Journal of Neurophysiology, 31*, 428–441.

Wong, Y. S. W., & Stapells, D. R. (2004). Brain stem and cortical mechanisms underlying the binaural masking level difference in humans: An auditory steady-state response study. *Ear and Hearing, 25*, 57–67.

CHAPTER 4

Neural Generators of the Auditory Steady-State Response

ANDREW DIMITRIJEVIC
BERNHARD ROSS

Introduction

The auditory steady-state response (ASSR) is becoming an increasingly popular tool in both clinical and research settings. From a research point of view, some knowledge of ASSR generation sites will provide insights for the basic auditory neurophysiological processing. From the clinical point of view, knowledge of the generators can potentially reveal site of lesion indications and help guide clinicians to the most efficient rehabilitation approach.

Although ASSRs share some qualities with classical "transient" evoked poten-

tials, in many ways there are some key differences. Ideally, transient responses represent neural activity that has occurred in response to one stimulus and subsequently reverts to a "baseline" state, and the next-occurring stimulus should evoke a subsequent brain response and be relatively independent of the previous response (obviously, this is not the case in reality, because the nervous system does retain some trace of previous stimuli). The ASSR, on the other hand, represents neural activation to repeated stimulation, and the stimulus rates are often high enough that the transient response does not have enough time to "revert" to baseline levels. After a few cycles of stimuli, the brain enters a "steady state" wherein the repeated stimuli evoke responses that remain unchanged throughout the duration of the stimulus presentation. Therefore, although transient and steady-state responses are related, the waveform morphology and subsequently the brain areas generating these responses are different.

ASSRs can be evoked by any repeating stimulus. In fact, early (Linden, Campbell, Hamel, & Picton, 1985) and later (Purcell, John, Schneider, & Picton, 2004) studies showed that if the stimulus is allowed to slowly change in modulation rates ranging from 2 Hz all the way up to 200 Hz ASSRs,[1] inherent peaks occur near 40 Hz and 80 Hz. These peaks in the electroencephalogram (EEG) spectrum form the basis of the two general types of responses under discussion here: 40 Hz and 80 Hz. It may be convenient to think of 40-Hz and 80-Hz ASSRs as homologues to transient cortical and brainstem responses, respectively; however, as described later, there are some inherent differences. Nonetheless, the basic idea that the higher modulation rates (80 Hz and above) are generated predominantly by subcortical structures and the lower modulation rates (40 Hz and below) are generated predominantly by the cortex is well accepted and depicted schematically in Figure 4–1.

Although a continuum exists between modulation rate and ASSR, the cortical responses, which are referred to in this chapter as 40-HZ ASSRs, and the subcortical responses, which are refer to as 80-Hz ASSRs, are indeed distinct, with their own physiology and as such, deserve their own consideration in the following two sections.

80-Hz Auditory Steady-State Responses

As one progresses along the auditory system from auditory nerve all the way up to the cortex, neurons show a decreased ability to follow high modulation rates. Neurons in the auditory nerve display phase-locked responses to stimulus frequencies of up to about 1 to 2 kHz. After that the signal is presumably converted from a rate code to a place code further along in the auditory system (Langer & Schreiner, 1988). Because the cortex has difficulty responding at high rates (above 80 Hz), a number of investigators have suggested that subcortical structures are predominantly involved in ASSR generation at these rates. Many lines of converging evidence suggest that ASSRs elicited by stimuli near 80-Hz modulation are generated predominantly by the brainstem, as opposed to the cortex; these include animal unit recordings, evaluation of ASSR latencies, human dipole source estimations, arousal states and functional magnetic resonance imaging (MRI).

The first obligatory stage of processing modulated signals involves transduction at the level of the cochlea and auditory nerve. Lins, Picton, Picton, Champagne, and Durieux-Smith (1995) proposed a model of this early-stage processing whereby the sound stimulus undergoes

---

[1]Technically these responses are not "ASSRs" because, by definition, the ASSR stimulus is unchanging. The stimuli in these studies are slowly changing in repetition rate and therefore should be termed "envelope following responses." For the purposes of clarity, however, these responses can be thought of as ASSRs at a particular rate.

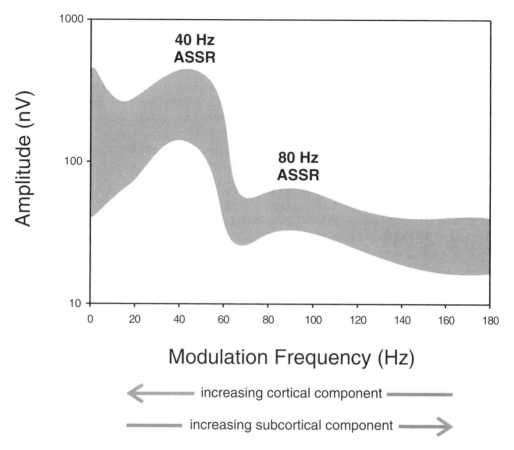

Figure 4–1. ASSR amplitude as a function of modulation frequency. The two major peaks in the function are at 40 and 80 Hz. 40-Hz ASSRs are generated predominantly by cortical generators, and 80-Hz ASSRs are generated predominantly by subcortical structures.

a half-wave rectification that ultimately creates a rhythmic firing of the auditory nerve at the rate of modulation. When the sound signal impinges on the cochlea, neurotransmitter is only released when the stereocilia on the hair cells are deflected in a particular direction. This process results in rhythmic neurotransmitter release at the modulation rate, as shown schematically in Figure 4–2, which illustrates the idea that although this signal is amplitude modulated at 80 Hz, there is no energy at 80 Hz in the stimulus itself. The half-wave rectification is

the first stage of processing that introduces energy at the modulation rate to the nervous system. This does not suggest that the sources of 80-Hz ASSRs are necessarily in the auditory nerve; rather, that the auditory nerve is able to follow rhythmic stimulation at these rates, (illustrating the general idea that 80-Hz ASSRs can be coded at multiple levels along the auditory neuraxis). Accordingly, human scalp-recorded responses most likely represent an overall summed activity across all "stations" along the ascending auditory system. This, however, does not preclude

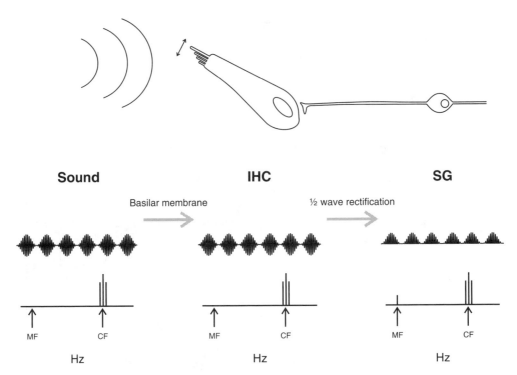

Figure 4–2. Simple model showing transduction of an amplitude-modulated sound into auditory nerve impulses that rhythmically fire at the modulation rate. As the sound enters the ear, stereocilia on inner hair cells are moved back and forth. Neurotransmitter release is initiated only with depolarization, so the signal undergoes half-wave rectification. This results in activity that can be recorded at modulation frequency. CF, **carrier frequency**; IHC, **inner hair cells**; MF, **modulation frequency**; SG, **spiral ganglion**.

the idea that some stations with more "dominant" sources contribute more to the overall response.

Animal Studies

One approach to describe the generators of the 80-Hz ASSR is to examine the cortical and subcortical structures that can support modulations at rates near 80 Hz. Much of our detailed understanding of the neurophysiology underlying coding of amplitude modulation comes from animal recordings. The detailed neuro-

physiology of AM coding along the entire auditory system is beyond the scope of this chapter; however, the interested reader is referred to a recent review of neurophysiology coding of amplitude modulation (Joris, Schreiner, & Rees, 2004).

Figure 4-2 summarizes how, at the level of the auditory nerve, an AM signal is converted to neural activity at the modulation frequency. The place of maximal stimulation along the cochlear basilar membrane is determined by carrier frequency, and the rhythmic activity is driven by the modulation frequency. Using stimuli that are commonly used in humans (100% AM signal modulated at 98 Hz with a carrier of 996 Hz), Khanna and Teich (1989) recorded rabbit auditory nerve fiber activity and,using Fourier transform histogram activity, showed components at the modulation rate. The upper limit of following modulation may be near 800 Hz (Joris & Yin, 1992). Therefore, ASSRs can potentially be generated as "early" in the auditory pathway as the auditory nerve.

Progressing along the auditory system, neurons in the cochlear nucleus faithfully preserve and enhance input from the auditory nerve (Moller, 1972). A necessary relay station for the auditory input is the inferior colliculus. Here, neurons are tuned to particular modulation frequencies. In a rabbit model, Kuwada and colleagues (2002) recorded ASSRs to AM stimuli at the level of the superior olivary complex (SOC), inferior colliculus (IC), and auditory cortex. Ranges of peak amplitudes progressively decreased with modulation frequency at higher stations along the auditory pathway. At the level of the SOC, peaks occurred near 200 Hz, near 100 Hz at the IC, and at 10 to 20 Hz for the auditory cortex. In the same study, cortical components of the ASSR were manipulated in a number of ways, including pentobarbital anesthesia, arousal (cocaine administration and tactile input), and potassium chloride (KCl)-induced cortical depression. All of these manipulations caused increased or decreased activity at rates near 40 Hz, but with no change at higher modulation rates. In species such as the rat, cat, guinea pig, and gerbil, the best modulation frequencies in the IC ranged from 30 to 100 Hz (reviewed by Joris et al., 2004). Relatively few studies have examined the thalamic responses to AM stimuli. Preuss and Muller-Pruess (1990) showed that medial geniculate neurons have the best modulation frequencies near 32 Hz. These results suggest a progressive shift of dominant generators at lower stations of the auditory system with increasing modulation frequency.

Human Studies

As shown in the preceding section, both cortical and subcortical areas can potentially support ASSR generation at rates near 80 Hz. However, because of species differences and electrode placement issues, it is problematic to directly relate animal findings to ASSRs recorded from the human scalp.

The previous section showed that many structures have the potential to follow modulation rates near 80 Hz. ASSRs recorded using scalp electrodes in humans, however, represent an overall summed activity of many overlapping generators. Therefore, rather than asking what specific brain regions code for 80 Hz ASSRs, the question is which of these generators is the "dominant" one. It appears that the dominant generator can change with behavioural state. For example, a 40-Hz ASSR contains both cortical and subcortical components. During wakefulness, the cortical component of the 40-Hz ASSR is the dominant source, whereas the underlying brainstem component is relatively small. During sleep, the roles are reversed as the cortical component diminishes while the underlying brainstem source remains unchanged. These results parallel those in the ASSR rabbit study (Kuwada et al., 2002) described previously.

Latency Estimates

Latency analysis of the 80 Hz ASSR can provide insight into where the responses are generated. Following a similar logic to "classical" cortical event–related potentials, ASSRs with short latencies point to lower relay stations in the auditory system compared with longer-latency responses. The measurement of ASSR latency is complicated because of an inherent ambiguity—that is, it is impossible to know how many cycles of the stimulus occurred before the ASSR was actually recorded. In recording ASSRs, the amplitude and phase of the response usually are derived (see Chapter 2). The phase of the response usually is expressed as a value ranging from 0 to 360 degrees. However, the circular nature of phase means that 10 degrees is effectively the same as 370 degrees. Despite these constraints, it is possible to get an estimate of latency given certain assumptions; the interested reader is referred to the work of John and Picton (2000) for a more detailed explanation.

The latency of the 80-Hz ASSR will decrease with (1) increases in intensity, (2) increases in carrier frequency, and (3) increases in modulation rate. The literature on ASSR latencies has been reviewed by Picton, John, Dimitrijevic, and Purcell (2003). In Table 1 of this summary, mean values for modulation rates near 80 Hz and at intensities near 50 dB HL revealed latencies of 27, 21, 15, and 16 ms for 500, 1000, 2000, and 4000 Hz, respectively. In another study by this group, modulation rates in the range of 150 to 190 Hz revealed latencies of 6 to 12 ms (John & Picton, 2000). These results suggest that 80-Hz ASSRs are generated by a source high in the brainstem and that ASSRs in the range of 150 to 190 Hz are generated by sources similar to those underlying wave V in the auditory brainstem response.

Dipole Source Analysis

Much of the work on dipole analysis in ASSR research has been dominated by magnetic encephalography (MEG) recordings at stimulation rates near 40 Hz. MEG recordings show good signal-to-noise ratios, in part because they are unaffected by the impedance volume conduction. However, the MEG dipoles are relatively "blind" to deep sources. Therefore, although good dipole signal-to-noise ratios may be achieved for superficial sources, brainstem sources are harder to measure using MEG. In addition, 40-Hz ASSRs can be up to five times larger than 80-Hz responses (Herdman et al., 2002). Thus, poor signal-to-noise ratios for 80-Hz responses make it difficult to obtain stable dipole fits.

It is surprising that only one study has examined dipole sources of 80-Hz ASSRs using scalp-recorded EEG in humans (Herdman et al., 2002). In this study, both 40- and 80-Hz ASSRs were examined using 46 surface electrodes. Six dipoles were fitted for each of the modulation rates. The first two were near the brainstem; two were placed at the ipsilateral and two at the contralateral auditory cortex. As can be seen in Figure 4–3, the largest source activity for the 80 Hz dipole fits was seen in the brainstem source (1.8 to 2.1 nA), with minimal amplitudes at the auditory cortices (0.3 to 0.7 nA).

Arousal

Another line of evidence suggesting that 40- and 80-Hz ASSR generators are dominated by cortical and subcortical pro-

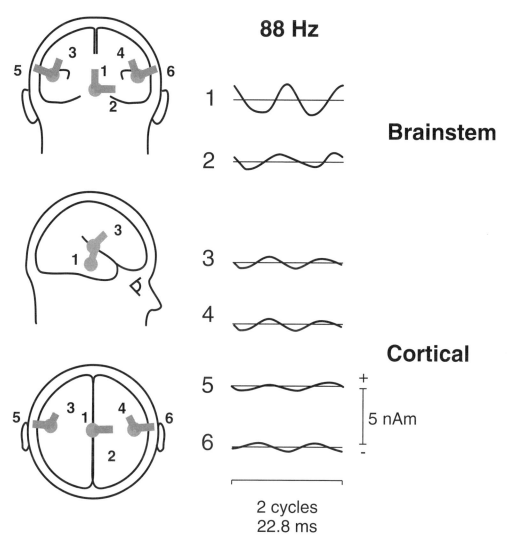

Figure 4–3. Brain electrical source analysis of an 88-Hz AM signal. Dipoles 1 and 2 are in the brainstem, and dipoles 3 to 6 are in auditory cortex. Although some activity is evident at the level of cortex, most of the activity occurs in the brainstem. (Adapted from Herdman et al., 2001)

cesses, respectively, is the reduction of 40-Hz ASSRs in sleep and anesthesia with no changes in 80-Hz ASSRs. The transition from wakefulness to sleep is in part related to the degree of hyperpolarization of thalamocortical neurons (Steriade, McCormick, & Sejnowski, 1993). Tonic hyperpolarization during sleep and anes-thesia reduces the flow of information reaching cortex. 40-Hz ASSRs presumably are mediated through the thalamocortical system (see later) and therefore are greatly reduced in sleep (Jerger, Chmiel, Frost, & Coker, 1986; Linden et al., 1985) and anesthesia (Plourde & Picton, 1990). However, the 80-Hz ASSR is still very robust during sleep and in fact is the preferable subject state during recordings.

Functional Magnetic Resonance Imaging

Functional MRI (fMRI) data have revealed progressive decreasing shifts of "best modulation frequencies" along the ascending auditory system. In the study by Giraud and colleagues (2000), white noise was modulated at rates varying from 4 to 256 Hz. Maximal blood flow was seen for high modulation rates (256 Hz) at lower brainstem regions; as the modulation rate decreased, maximal activity subsequently increased at higher relay stations such as the inferior colliculus, medial geniculate, and Heschl's gyrus. Although the investigators did not use "typical" ASSR stimuli, the idea nonetheless is consistent with electrophysiological data suggesting that on progression along the auditory neuroaxis, slower modulation rates are preferentially coded by the cortex, and fast modulation rates are preferentially coded by subcortical structures.

40-Hz Auditory Steady-State Responses

Studying the neural origin of ASSRs in the 40-Hz range is closely related to the understanding of the underlying generation mechanism. The goal is to determine which part of the brain produces the 40-Hz ASSR and which parts of the auditory pathway they represent. The latter is most important for interpretation of implications for auditory function and for interpretation of the results of clinical application of the 40-Hz ASSR.

Two main principles of ASSR generation have been discussed over the course of almost 30 years. The *superimposition hypothesis* postulates that repeatedly evoked transient responses accumulate to form the ASSR. This is not entirely in contrast with the second hypothesis, the *hypothesis of intrinsic oscillations in neural networks,* which states that oscillatory neural networks are driven by periodic stimuli and respond with steady-state oscillations. Both of these hypotheses are discussed in this section.

The Superimposition Hypothesis

The hypothesis that ASSRs with maximal amplitudes around 40 Hz result from superimposition of repeatedly evoked middle-latency responses (MLRs) was inaugurated by a report by Galambos, Makeig, and Talmachoff (1981), which inspired a large number of studies about this phenomenon. These researchers recorded auditory evoked responses to repeated click stimuli at various stimulation rates. A slow click rate (up to 10 clicks/s) evoked isolated groups of MLRs with interpeak latencies of about 25 ms between the vertex-negative N_a and N_b waves as well between the positive P_a and P_b waves. Both the N_a/P_a and N_b/P_b waves of the MLRs were described as resembling single waves of a 40-Hz sinusoid. At 20-Hz stimulation, N_a/P_a and N_b/P_b cycles followed each other periodically and formed a stream of continuous 40-Hz oscillation. The amplitude of oscillation was maximal with stimulation at 40 Hz, when the N_a/P_a wave of a response probably perfectly superimposes on the N_b/P_b wave of the response to the preceding click. With a sample waveform of MLRs, recorded at slow click rate, Galambos and colleagues (1981) demonstrated that repeated superimposition of multiple versions of the response, each shifted by 25 ms, resulted in a waveform like that of the recorded evoked response, which was observed at the 40-Hz stimulation rate (Figure 4–4).

Experimental results at various stimulation rates showed maximum response amplitude at 40 Hz. Moreover, minimum response amplitudes were reported close to 30 and 55 Hz in concordance with the model of MLR superimposition, which predicts that subsequent positive and negative responses would cancel out each other at these frequencies.

Sources of the Auditory Middle-Latency Response

If the model for the auditory 40-Hz response as proposed by Galambos and associates (1981) completely describes the response generation mechanism, the intracerebral sources of the ASSR must be assumed to be identical to the sources of the MLR. In a study using EEG, the

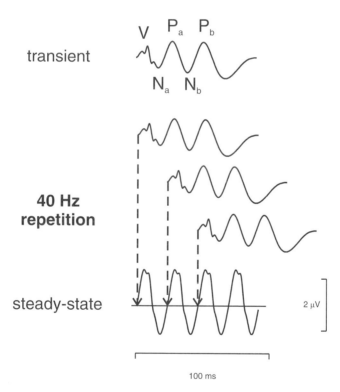

Figure 4–4. Superimposition of MLRs as a mechanism for generation of the 40-Hz ASSR. MLRs were recorded with a stimulus rate of 10 clicks per second (*top*). Samples of the MLR were shifted by multiples of 25 ms and averaged. The *arrows* denote the time of stimulus presentation.

MLR-generating system was described by Kraus and McGee (1995) as part of the thalamocortical pathway. Even though the amplitudes of MLRs are small, single components of the response were localized from data recorded with EEG or MEG. The first MEG study by Pellizzone, Hari, and coworkers (1987) demonstrated the cortical origin of the P_a wave, in a location slightly more anterior than the source of the N_1 response. Thus, P_a and N_a waves of the MLRs reflect the earliest part of primary auditory cortex activation. The origin of the N_a component was studied with click-evoked magnetic fields (Scherg, Hari, et al., 1989; Hashimoto, Mashiko, et al., 1995; Kuriki, Nogai, et al., 1995; Yoshiura, Ueno, et al., 1995) and was found mainly in the posterior medial part of Heschl's gyri. The P_a wave commonly was localized at the place of the N_a generator in several studies (Scherg, Hari, et al., 1989; Makela, Hamalainen, et al, 1994; Hashimoto, Mashiko, et al., 1995; Yoshiura, Ueno, et al., 1995; Gutschalk, Mase, et al., 1999). In a very precise localization study, based on simultaneous EEG and MEG recordings, the P_a was found in the medial portion of Heschl's gyri, N_b/P_b in the lateral aspect of the supratemporal gyrus (STG), and a later component of the P_b in the anterolateral portion of Heschl's gyri (Yvert, Crouzeix, et al., 2001). The localization of MLRs along the Heschl's gyri was confirmed by intracerebral and MEG recordings from the same subjects (Godey, Schwartz, et al., 2001). These studies showed consistently that MLRs represent early activation of bilateral auditory cortices. Because MLRs are generated in thalamocortical networks, it has to be considered that the activity seen in EEG and MEG recordings reflects mainly the cortical part, for which the recordings from the scalp surface (EEG) or even extracranially (MEG) are most sensitive.

The Hypothesis of Intrinsic Oscillations in Neural Networks

The hypothesis of intrinsic oscillations in neural networks predicts that 40-Hz ASSRs are produced by oscillatory neural populations, which are driven and synchronized by periodic auditory stimuli. The first requirement of the hypothesis is the presence of a neural mechanism that is capable of oscillating at a specific frequency. Such neural oscillations may result from firing properties of single neurons or from small local networks of neurons that are connected as a loop. Interactions between excitatory and inhibitory connections within such a loop result in local oscillations at a frequency that is determined mainly by conduction delay within the loop.

Both types of neural oscillators have been reported. For example, rhythmic bursts of discharges in single neurons in neocortex and thalamus in the cat showed a high temporal correlation with depth-EEG recordings (Steriade, 1997). Neurons with such intrinsic oscillatory properties may serve as pacemakers in thalamocortical networks (Llinas, Grace, et al., 1991), with a wide frequency range of responsiveness (Gray, Konig, et al., 1989). When the bursting neurons are embedded in a thalamocortical loop, as in the model proposed by Llinas and Ribary (2001), the network responds maximally at frequencies close to 40 Hz. Several modulating inputs in the model allow the network to start and stop the rhythmical activity. Thus, sensory input can reset the network, and the immediate restart after the reset then results in synchronized oscillatory activity, which can be recorded as mass activity in EEG and MEG studies (Llinas & Ribary, 1993).

Significance of 40-Hz Oscillatory Networks

Several studies indicate that oscillatory activity in the 40-Hz range is involved in sensory perception, as well in the integration of sensory modalities. In single-unit recordings from the visual cortex of the cat, local 40-Hz oscillations were observed that were tuned for a specific stimulus feature, as in a case reporting the orientation of the visual stimulus (Gray & Singer, 1989). The oscillations resulted from properties of cortical neurons and within cortex connections without involvement of thalamocortical networks. The important concept derived from those observations is that neurons that synchronously oscillate establish a local network. Thus the recorded oscillatory responses likely provide a general mechanism by which activity patterns in spatially separate regions of the cortex are temporally coordinated. In this sense, 40-Hz oscillations are an important mechanism for representation of the stimulus.

In contrast with a hard-wired neural network, a network established by oscillatory synchrony can be reconfigured dynamically through reset and restart of oscillation in a new configuration. Such reset mechanisms have been reported by Llinas and Ribary (1993). Using MEG recording, a stimulus-induced reset of 40-Hz oscillation was reported in alert subjects. The effect could be observed as a stimulus-locked burst of 40-Hz activity

in the averaged MEG recording. A similar type of activity was recorded in REM sleep. Llinas and Ribary interpreted their results as a correlate of cognitive processing resulting from coherent oscillation in thalamocortical loops. In a MEG experiment from the same group (Joliot, Ribary, et al., 1994), a pair of click stimuli evoked a burst of 40-Hz activity in response to the first click if the second click was delayed by no more than 14 ms. A wider separation of the clicks, inducing the percept of two items, resulted in additional 40-Hz activity. The results were interpreted as coexistence of primary sensory 40-Hz activity and 40-Hz activity reflecting temporal binding underlying cognition.

In recent years, a large number of EEG and MEG studies have addressed the relevance of high-frequency oscillations related to cognition. In contrast with strictly time-locked (or phase-locked) activity, as observed in sensory processing, mainly changes in the signal energy were observed and termed "induced gamma-band activity," in contrast with evoked responses (Tallon-Baudry & Bertrand, 1999; Kaiser & Lutzenberger, 2005).

Both hypotheses of 40-Hz ASSR generation—the MLR superimposition and the oscillatory network models—seem to be very distinct. However, they predict the same pattern of ASSRs as measured on EEG and MEG. A fair amount of studies have been carried out to probe both hypotheses.

Probing the Superimposition Hypothesis

Characteristics of the response amplitude and phase of the ASSR as functions of the stimulation rate have been investigated in several studies using click stimuli or AM sound. Azzena and associates. (1995) investigated the ASSR generation mechanism with click-evoked ASSRs at stimulation rates of 20 to 60 Hz (with 10-Hz increments) and compared amplitudes and phases of recorded responses with artificial ASSRs, which were derived from MLRs recorded at a 7.9-Hz repetition rate. The artificial ASSR replicated the recorded waveforms at 40 Hz; however, substantial differences were observed at lower and higher stimulation rates. In particular, the minima in the amplitude characteristic around 30 and 60 Hz, as reported by Galambos and co-workers (1981), could not be reproduced, and the phase of recorded responses could not be explained by the simulated responses. In a follow-up study by the same group, Santarelli, Maurizi, and colleagues (1995) modeled the recorded ASSRs sufficiently with isolated MLRs, as well as with the response to the last click in a stimulus train. However, the response to the last click showed additional oscillations compared with the MLRs; this finding was interpreted as a modification of MLRs at high stimulation rates, probably by additional activity in oscillatory networks. The conclusion from these results was that explanations of superimposed MLRs and oscillatory brain activity are not mutually exclusive.

Reconstruction of ASSRs by superimposition of MLRs, which were elicited with stimulation rates short enough to avoid any overlap from subsequent responses (typically around 10 Hz) as initially shown by Galambos and associates (1981) has been confirmed in several studies (Stapells, Galambos, et al., 1988; Hari, Hamalainen, et al., 1989; Plourde, Stapells, & Picton, 1991). Gutschalk, Mase, and colleagues (1999) went one step further and demonstrated that click-evoked ASSRs could be de-convolved into MLR waveforms. These investigators recorded ASSRs in the frequency range 32 to 52 Hz with MEG, performed a temporal deconvolution on all magnetic field waveforms, identified the N_a/P_a-N_b/P_b waves, and performed dipole source analysis of the reconstructed MLRs, which resulted in source locations consistent with previous observation of MLR sources.

Dissociation between Transient and Steady-State Responses

ASSRs are defined by their amplitude and phases and consequently are typically analyzed in the frequency domain. Time domain analysis may give additional insight into temporal dynamics of the ASSR. Ross, Picton, and Pantev (2002) compared the onset of auditory-evoked responses to tone bursts and to 40-Hz AM tone bursts. In nine subjects, averaged waveforms band pass–filtered between 24 and 60 Hz (Figure 4–5) showed a similar response pattern during the first 100 ms for both the pure tone and the AM tone bursts, which has been described as the *transient gamma band response* (tGBR) (Pantev, 1995). Most likely the tGBR and MLR describe the same phenomenon (Basar, Rosen, et al., 1987).

During the 100- to 250-ms latency interval, the 40-Hz oscillations developed for the AM stimulus and reached the steady-state value about 250 ms after stimulus onset. The ASSR offset, by contrast, showed a steeper slope and decayed within two cycles of the response. The group mean tGBR to the onset of the pure tone (Figure 4–6) resembled the N_a-P_a/N_b-P_b pattern in the model wave as used for explanation of response superimposition by Galambos and associates (1981).

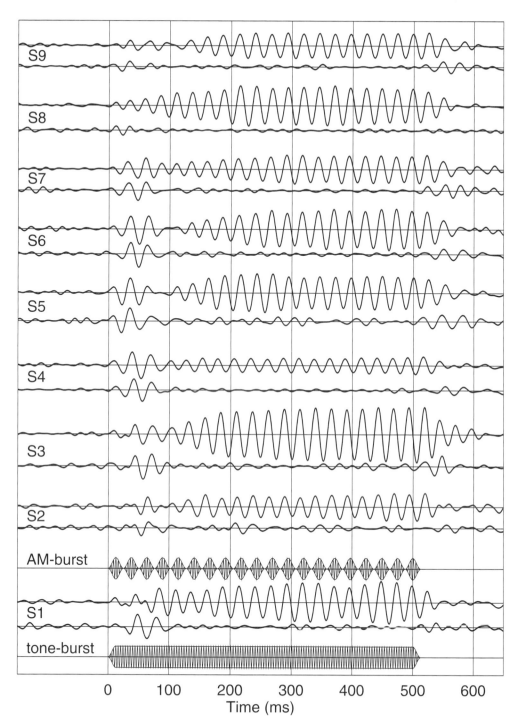

Figure 4–5. Transient and steady-state responses elicited by tone bursts and 40-Hz AM tone bursts, respectively, in nine subjects (S1 to S9) band pass-filtered between 24 and 60 Hz. For each subject, the response in the *upper trace* was elicited by the AM sound, and the response in the *lower trace* was elicited by the pure tone. Both stimuli evoked a similar transient response (latency less than 100 ms). The ASSR develops over a 200-ms time interval and continues for the duration of the stimulus. (From Ross et al. 2002.)

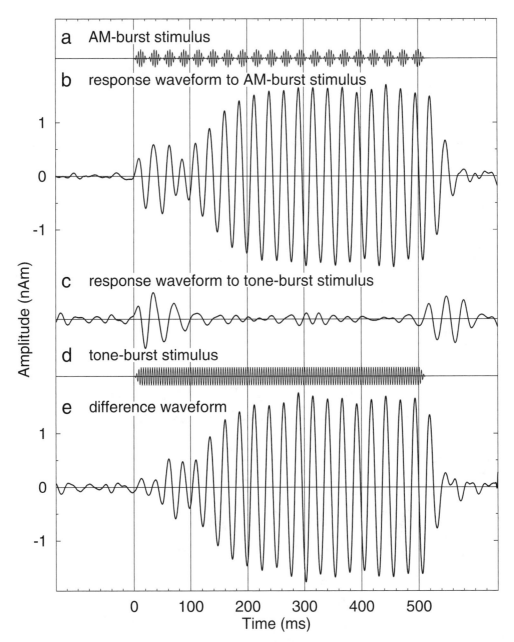

Figure 4–6. Grand averaged (*n* = 9) transient and steady-state waveforms: **a**, 40-Hz AM tone burst stimulus; **b**, response to the 40-Hz AM tone burst; **c**, response to non-modulated tone burst; **d**, tone burst stimulus; **e**, difference between responses to the AM sound and pure tone. The transient response is almost canceled out. The ASSR shows the characteristic 250-ms onset slope.

A same approach of ASSR reconstruction (Figure 4-7) successfully explained the steady-state part of the response; however, it failed to explain the onset dynamics. Although partially overlapping source locations for the tGBR and ASSR were found,

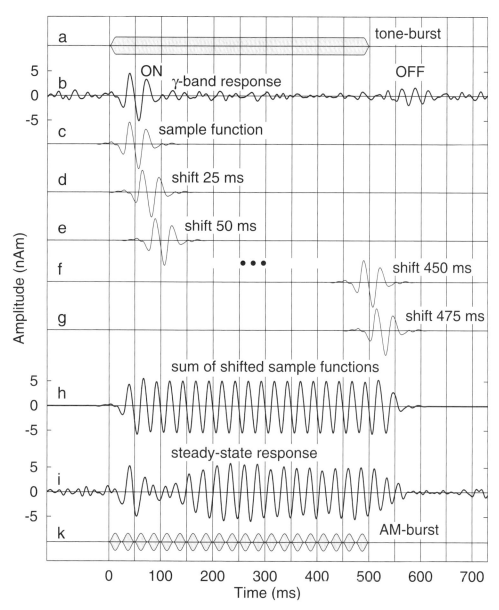

Figure 4–7. Reconstruction of ASSR waveform by linear superimposition of shifted transient response: **a**, tone burst stimulus; **b**, single subject's transient response in the gamma-frequency band; **c–g**, shifted versions of the transient response according to the periodicity of the modulation frequency, shown in half-scale compared with the original version in **a**; **h**, compound response signal from superimposition of shifted sample functions in **c–g**; **i**, response signal to AM tone burst stimulation obtained from the same subject; **k**, AM tone burst stimulus. (From Ross et al. 2002.)

the data were interpreted as distinct transient and steady-state responses.

Complete separation between transient and steady-state responses was demonstrated with AM stimuli having opposite polarity of the modulation during "odd and even" trials (Ross, Herdman, et al., 2005a). In the sum of responses to odd and even trials, the ASSR was canceled out and the tGBR remained, whereas in the difference the tGBR was canceled out but the ASSR was summed with equal polarity. This study revealed another difference in the characteristics of the tGBR and ASSR: The ASSR was lateralized in the right hemisphere, whereas the tGBR did not show a hemispheric dominance.

Reset Mechanism of 40-Hz Auditory Steady-State Responses

Increasing insight into the temporal dynamics of 40-Hz ASSRs came from a study about the detection of amplitude modulation gaps (Ross & Pantev, 2004). The stimuli were brief gaps inserted at the minimum of 40-Hz AM stimuli of 500-Hz tones. The behavioural threshold for detection of such AM gaps was close to 3 ms. ASSR MEG recordings showed substantial decrease in amplitude after a gap. The duration of the ASSR amplitude perturbation was clearly longer than the gap itself. Detailed analysis of the time course of amplitudes and phases revealed that a gap stimulus induced a reset of the ASSR. The onset of ASSR after the gap was widely independent of the gap duration and required about 250 ms, the same time as that found for the onset of 40-Hz ASSRs (Ross, Picton, et al., 2002). Also, the time course of ASSR phase changes after the gap stimulus resembled the time course of ASSR phase changes after stimulus onset. The observation of a new ASSR onset after each gap stimulus supported the hypothesis of an ASSR reset, which was induced by a change in the periodicity of the stimulus.

A generalization of the concept of stimulus-induced reset of 40-Hz ASSRs has been demonstrated in an experiment in which a 40-Hz AM sound was presented to the right ear and a narrow band noise impulse to the left ear (Ross, Herdman, et al. 2005b). The click-like stimulus caused a reset of the 40-Hz ASSR, with a characteristic recovery time of about 250 ms for the ASSR amplitude and phase. The ASSR reset was observed even when the ASSR-generating AM sound continued over time and the interfering click stimulus was in different perceptual channels, such as a different frequency band and a different ear. The results were interpreted as indicating that the ASSR reflected a strong representation of the AM sound stimulus after sensory integration. A too-strong representation of sensory input might be disadvantageous for the detection of small environmental changes or changes of very brief duration. The reset mechanism demonstrated in this study resolved the strong representation of previous sensory input in favour of a stimulus change. Such encoding of sensory information allows simultaneously temporal integration over several hundred milliseconds and high temporal acuity. Clearly, the described temporal dynamics of 40-Hz ASSRs are not compatible with the hypothesis of repeatedly superimposed transient responses.

A Single Case Lesion Study

Evidence for dissociation between MLRs and 40-Hz ASSRs came from recordings in a patient with multiple lesions in bilateral external capsules but intact auditory cortices (Santarelli & Conti, 1999). Click-evoked MLRs were robustly recorded from both hemispheres in this patient;

however, 40-Hz ASSRs were completely absent. It can be assumed that the afferent auditory pathway up to primary auditory cortex was intact in this patient, as indexed by the MLR. However the lesions in white matter connecting the cortex and thalamus disrupted the generation of the ASSRs. Missing 40-Hz ASSRs in this patient strongly supports the hypothesis that corticothalamic connections are necessary for the ASSR-generating system in addition to the afferent pathway, which is sufficient for MLR generation. The fact that the patient was profoundly deaf despite the presence of ABRs and MLRs sheds light on the potential importance of 40-Hz responses for diagnostic assessment.

Dipole Source Localization of the Auditory Steady-State Response

Source analysis using the model of a small number of dipole sources was mainly performed from MEG data. MEG recordings of the magnetic field of 40-Hz ASSRs result in magnetic field maps with distinct dipolar patterns above the temporal brain regions (Figure 4–8). That such a magnetic field distribution can be explained largely with single equivalent dipoles in the left and right hemisphere had been shown in early MEG studies using click (Romani, Williamson, et al., 1982) or AM stimuli (Hari, Hamalainen, et al., 1989). Pantev, Roberts, and associates (1996) demonstrated tonotopic organization of an equivalent dipole model of tone pip-evoked ASSRs. ASSR sources for higher frequencies (4000 Hz) were found more medial than for lower frequencies (250 Hz), which is consistent with the tonotopic organization of N_1 sources (Pantev, Bertrand, et al., 1995).

The finding of tonotopic organization of the ASSR sources was recently corroborated by Wienbruch, Paul, and colleagues (2006), who also showed attenuated tonotopy in tinnitus patients. Individual anatomical information, commonly obtained with MRI, was not available in some MEG studies. In those cases, the relative location between sources of the auditory evoked N_1 response and the ASSR was reported. Consistently reported findings are more medial and more anterior ASSR sources (Ross, Borgmann, et al., 2000; Draganova, Ross, et al., 2002; Ross, Picton, et al., 2002) . If the N_1 source locations represent the center of gravity of multiple sources in primary and secondary auditory cortices, the ASSR sources located more medially and anteriorly would be likely to be found deep in Heschl's gyri, which is accepted as the location of primary auditory cortices (Penhune, Zatorre, et al., 1996).

A common result of the MEG studies of 40-Hz ASSR dipole source localization is that a single dipole or a small number of dipoles in the left and right auditory cortices explain the recorded magnetic fields. In most studies, dipole modeling was possible even for individual subjects. Thus, the model of single dipoles in the auditory cortex seems to be a robust explanation for the MEG-recorded responses. However, such results are not completely compatible with the hypothesis that ASSRs are generated in widespread neural networks involving subcortical structures. The dipole results probably represent centers of activation and current recording techniques that are unable to separate adjacently located sources. Also, dipole source analysis does not seem sufficiently sensitive for deeper sources in the presence of dominant superficial sources.

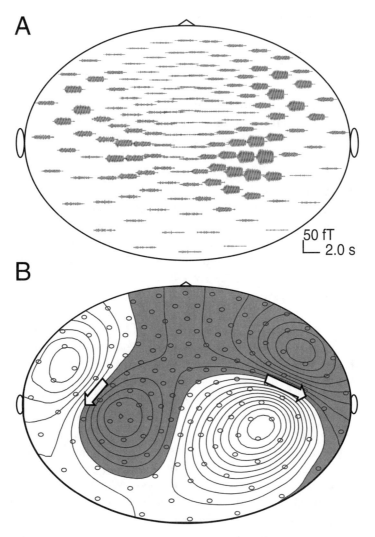

Figure 4–8. MEG-recorded magnetic field of the 40-Hz ASSR elicited with AM sound of 2-s duration. **A**, ASSR waveforms from 150 MEG channels above the head (*front*, on *top*). Two groups of channels with maximal response amplitudes can be seen above the left and right temporal regions. **B**, Magnetic field map of 40-Hz ASSR amplitude. *Gray* and *white areas* denote regions of opposite polarity. The *contour lines* (equally spaced lines of constant magnetic field strength) indicate maxima for each polarity above the left and right hemispheres. Such magnetic field distribution is characteristic of the field of single dipoles. The *arrows* indicate the position and orientation of dipoles in the left and right hemispheres.

Analysis of Continuously Distributed Auditory Steady-State Response Sources

Several approaches using EEG and MEG data analysis overcome the limitation of dipole modeling. One approach is to model the observed scalp potential distribution in the EEG or the extracranial magnetic field in MEG with a continuous distribution of source activity (Michel, Murray, et al., 2004). Other approaches, such as "beamformer" techniques, do not apply a source model at all and construct virtual sensors for each brain volume element (Hillebrand & Barnes, 2005).

Using the distributed source approach and additional information from a positron emission tomography (PET) study, Reyes, Lockwood, and coworkers (2005) found widespread activation in frontal cortex and even in the cerebellum, in addition to left and right temporal activation. Their interpretation was that the ASSRs result from synchronization of

gamma band activity across a wide spatial range of brain areas.

Using the beamformer approach, Herdman and colleagues (2003) showed left and right auditory cortex activation and corroborated previous dipole modeling with the finding of more lateral sources of 40-Hz ASSRs than the N_1 sources (Figure 4–9). However, the method was not sensitive enough, showing additional sources as predicted by the ongoing discussion. The beamformer method used by Herdman and co-workers (2003) compared the MEG signal power during stimulation with AM sound with the MEG signal power in a stimulus-free interval (Vrba & Robinson, 2001). Signal power changes are small, however, and the ASSR is better characterized by phase synchronization (Ross et al., 2005). Using the same beamformer but a measure of phase coherence instead of the measure of signal power change results in volumetric mapping of 40-Hz activity shown in Figure 4–10. In addition to left and

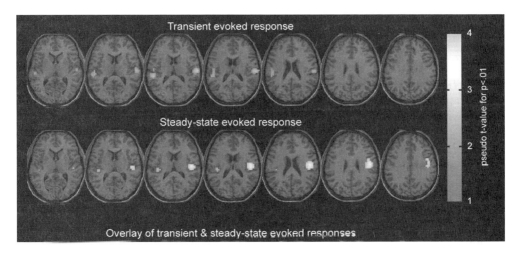

Figure 4–9. Brain regions activated by the onset of a tone burst (*top row*) and 40-Hz AM sound (*middle row*) observed with volumetric statistical mapping of the MEG response. The overlay of transient and steady-state responses (*bottom row*) indicates more medially localized ASSR sources. (From Herdman et al. 2003.)

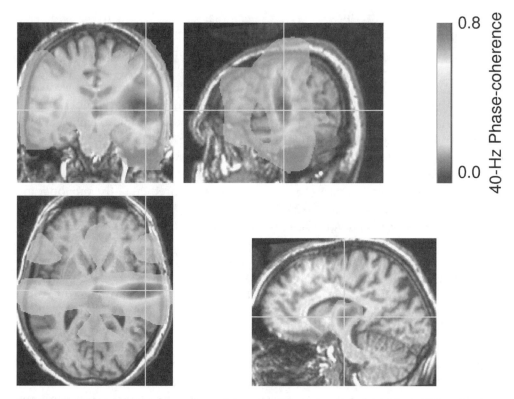

0.8

0.0

40-Hz Phase-coherence

Figure 4–10. Volumetric mapping of the phase coherence of 40-Hz ASSRs obtained from MEG recording with binaural stimulation. The first three sections through the right auditory cortex (*blue cursor*) show activation of the auditory cortices, left and right thalamus, anterior and posterior cingulate cortices, and frontal areas. The insert (*bottom right*) is a more medial sagittal slice showing activation of the right thalamus.

right auditory cortex activation of the left and right thalamus, anterior and posterior cingulated cortex and frontal cortices can be identified.

Other Imaging Modalities for Localization of 40-Hz Auditory Steady-State Responses

Although other neuroimaging methods such as fMRI and PET do not show the high temporal resolution of EEG and MEG, both fMRI and PET can be used

because of their high temporal resolution for localization of 40-Hz ASSR activity. In one PET study, Reyes and associates. (2004) compared brain activation with a pure 1000-Hz tone and 40-Hz AM sound. Both monaural, right ear stimuli activated bilateral auditory cortices and the left thalamus. The difference between the activation patterns for the AM sound and the pure tone showed activation of the right auditory cortex and the anterior cingulate cortex, which are areas that specifically respond to 40-Hz modulation. The study did not include a control condition with left ear stimulation and could not determine whether the lateralization of activity was caused by the side of stimulation or was an effect of lateralized brain organization. However, the observation that the AM sound dominantly activated the right hemisphere, which was ipsilateral to the stimulation, is consistent with right hemispheric dominance for the 40-Hz ASSR found in another study (Ross et al., 2005).

In an fMRI study by Giraud, Lorenzi, and associates (2000), the contrast in brain activation observed with continuous noise stimulation and AM noise showed a spatial organization involving both auditory cortices for a wide range of modulation frequencies. In another fMRI study with AM sounds of various modulation frequencies (Pastor, Artieda, et al., 2002), activation of the cerebellum was found for 40-Hz stimulation but not for other modulation rates, which was interpreted as an indication of the special role of 40-Hz activity in auditory processing. These studies demonstrate that PET and fMRI studies image, with high resolution, those brain areas that are activated specifically by AM sound. The limited temporal resolution, however, leaves open the question of whether those activations are identical to the ASSRs recorded with EEG and MEG.

Summary

Converging evidence from a number of studies support the hypothesis that ASSRs in the 40-Hz frequency range are generated primarily in thalamocortical oscillatory networks and may synchronize higher auditory associative areas and nonauditory cortices. EEG and MEG recordings of 40-Hz ASSRs show mainly the contribution from primary auditory cortices and dipole source localization in bilateral auditory cortices. The temporal dynamics of 40-Hz ASSRs dissociate transient MLRs and sustained ASSRs.

During the discussion of 40-Hz ASSR generation mechanisms, it has been argued that the transient superimposition and the intrinsic oscillation hypotheses of ASSR generation are not mutually exclusive, but rather that they are just different descriptions of the same phenomenon. This argument is inspired by a concept in engineering science stating that a linear time invariant system can be completely described by its impulse response (the transient response) or its transfer function in the frequency domain (the frequency characteristics of ASSRs). However, the assumption of time invariance does not seem to be fulfilled for brain function. The dissociation between transient and steady-state 40-Hz responses is an important step because it addresses different functional implications for MLRs and ASSRs.

References

Azzena, G. B., Conti G., Santarelli, R., Ottaviani, F., Paludetti, G., & Maurizi, M. (1995). Generation of human auditory steady-state responses (SSRs). I: Stimulus rate effects. *Hearing Research, 83*(1–2), 1–8.

Basar, E., Rosen, B., Basareroglu, C., & Greitschus, F. (1987). The associations between 40 Hz-EEG and the middle latency response of the auditory evoked potential. *International Journal of Neuroscience, 33*(1–2), 103–117.

Draganova, R., Ross, B., Borgmann, C., & Pantev, C. (2002). Auditory cortical response patterns to multiple rhythms of AM sound. *Ear and Hearing, 23*(3), 254-265.

Galambos, R., Makeig, S., & Talmachoff, P. (1981). A 40-Hz auditory potential recorded from the human scalp. *Proceedings of the National Academy of Science of the United States of America, 78*(4), 2643-2647.

Giraud, A. L., Lorenzi, C., Ashburner, J., Wable, J., Johnsrude, I., Frackowiak, R., & Kleinschmidt, A. (2000). Representation of the temporal envelope of sounds in the human brain. *Journal of Neurophysiology, 84*(3), 1588-1598.

Godey, B., Schwartz, D., de Graaf, J. B., Chauvel, P., & Leigeois-Chauvel, C. (2001). Neuromagnetic source localization of auditory evoked fields and intracerebral evoked potentials: A comparison of data in the same patients. *Clinical Neurophysiology, 112*(10), 1850-1859.

Gray, C. M., Konig, P., Engel, A. K., & Singer, W. (1989). Oscillatory responses in cat visual cortex exhibit inter-columnar synchronization which reflects global stimulus properties. *Nature 338*(6213), 334-337.

Gray, C. M., & Singer, W. (1989). Stimulus-specific neuronal oscillations in orientation columns of cat visual cortex. *Proceedings of the National Academy of Science of the United States of America, 86*(5), 1698-1702.

Gutschalk, A., Mase, R., Roth, R., Ille, N., Rupp, A., Hahnel, S., Picton, T. W., & Scherg, M. (1999). Deconvolution of 40 Hz steady-state fields reveals two overlapping source activities of the human auditory cortex. *Clinical Neurophysiology, 110*(5), 856-868.

Hari, R., Hamalainen, M., & Joutsiniemi, S. L. (1989). Neuromagnetic steady-state responses to auditory stimuli. *Journal of the Acoustical Society of America, 86*(3), 1033-1039.

Hashimoto, I., Mashiko, T., Yoshikawa, K., Mizuta, T., Imada, T., & Hayashi, M. (1995). Neuromagnetic measurements of the human primary auditory response. *Electroencephalography and Clinical Neurophysiology, 96*(4), 348-356.

Herdman, A. T., Lins, O., Van Roon, P., Stapells, D. R., Scherg, M., & Picton, T. W. (2002). Intracerebral sources of human auditory steady-state responses. *Brain Topography, 15*(2), 69-86.

Herdman, A. T., Wollbrink, A., Chau, W., Ishii, R., Ross, B., & Pantev, C. (2003). Determination of activation areas in the human auditory cortex by means of synthetic aperture magnetometry. *Neuroimage, 20*(2), 995-1005.

Hillebrand, A., & Barnes, G. R. (2005). Beamformer analysis of MEG data. *International Review of Neurobiology, 68*, 149-171.

Jerger, J., Chmiel, R., Frost, J. D., & Coker, N. (1986). Effect of sleep on the auditory steady-state evoked potential. *Ear and Hearing, 7*(4), 240-245.

John, M. S., & Picton, T. W. (2000). Human auditory steady-state responses to amplitude-modulated tones: Phase and latency measurements. *Hearing Research, 141*(1-2), 57-79.

Joliot, M., Ribary, U., & Llinas, R. (1994). Human oscillatory brain activity near 40 Hz coexists with cognitive temporal binding. *Proceedings of the National Academy of Science of the United States of America, 91*(24), 11748-11751.

Joris, P. X., Schreiner, C. E., & Rees, A. (2004). Neural processing of amplitude-modulated sounds. *Physiology Reviews, 84*(2), 541-577.

Joris, P. X., & Yin, T. C. (1992). Responses to amplitude-modulated tones in the auditory nerve of the cat. *Journal of the Acoustical Society of America, 91*(1), 215-232.

Kaiser, J., & Lutzenberger, W. (2005). Human gamma-band activity: A window to cognitive processing. *Neuroreport, 16*(3), 207-211.

Khanna, S. M., & Teich, M. C. (1989). Spectral characteristics of the responses of primary auditory-nerve fibers to amplitude-modulated signals. *Hearing Research, 39*(1-2), 143-157.

Kraus, N., & McGee, T. (1995). The middle latency response generating system. *Electroencephalography and Clinical Neurophysiology. Supplement, 44*, 93-101.

Kuriki, S., Nogai, T., & Hirata, Y. (1995). Cortical sources of middle latency responses of auditory evoked magnetic field. *Hearing Research, 92*(1-2), 47-51.

Kuwada, S., Anderson, J. S., Batra, R., Fitzpatrick, D. C., Teissier, N., & D'Angelo, W. R. (2002). Sources of the scalp-recorded amplitude-modulation following response. *Journal of the American Academy of Audiology, 13*(4), 188-204.

Langner, G., & Schreiner, C. E. (1988). Periodicity coding in the inferior colliculus of the cat. I. Neuronal mechanisms. *Journal of Neurophysiology, 60*(6), 1799-1822.

Linden, R. D., Campbell, K. B., Hamel, G., & Picton, T. W. (1985). Human auditory steady state evoked potentials during sleep. *Ear and Hearing, 6*(3), 167-174.

Lins, O. G., Picton, P. E., Picton, T. W., Champagne, S. C., & Durieux-Smith, A. (1995). Auditory steady-state responses to tones amplitude-modulated at 80-110 Hz. *Journal of the Acoustical Society of America, 97*(5 Pt 1), 3051-3063.

Llinas, R., & Ribary, U. (1993). Coherent 40-Hz oscillation characterizes dream state in humans. *Proceedings of the National Academy of Science of the United States of America, 90*(5), 2078-2081.

Llinas, R., & Ribary U. (2001). Consciousness and the brain. The thalamocortical dialogue in health and disease. *Annals of the New York Academy of Sciences, 929*, 166-175.

Llinas, R. R., Grace, A. A., & Yarom, Y. (1991). In vitro neurons in mammalian cortical layer 4 exhibit intrinsic oscillatory activity in the 10- to 50-Hz frequency range. *Proceedings of the National Academy of Science of the United States of America, 88*(3), 897-901.

Makela, J. P., Hamalainen, M., Hari, R., & McEvoy, L. (1994). Whole-head mapping of middle-latency auditory evoked magnetic fields. *Electroencephalography and Clinical Neurophysiology, 92*(5), 414-421.

Michel, C. M., Murray, M. M., Lantz, G., Gonzalez, S., Spinelli, L., & Grave de Peralta, R. (2004). EEG source imaging. *Clinical Neurophysiology, 115*(10), 2195-2222.

Moller, A. R. (1972). Coding of amplitude and frequency modulated sounds in the cochlear nucleus of the rat. *Acta Physiologica Scandinavica, 86*(2), 223-238.

Pantev, C. (1995). Evoked and induced gamma-band activity of the human cortex. *Brain Topography, 7*(4), 321-330.

Pantev, C., Bertrand, O., Eulitz, C., Verkindt, C., Hampson, S., Schuierer, G., & Elbert, T. (1995). Specific tonotopic organizations of different areas of the human auditory cortex revealed by simultaneous magnetic and electric recordings. *Electroencephalography and Clinical Neurophysiology, 94*(1), 26-40.

Pantev, C., Roberts, L. E., Elbert, T., Ross, B., & Wienbruch, C. (1996). Tonotopic organization of the sources of human, auditory steady-state responses. *Hearing Research, 101*(1-2), 62-74.

Pastor, M. A., Artieda J., Arbizu, J., Marti-Climent, J. M., Penuelas, L., & Masdeu, J. C., (2002). Activation of human cerebral and cerebellar cortex by auditory stimulation at 40 Hz. *Journal of Neuroscience, 22*(23), 10501-10506.

Pelizzone, M., Hari, R., Makela, J. P., Huttunen, J., Ahlfors, S., & Hamalainen, M. (1987). Cortical origin of middle-latency auditory evoked responses in man. *Neuroscience Letters, 82*(3), 303-307.

Penhune, V. B., Zatorre, R. J., MacDonald, J. D., & Evans, A. C. (1996).Interhemispheric anatomical differences in human primary auditory cortex: Probabilistic mapping and volume measurement from magnetic resonance scans. *Cerebral Cortex, 6*(5), 661-672.

Picton, T. W., John, M. S., Dimitrijevic, A., & Purcell, D. (2003). Human auditory steady-state responses. *International Journal of Audiology, 42*(4), 177-219.

Plourde, G., & Picton, T. W. (1990). Human auditory steady-state response during general anesthesia. *Anesthesia and Analgesia, 71*(5), 460–468.

Plourde, G., Stapells, D. R., & Picton, T. W. (1991). The human auditory steady-state evoked potentials. *Acta Otolaryngologica Supplementum, 491*, 153–159.

Preuss, A., & Muller-Preuss, P. (1990). Processing of amplitude modulated sounds in the medial geniculate body of squirrel monkeys. *Experimental Brain Research, 79*(1), 207–211.

Purcell, D. W., John, S. M., Schneider, B. A., & Picton, T. W. (2004). Human temporal auditory acuity as assessed by envelope following responses. *Journal of the Acoustical Society of America, 116*(6), 3581–3593.

Reyes, S. A., Lockwood, A. H., Salvi, R. J., Coad, M. L., Wack, D. S., & Burkard, R. F. (2005). Mapping the 40-Hz auditory steady-state response using current density reconstructions. *Hearing Research, 204*(1–2), 1–15.

Reyes, S. A., Salvi, R. J., Burkard, R. F., Coad, M. L., Wack, D. S., Galantowicz, P. J., & Lockwood, A. H. (2004). PET imaging of the 40 Hz auditory steady state response. *Hearing Research, 194*(1–2), 73–80.

Romani, G. L., Williamson, S. J., Kaufman, L., & Brenner, D. (1982). Characterization of the human auditory cortex by the neuromagnetic method. *Experimental Brain Research, 47*(3), 381–393.

Ross, B., Borgmann, C., Draganova, R., Roberts, L. E., & Pantev, C. (2000). A high-precision magnetoencephalographic study of human auditory steady-state responses to amplitude-modulated tones. *Journal of the Acoustical Society of America, 108*(2), 679–691.

Ross, B., Herdman, A. T., & Pantev, C. (2005a). Right hemispheric laterality of human 40 Hz auditory steady-state responses. *Cerebral Cortex, 15*(12), 2029–2039.

Ross, B., Herdman, A. T., & Pantev, C. (2005b). Stimulus induced desynchronization of human auditory 40-Hz steady-state responses. *Journal of Neurophysiology, 94*(6), 4082–4093.

Ross, B., & Pantev, C. (2004). Auditory steady-state responses reveal amplitude modulation gap detection thresholds. *Journal of the Acoustical Society of America, 115*(5 Pt 1), 2193–2206.

Ross, B., Picton, T. W., & Pantev, C. (2002). Temporal integration in the human auditory cortex as represented by the development of the steady-state magnetic field. *Hearing Research, 165*(1–2), 68–84.

Santarelli, R., & Conti, G. (1999). Generation of auditory steady-state responses: Linearity assessment. *Scandinavian Audiology. Supplementum, 51*, 23–32.

Santarelli, R., Maurizi, M., Conti, G., Ottaviani, F., Paludetti, G., & Pettorossi, V. E. (1995). Generation of human auditory steady-state responses (SSRs). II: Addition of responses to individual stimuli. *Hearing Research, 83*(1–2), 9–18.

Scherg, M., Hari, R., et al. (1989). Frequency specific sources of the auditory N19-P30-P50 response detected by a multiple source analysis of evoked magnetic fields and potentials. In S. J. Williamson, et al. (Eds.), *Advances in biomagnetics* (pp. 97–100). New York: Plenum Press.

Stapells, D. R., Galambos, R., Costello, J. A. & Makeig, S. (1988). Inconsistency of auditory middle latency and steady-state responses in infants. *Electroencephalography and Clinical Neurophysiology, 71*(4), 289–295.

Steriade, M. (1997). Synchronized activities of coupled oscillators in the cerebral cortex and thalamus at different levels of vigilance. *Cerebral Cortex, 7*(6), 583–604.

Steriade, M., McCormick, D. A., & Sejnowski, T. J. (1993). Thalamocortical oscillations in the sleeping and aroused brain. *Science, 262*(5134), 679–685.

Tallon-Baudry, C., & Bertrand, O. (1999). Oscillatory gamma activity in humans and its role in object representation. *Trends in Cognitive Science, 3*(4),151–162.

Vrba, J., & Robinson, S. E. (2001). Signal processing in magnetoencephalography. *Methods, 25*(2), 249–271.

Wienbruch, C., Paul, I., Weisz, N., Elbert, T., & Roberts, L. E. (2006). Frequency organization of the 40-Hz auditory steady-state response in normal hearing and in tinnitus. *Neuroimage*, *33*(1), 180–194.

Yoshiura, T., Ueno, S., Iramina, K., & Masuda, K. (1995). Source localization of middle latency auditory evoked magnetic fields. *Brain Research*, *703*(1–2), 139–144.

Yvert, B., Crouzeix, A., Bertrand, O., Seither-Preisler, A., & Pantev, C. (2001). Multiple supratemporal sources of magnetic and electric auditory evoked middle latency components in humans. *Cerebral Cortex*, *11*(5), 411–423.

CHAPTER 5

Subject Variables in Auditory Steady-State Response Testing: State, Anesthesia, Age, and Attention

BARBARA CONE-WESSON

Subject variables such as state of consciousness, age, and attention can affect the auditory steady-state response (ASSR). Of course, hearing loss or other neuropathologic conditions will have the most profound effect on the ASSR, but these are dealt with in Chapters 7 and 14. This chapter focuses on the effects of subject state and age, anesthesia, and attention.

State of Consciousness

Adults

Although the modulation and carrier frequencies (MF and CF) are the primary determinants of ASSR stimulus response properties, significant interactions between these stimulus response properties are observed with subject state. These effects in adults were evaluated by Cohen, Rickards, and Clark (1991), in a parametric study of CF, MF, and sleep versus wakefulness. These investigators showed that background electroencephalogram (EEG) noise levels were much higher in awake adults, compared to sleeping adults, regardless of MF, but the difference in background noise in the two states was greatest for modulation frequencies above 80 Hz. Given the fact that the amplitude of the ASSR decreases as MF increases, the higher background noise during wakefulness means that very long averaging times would be needed to obtain an adequate (ASSR) signal-to-noise ratio. Cohen and associates used CFs of 250 to 4000 Hz (in octave steps) presented at 55 dB HL to evoke ASSRs in awake adults at MFs of 30 to 185 Hz. MFs of 60 Hz or lower resulted in response latencies (calculated from phase delay data) in the range of 28 to 33 ms, clearly similar to the range for auditory middle latency responses (AMLRs), and thus suggesting a cortical contribution to the ASSR at these modulation frequencies. For MFs at 90 Hz and above, the latencies ranged from 11.6 ms for a CF of 250 Hz to 8.9 ms for a CF of 4000 Hz. The latencies at these MFs indicated a likely homology to tone-burst evoked ABRs. Again, this has implications for the effects of subject state. Auditory evoked potentials from the cortex, such as the AMLR, are sensitive to sleep stage, whereas ABRs are not. ASSRs with a large signal-to-noise ratio were obtained for an MF of 45 Hz during testing in both awake and asleep conditions, using a stimulus level of 30 dB HL, and CFs at 1000 Hz or lower. The advantage for the MF at 45 Hz was not however apparent for sleeping subjects tested with CFs at 2 kHz or 4 kHz. For these carrier frequencies, and at MFs at 80 Hz and above, the signal-to-noise ratios were equivalent to those found at lower MFs (less than 60 Hz) in sleeping subjects. These results can be used to optimize ASSR recording parameters in adults. If the CF is 1000 Hz or below, and the (adult) subject is sleeping, then MFs in the range of 40 to 45 Hz should be used. If the CF is above 1500 Hz, MFs of greater than 70 Hz should be used. If the (adult) subject is awake, then the best results will be obtained using MFs in the 40- to 45-Hz range, regardless of CF.

Dobie and Wilson (1998) also determined the detectability of ASSRs in adults tested both in the awake state and during sedated sleep. They used a low-frequency carrier (640 Hz) presented at 40 and 20 dB SL (58 dB SPL and 38 dB SPL, respectively), to assess a group of normal-hearing listeners. The ASSR tests at these levels were given using MFs at 40 to 90 Hz. The number of ASSRs meeting an *a priori* statistical criterion (based on response phase coherence and amplitude) was used to determine the best MFs as a function of stimulus level and subject state.

Amplitude MFs of 40 and 90 Hz yielded peaks in the response detection function for both awake and sedated sleep states when the stimulus level was 40 dB SL. Less than 75% of the trials conducted at 20 dB SL resulted in a detectable response, regardless of the MF. Overall, detectability was considerably reduced in the sedated sleep state compared with that in the awake state, particularly for MFs below 50 Hz. The results obtained by Dobie and Wilson (1998) indicate that both low (40-Hz) and high (90-Hz) MFs are effective in evoking an ASSR for CFs below 1000 Hz in awake or sleeping adults, at least when stimuli are presented at suprathreshold levels.

Adults with normal hearing were tested during natural sleep by Aoyagi, Furuse, Yokota, Kiren, Suzuki, and Koikel (1994), using CFs of 500, 1000, 2000, and 4000 Hz presented at 50 dB HL, at MFs of 20 to 120 Hz. Results were similar to those of Cohen and coworkers (1991), with peaks in the ASSR detectability functions found at 40 and 80 Hz for CFs at 500 and 1000 Hz, and at MFs of 80 Hz or higher for CFs at 2000 and 4000 Hz. It should be noted that responses were detected at all MFs except for 20 Hz.

Results from these studies indicate that when testing adults who are asleep, the MF should be close to 40 Hz for CFs below 1500 Hz, and near 80 Hz for CFs at 2 to 8 kHz. If adults are tested during quiet wakefulness, then an MF of 40 Hz should yield the best response-to-noise ratios, regardless of carrier frequency.

Lins and Picton (1995) demonstrated that it was possible to measure ASSRs using the same CF (1.0 kHz) and up to four different modulation rates presented simultaneously, with modulation rates in the low (39 and 49 Hz) and high (81 and 97 Hz) range. This would appear to be a beneficial technique for testing patients who may be in a variable state of arousal, from alert to deep (stage 4) sleep, as might occur during a typical clinical test session. When adults were tested during an awake state, the amplitudes of the responses to the low MFs (presented individually) were up to three times those of the responses for high MFs (presented individually). When two different MFs were used in each ear, the responses to each MF were decreased by about 20%. In sleeping adults, when four different

MFs were presented simultaneously (39, 49, 81, and 97 Hz) the ASSR amplitudes for MFs at 39 and 49 Hz decreased with sleep stage, whereas the amplitudes at 81 and 97 Hz remained unchanged. Although only a small group of adults were tested in each of these conditions, and the 1000-Hz CF was at a suprathreshold level, the implications for a clinical test protocol are compelling. That is, each carrier could be presented at 39 Hz and 81 Hz, simultaneously. If threshold estimates are needed and the patient is in an awake state, the low-MF responses may be best, but at the same time, high MF components also can be tested. If the patient is drifting from wakefulness to drowsiness and sleep, the stability of the high-MF components will yield adequate information. In this case, the lower of the two thresholds could be used as the threshold estimate. It should be possible to implement this protocol on instruments that allow for simultaneous presentation of two or more carrier and modulation frequencies.

Infants

The effect of sleep versus wakefulness on the ASSR in infants has never been investigated. All published findings of infant-specific data have been obtained while infants were in natural or sedated sleep. Findings of Levi, Folsom, and Dobie (1993) indicate that modulation frequencies above 40 Hz, and particularly at 80 Hz, are preferable for testing sleeping infants. Using amplitude-modulated (AM) tones at 500 and 2000 Hz, presented at 60 dB HL (78 dB SPL), these investigators measured response coherence, which is an estimate of response power relative to overall response plus noise power (similar to a signal-to-noise ratio), as a function of modulation frequency. The largest coherence values in sleeping infants were obtained at 80 Hz, regardless of carrier frequency. When a 500-Hz CF was used, coherence values indicating statistical significance (response detected from background noise) were obtained at MFs of 40, 50, and 80 Hz, but not at 10, 20, or 30 Hz. For the 2000-Hz CF, only the 80-Hz MF yielded statistically significant results (response present) for all infants. When a cohort of adult subjects were tested in the sedated-sleep state, the largest mean coherence values for responses to 500- and 2000-Hz CF also were obtained at a MF of 80 Hz; however, coherence values also were well above statistical significance for MFs at 30 and 40 Hz. When the coherence values as a function of MF were compared for sleeping infants and sleeping adults, coherence values were greater for the sleeping adults, but the trend for growth of coherence with increasing MF was clear for both groups. The results for adults are similar to those obtained by Cohen and colleagues (1991) and Dobie and Wilson (1998). These findings of Levi et al were the first to demonstrate a clear advantage for a high MF (greater than 60 Hz) for infants.

Aoyagi and associates also showed that MFs in the 80-Hz range resulted in the most stable and reliable ASSR results among normal-hearing infants and children (aged 4 months to 15 years), tested during sedated sleep (Aoyagi, Kiren, Furuse, Fuse, Suzuki, Yokota, Furuse, et al., 1994). Although only one CF (1000 Hz), and one level (50 dB HL) were used, the MF was varied from 20 to 200 Hz. Measures of phase coherence were highest for 80 Hz, although peaks also were found at 120 and 160 Hz for infants and children less than 4 years of age; these additional peaks in the coherence functions were not clear for older children or for a group of normal-hearing adults. There was a clear advantage for the 80 Hz MF compared with the 40 Hz MF for ASSR tests in infants and young children. This advantage was not seen for children older than 9 years or for adults; peaks in the coherence functions in these older subjects were found at MFs of 40 and 80 Hz.

A large-scale study of newborns completed by Rickards, Tan, Cohen, Wilson, Drew, and Clark (1994) provides compelling evidence for the efficacy of ASSR tests using modulation rates higher than 60 Hz in this age group. CFs of 500, 1500, and 4000 Hz (at 55 dB HL) were used to obtain ASSRs at MFs ranging from 35 to 185 Hz. As CF increased, so did the best MF for response detection. MFs in the 65- to 100-Hz range yielded the best detection efficiencies in sleeping newborns (see Figure 9–2). In addition, latencies calculated from the response phase were in the 11- to 14-ms range, with a systematic decrease in latency with increased frequency. Both the range and the type of latency change suggest that the ASSRs recorded at high MFs in sleeping newborns are generated by the brainstem.

In summary, studies in sleeping infants and young children indicate that MF should be varied with CF to obtain the largest ASSRs. They further show that for CFs less than 1.0 kHz, and for MFs at 30 to 50 Hz, ASSR latency estimates are similar to those of the AMLR, and that they are of larger amplitude than those obtained at MFs greater than 80 Hz. This may be because at lower MFs, the modulation envelope is of longer duration, allowing greater temporal summation and thus a larger response. It also is likely because the ASSRs from the cortex (i.e., evoked at MFs less than 50 Hz) are larger than those from the brainstem (evoked at MFs greater than 80 Hz). Although Levi and colleagues (1993) were able to obtain ASSRs for low-frequency MF-CF combinations in very young infants, the ASSRs for the 0.5-Hz CF at 80-Hz MFs were more consistently present and of larger amplitude than those obtained at lower MFs. Previous research on ASSRs for 40-Hz MFs in sleeping infants and young children indicates that ASSRs are unstable at this MF (Stapells, Galambos, Costello, & Makeig, 1988). This is not the case, however, for adults, in whom ASSRs for low- (less than 1.0 kHz) CF and low- (less than 50 Hz) MF stimuli are present during sleep and wakefulness.

Effects of Anesthesia

The rationale for using the 40-Hz ASSR to monitor the effects of general anesthetics on consciousness is based on two premises. First, endogenous thalamocortical activity, gamma rhythms, are necessary for, and their presence indicates consciousness. Second, the 40-Hz ASSR and the gamma rhythms probably share the same thalamocortical generators. The robust association between attenuation of 40-Hz ASSR and anesthesia-induced unconsciousness with general anesthesia provides a reasonable basis for using the 40-Hz ASSR to monitor anesthesia.

Plourde and Picton (1990) demonstrated a reduction in the 40-Hz ASSR during the use of such anesthetic agents as thiopental, fentanyl, and isoflurane.

They also observed a recovery of amplitude as the subjects recovered from the effects of anesthesia. These investigators suggested that the mechanism for these effects was the shared thalamocortical activity (at 40 Hz) that is present during consciousness and also necessary for the 40-Hz ASSR. Other agents that have been investigated are sufentanil (Gilron, Plourde, Marcantoni, & Varin, 1998), enflurane (Plourde & Villemure, 1996), and propofol (Plourde, 1996), and all result in a reduction of ASSR amplitude. Because certain surgical techniques may affect peripheral hearing sensitivity, such as intubation or a change in middle ear pressure caused by prolonged anesthesia or artificial respiration, Picton, John, Dimitrijevic, and Purcell (2003) caution that it is necessary to monitor peripheral hearing status at the same time as the 40-Hz response using transient evoked ABRs or ASSRs at 80 Hz, which would be unaffected by anesthesia.

Ketamine-induced anesthesia has a paradoxical effect on the 40-Hz ASSR—that is, the responses are enhanced, rather than diminished, when this agent is used (Plourde et al., 1997). This effect of ketamine is known as "dissociative" anesthesia, which is defined as "a form of general anesthesia characterized by catalepsy, catatonia, and amnesia but not necessarily involving complete unconsciousness" (http://medical-dictionary.thefree dictionary.com/dissociative+anesthesia; retrieved 18 June 2007). The mechanism of ketamine-induced anesthesia is different from that for agents that cause reduction or absence of the 40-Hz ASSR.

Anesthesia per se does not appear to affect the ASSR obtained at high MFs (greater than 70 Hz) but would be expected to decrease the background EEG noise, such that the ASSR threshold may be achieved in fewer sweeps than in a natural sleep or quiet wakefulness condition. Picton, John, Purcell, and Plourde (2003) demonstrated no effects of drowsiness and sedation on the 80-Hz ASSR, confirming the results of Dobie and Wilson (1998).

Rance and associates (1995) compared ASSR thresholds in subjects assessed in natural sleep or sedated sleep (chloralhydrate) or under general anesthesia and found no differences. Investigations of neural generators of ASSRs (Kuwada, Anderson, Batra, Fitzpatrick, Teissier, & D'Angelo, 2002; Szalda & Burkard, 2005) in experimental animals use various anesthetic agents to reduce or eliminate the effects of the cortex. This research indicates that the ASSR at 80 Hz or higher is generated largely by the brainstem and therefore is not subject to the effects of these drugs.

Effects of Age on the Auditory Steady-State Response

The 40-Hz ASSR does not change significantly with increasing age in adulthood (Boettcher, Poth, Mills, & Dubno, 2001; Johnson, Weinberg, Ribary, Cheyne, & Ancill, 1988; Muchnik, Katz-Putter, Rubinstein, & Hildesheimer, 1993), although even slight-to-mild hearing loss among older adults may be a confounding variable. Larger amplitudes for the ASSR have been found among elderly persons who have hearing levels at the "lower" end of normal (e.g., 20 to 25 dB HL), probably owing to a recruitment-like phenomenon (Muchnik et al., 1993). Picton et al. (2003) report no age-related changes in

the amplitude or phase of ASSRs for a 1000-Hz pure tone modulated at 3, 43, and 95 Hz in a group of normal-hearing adults aged 20 to 81 years. These investigators do, however, report high intersubject variability in amplitude and phase measures that may have precluded finding statistically significant age-related differences. Significant age-related findings in infants as a result of auditory system development are discussed in Chapter 9.

Effects of Attention

The effects of attention on ASSR have been evaluated by several groups. Linden, Picton, Hamel, and Campbell (1987) presented a train of tone bursts to each ear, with the trains differing in rate (37 and 41 Hz) and in tonal frequency (500 and 1000 Hz). The subjects were instructed to attend to one of the trains and to detect low-probability, brief changes in frequency. ASSRs elicited by the tone-burst trains were not affected by engaging attention. These findings were unlike those of Woldorff, Hansen, and Hillyard (1987), who found that attention had a dramatic effect on the transiently evoked AMLR.

By contrast, Makeig and Galambos (1989) observed a decrease in the ongoing ASSR amplitude in response to amplitude or frequency changes in a 40-Hz tone-burst train, or to omissions of a single tone burst within the series. The depression of ASSR amplitude persisted for 200 ms. When a 40-Hz steady-state stimulus was used as a background, and subjects were asked to listen for changes in a train of repeating tones in the foreground, a decrease in amplitude caused a decrease in the amplitude of the ASSR (Rohrbaugh,

Varner, Paige, Eckardt, & Ellingson, 1989, 1990). Similarly, Rockstroh, Muller, Heinz, Wagner, Berg, and Elbert (1996) demonstrated a decrease in the ASSR when a P300 event-related-potential was evoked during the detection of a low-probability stimulus change.

In these experiments, it was apparent that the 40-Hz ASSR could be affected by attentional changes that were not related to the stimuli being used to evoke the ASSR. Ross, Picton, Herdman, Hillyard, and Pantev (2004) tested whether attention directed to the ASSR-evoking stimuli would affect the response. The ASSRs were recorded using magnetoencephalography (MEG). The standard stimuli were 800-ms duration trains of 500-Hz tone bursts presented at 40 Hz. The target stimuli, presented at a probability of 10%, were also 800 ms in duration; however, the toneburst rate within the train was 30 Hz. The subjects signaled their detection of the stimulus change by pressing a response button. A visual attention task was also used as a control condition during ASSR recordings. During the auditory attention task, the amplitude of the ASSR (that is the "sustained field potential" in the averaged MEG) increased during the first 200 ms following the presentation of a target, and then the amplitude increase was sustained for 300 to 800 ms. ASSR amplitude had a fast decline at the offset of the target stimulus. In addition, the MEG technique allowed localization of the ASSR to the primary auditory cortex at a site more medial than that which generates the transient cortical auditory evoked potential N1. This experiment provided evidence that the ASSR amplitude can reflect sensory perception and discrimination during an attention task.

Conclusions

Clinical applications of ASSR include estimation of threshold and also monitoring of anesthesia. Subject state and certain stimulus variables interact, and awareness of these interactions is necessary for optimizing ASSR test results. Modulation rates at 80 Hz and above are best for using ASSRs to estimate threshold in sleeping infants and young children, while for older children or adults, 40 Hz may be used for testing CFs below 2.0 kHz during sleep, or when the subject is awake. Anesthesia will diminish or abolish the 40-Hz ASSR and can be used to indicate unconsciousness; however, monitoring peripheral hearing status apart from consciousness is necessary. The 40-Hz ASSR shows some effects of selective attention, but a clinical application for this phenomenon is not yet apparent.

References

Aoyagi, M., Furuse, H., Yokota, M., Kiren, T., Suzuki, Y., & Koike, Y. (1994). Detectability of amplitude-modulation following response at different carrier frequencies. *Acta Otolaryngologica, 511*(Suppl.), 23–27.

Aoyagi, M., Kiren, T., Furuse, H., Fuse, T., Suzuki, Y., Yokota, M., et al. (1994). Effects of aging on amplitude modulation-following response. *Acta Otolaryngologica, 511*(Suppl.), 15–22.

Boettcher, F. A., Poth, E. A., Mills, J. H., & Dubno, J. R. (2001). The amplitude-modulation following response in young and aged human subjects. *Hearing Research, 153,* 32–42.

Cohen, L. T., Rickards, F. W., & Clark, G. M. (1991). A comparison of steady-state evoked potentials to modulated tones in awake and sleeping humans. *Journal of the Acoustical Society of America*, *90*, 2467–2479.

Dobie, R. A., & Wilson, M. J. (1998). Low-level steady-state auditory evoked potentials: Effects of rate and sedation on detectability. *Journal of the Acoustical Society of America*, *104*, 3482–3488.

Gilron, I., Plourde, G., Marcantoni, W., & Varin, F. (1998). 40 Hz auditory steady-state response and EEG spectral edge frequency during sufentanil anaesthesia. *Canadian Journal of Anaesthia*, *45*, 115–121.

Johnson, B. W., Weinberg, H., Ribary, U., Cheyne, D. O., & Ancill, R. (1988). Topographic distribution of the 40 Hz auditory evoked-related potential in normal and aged subjects. *Brain Topography*, *1*, 117–121.

Kuwada, S., Anderson, J. S., Batra, R., Fitzpatrick, D. C., Teissier, N., & D'Angelo, W. R. (2002). Sources of the scalp-recorded amplitude-modulation following response. *Journal of the American Academy of Audiology*, *13*, 188–204.

Levi, E. C., Folsom, R. C., & Dobie, R. A. (1993). Amplitude-modulation following response (AMFR): Effects of modulation rate, carrier frequency, age and state. *Hearing Research*, *68*, 42–52.

Linden, R. D., Picton, T. W., Hamel, G., & Campbell, K. B. (1987). Human auditory steady state evoked potentials during selective attention. *Electroencephalography and Clinical Neurophysiology*, *66*, 145–159.

Lins, O. G, & Picton, T. W. (1995). Auditory steady-state responses to multiple simultaneous stimuli. *Electroencephalography and Clinical Neurophysiology*, *96*, 420–432.

Makeig, S., & Galambos, R. (1989). The CERP: Event-related perturbations in steady-state responses. In E. Basar (Ed.), *Brain dynamics: Progress and perspectives* (pp. 373–400). Berlin/Heidelberg: Springer.

Muchnik, C., Katz-Putter, H., Rubinstein, M., & Hildesheimer, M. (1993). Normative data for 40-Hz event-related potentials to 500-Hz tonal stimuli in young and elderly subjects. *Audiology*, *32*, 27–35.

Picton, T. W., John, M. S., Dimitrijevic, A., & Purcell, D. (2003). Human auditory steady-state responses. *International Journal of Audiology*, *42*, 177–219.

Picton, T. W., John, M. S., Purcell, D. W., & Plourde, G. (2003). Human auditory steady-state responses: The effects of recording technique and state of arousal. *Anesthesia and Analgesia*, *97*, 1396–1402.

Plourde, G. (1996). The effects of propofol on the 40-Hz auditory steady-state response and on the electroencephalogram in humans. *Anesthesia and Analgesia*, *82*, 1015–1022.

Plourde, G,. Baribeau, J., & Bonhomme, V. (1997). Ketamine increases the amplitude of the 40-Hz auditory steady-state response in humans. *British Journal of Anaesthesia*, *78*, 524–529.

Plourde, G., & Picton, T. W. (1990). Human auditory steady state responses during general anesthesia. *Anesthesia and Analgesia*, *71*, 460–468.

Plourde, G., & Villemure, C. (1996). Comparison of the effects of enflurane/N$_2$O on the 40-Hz auditory steady-state response versus the auditory middle-latency response. *Anesthesia and Analgesia*, *82*, 75–83.

Rickards, F. W., Tan, L. E., Cohen, L. T., Wilson, O. J., Drew, J. H., & Clark, G. M. (1994). Auditory steady-state evoked potential in newborns. *British Journal of Audiology*, *28*, 327–337.

Rockstroh, B., Muller, M., Heinz, A., Wagner, M., Berg, P., & Elbert, T. (1996). Modulation of auditory responses during oddball tasks. *Biology and Psychology*, *43*, 41–55.

Rohrbaugh, J. W., Varner, J. L., Paige, S. R., Eckardt, M. J., & Ellingson, R. J. (1989). Event-related perturbations in an electrophysiological measure of auditory function: A measure of sensitivity during orienting? *Biology and Psychology*, *29*, 247–271.

Rohrbaugh, J. W., Varner, J. L., Paige, S. R., Eckardt, M. J., & Ellingson, R. J. (1990). Auditory and visual event-related perturbations in the 40 Hz auditory steady-state response. *Electroencephalography and Clinical Neurophysiology*, *76*, 148–164.

Ross, B., Picton, T. W., Herdman, A. T., Hillyard S. A., & Pantev, C. (2004). The effect of attention on the auditory steady-state response. *Neurology and Clinical Neurophysiology*, *22*, 1–4.

Stapells, D. R., Galambos, R., Costello, J. A., & Makeig, S. (1988). Inconsistency of auditory middle latency and steady-state responses in infants. *Electroencephalography and Clinical Neurophysiology*, *71*, 289–295.

Szalda, K., & Burkard, R. (2005). The effects of nembutal anesthesia on the auditory steady state response (ASSR) from the inferior colliculus and auditory cortex of the chinchilla. *Hearing Research*, *203*, 32–44.

Woldorff, M. G., Hansen, J. C., & Hillyard, S. A. (1987). Evidence for effects of selective attention in the middle latency range of the human auditory event–related brain potential. *Electroencephalography and Clinical Neurophysiology Supplement*, *40*, 146–154.

CHAPTER 6

Clinical Application of Auditory Steady-State Responses

GARY RANCE
BARBARA CONE-WESSON

Auditory Evoked Potentials in Clinical Practice

Since auditory evoked potentials (AEPs) were first identified, attempts have been made to incorporate the auditory pathway insights they offer into clinical practice. Current applications can essentially be divided into three categories:

■ Estimation of hearing threshold

■ Differential diagnosis

■ Auditory processing

Estimation of Hearing Threshold

To date, the major clinical application for the auditory steady-state response (ASSR) has been the objective estimation of hearing levels. The clinical populations that may potentially require this form of assessment fall broadly into two groups: (1) adults and children older than 6 to 9 months of age who are unable (as a result of physical, intellectual, or emotional problems) or unwilling (for financial or other reasons) to provide accurate audiometric results and (2) infants and young children who are too immature to be conditioned for audiometric assessment. Evaluation of the second of these groups has been the primary focus of much of the clinical ASSR research effort over the past decade. The importance of early identification and management of congenital hearing loss is now well established. Provision of sound at audible levels (through hearing aids or other means) in the first months of life can minimize degenerative processes in the central auditory pathways (Sharma, Dorman, & Spahr, 2002) and can, in combination with appropriate family and educational support, maximize long-term speech and language outcomes (Moeller, 2000; Yoshinga-Itano, Sedley, Coulter, & Mehl, 1998). Newborn hearing screening programs have resulted in an increase in the number of newborns diagnosed with hearing loss (Kennedy & McCann, 2004; Thompson, McPhillips, Davis, Lieu, Homer, & Helfand, 2001). Identification of affected children is of course only the first step in the diagnostic process, and the significant challenge currently facing auditory clinicians is to accurately quantify hearing levels in these very young babies so that appropriate intervention strategies can be implemented. Various aspects of ASSR generation and recording make the response a good candidate (in theory at least) for an objective measure of hearing. First, there are a number of potential advantages related to the types of stimuli used to generate the response. Unlike some transient AEPs that require short-duration signals (such as acoustic clicks or brief tone bursts) to produce sufficiently synchronized neural activity, the ASSR can be elicited by reasonably frequency-specific stimuli such as continuous-amplitude or amplitude- and frequency-modulated

(AM-FM) tones. This frequency specificity, coupled with the fact that ASSRs can be evoked by carrier tones across the audiometric range, allows the possibility of generating "evoked potential audiograms" that reflect the audiometric configuration of the subject. The ability to elicit the ASSR with continuous stimuli has a number of other potential advantages. Continuous modulated tones more closely resemble the pure tones used in audiometric testing (than do brief tone bursts or click stimuli). Behavioural detection thresholds for continuous modulated tones, for example, are typically within 1 to 2 dB of American National Standards Institute (ANSI) reference levels and, as such, are usually presented in the same units (dB HL). Brief stimuli, by contrast, require a correction factor (to compensate for their brevity), which creates the potential for calibration error if the correction (which is based on average behavioural detection thresholds in normal-hearing adults) is not appropriate for every subject.

Furthermore, continuous AM or AM/ FM tones may be delivered with a presentation level range similar to that of pure tones. Maximum presentation levels for most test frequencies in the audiometric range may be as high as 120 dB HL, allowing for the possibility of assessment of hearing levels in the profound range (Rance, Dowell, Beer, Rickards, & Clark, 1998). By contrast, calibration corrections (accounting for differences in temporal summation for brief- versus long-duration stimuli) limit the maximum presentation levels available for tone-burst testing to approximately 100 to 110 dB nHL (Stapells, Picton, Durieux-Smith, Edwards, & Moran, 1990). Although 100 dB nHL is equivalent to a peak equivalent SPL of 120 or 125 dB, it appears that the AM-FM tones used for ASSRs may be more effective than transients for estimating minimal residual hearing.

As discussed in previous chapters, the ASSR can be extracted mathematically from within the electroencephalogram (EEG), and response presence or absence can be determined statistically using measures such as phase- or magnitude-squared coherence or analysis of variance of the response spectrum. These features obviously are desirable from a clinical implementation perspective in that they offer the possibility of truly objective assessment procedures, removing the need for clinicians (with varying degrees of experience in waveform detection) to visually interpret averaged EEG tracings. When coupled with algorithms or regression formulae for estimating behavioural threshold from ASSR threshold, it is plausible that the ASSR test and its interpretation could be completely automated.

Another potential advantage afforded by the ASSR analysis technique relates to the ability to record more than one response at the same time. Independent ASSRs to a number of stimulus tones can be elicited simultaneously, provided that the center frequencies of the signals are sufficiently different (i.e., separated by at least one octave) and that the tones are modulated at different rates (Lins & Picton, 1995). Up to eight stimuli configured in this way (four tones presented to each ear) have been used to simultaneously elicit ASSRs (John, Lins, Boucher, & Picton, 1998). Although this does not necessarily allow an eightfold reduction in test time, the ability to record multiple responses offers the potential for significant clinical efficiencies that have great appeal, particularly for assessing subjects in natural or sedated sleep.

Differential Diagnosis

Determining the site (or sites) of abnormality for patients presenting with hearing-related problems is one of the particular challenges facing auditory clinicians. Differentiating between pathologic conditions occurring at different points along the auditory pathway—from peripheral disorders affecting the external or middle ear conductive mechanisms to cochlear abnormalities and central nervous system disturbances—has been the focus of a substantial body of transient AEP research over the past decades. Assessment techniques using compound action potentials, auditory brainstem response, auditory middle latency response, and cortical AEPs can be used to evaluate the afferent auditory nervous system. By contrast, application of the ASSR as a tool for differential diagnosis, or even the development of a working understanding of how different (central) pathologies might affect the response, is only just beginning. Recent work has considered the distinction between peripheral and cochlear dysfunction (see Chapter 11 for details) and the influence of neural synchrony disorders such has auditory neuropathy/dyssynchrony on the response has been noted (Rance et al., 1999). Shinn (2005) found large discrepancies between behavioural threshold and ASSR threshold in 11 adults with neurologic lesions of the brainstem or cortex confirmed by magnetic resonance imaging (MRI). In neonates with a history of extreme prematurity and risk for neurologic impairment, Cone-Wesson, Parker, Swiderski, and Rickards (2002) also found an exceptionally high incidence of elevated ASSR thresholds. However, detailed and extensive investigation of the effects on the

ASSR of central disorders such as intracranial tumors and neoplasms and the various disease processes that affect the central auditory pathways is yet to be undertaken.

Auditory Processing

The ability to objectively measure auditory processing skills is highly desirable in clinical populations involving subjects unable to provide reliable volitional responses to auditory stimuli. Transient AEPs such as the P300 and mismatched negativity (MMN) response have been used (with varying degrees of success) in such groups as metrics for a range of abilities including auditory discrimination, information processing, memory, and attention (Davis, 1964; Näätänen, Gaillard, & Mäntysalo, 1978; Sutton, Tueting, Zubin, & John, 1965).

Assessment of auditory processing abilities using the ASSR is another area yet to be fully explored. Preliminary work has, however, pointed to potential applications involving both basic feature level discrimination and processing of complex stimuli. A number of authors have for example, measured ASSRs to AM stimuli with different modulation depths and rates (John, Dimitrijevic, Van Roon, & Picton, 2001; Purcell, John, Schneider, & Picton, 2004) with a view to providing objective correlates of temporal resolution ability. ASSRs also may provide insights into spectral processing when responses are elicited by frequency rather than by amplitude modulation or when dynamic response changes are generated by variations in carrier frequency (Patel & Balaban, 2004). In addition to these auditory discrimination

applications, the ASSR technique, by virtue of its ability to elicit multiple responses to complex stimuli, may offer insights into a subject's overall processing capacity. For example, Dimitrijevic and colleagues (2002) presented multiple simultaneous tones and considered the number of independent responses obtained to be a reflection of the amount of information available in the central auditory pathways for processing of complex signals (such as speech).

A comprehensive discussion of the current research relating to ASSR assessment of suprathreshold hearing in both adults and children is provided in Chapter 12 of this book.

From the Laboratory to the Clinic

Translating the insights obtained in the laboratory setting into clinical practice poses a number of challenges. Where assessment in an experimental context typically involves relaxed and cooperative subjects of well-defined hearing status, clinicians are faced with patients of all ages presenting with a range of (often undiagnosed) dysfunctions. Assessment techniques need to be robust and able to provide accurate (or at least predictable) results in a wide range of circumstances. In particular, successful clinical application of the ASSR (as with any AEP technique) requires answers to the following questions:

■ Can the ASSR be reliably recorded in subjects of all ages?

■ What effect does auditory pathway maturation have on the ASSR, and what is the time course of developmental effects?

▨ How does subject state (natural sleep/sedation/general anesthesia) affect the response?

▨ What are the optimal test parameters (e.g., modulation rate, stimulus type) for response generation in different subject groups?

▨ What is the most reliable way to predict hearing threshold from ASSR findings (e.g., correlation of ASSR-behavioural hearing thresholds, extrapolation from amplitude/intensity functions)?

▨ Can reliable results be obtained within a manageable test time?

▨ What is the relationship between ASSR findings and behavioural hearing levels in normal-hearing adult subjects?

▨ Is this relationship different in hearing-impaired subjects, and does the accuracy of hearing level estimation vary with degree and type of hearing loss?

▨ Apart from hearing level, what factors (such as site of lesion, subject age, and so on) may affect the ASSR hearing threshold relationship?

▨ How does hearing threshold prediction using the ASSR compare with other (transient) AEPs in different populations?

▨ Does the ASSR have any neurodiagnostic value for identification of central auditory pathway disorders (e.g., acoustic tumors, auditory neuropathy/dys-synchrony)?

▨ Can the ASSR be used for auditory processing applications?

▨ Can the ASSR be used to measure device function (amplification/cochlear implant)?

Outlining the ways in which these questions have been approached over the last 2 decades, and the degree to which they have been satisfactorily answered is the focus of the remaining chapters in this book.

References

Cone-Wesson, B., Parker, J., Swiderski, N., & Rickards F. (2002). The auditory steady-state response: Full-term and premature neonates. *Journal of the American Academy of Audiology, 13*(5), 260–269.

Davis, H. (1964). Enhancement of evoked cortical potentials in humans related to a task requiring a decision. *Science, 145,* 182–183.

Dimitrijevic, A., John, M. S., Van Roon, P., Adamonis, J., Ostroff. J., Nedzelski, J. M., et al. (2002). Estimating the audiogram using multiple steady-state responses. *Journal of the American Academy of Audiology, 13,* 205–224.

John, M. S., Lins, O., Boucher, B., & Picton, T. W. (1998). Multiple auditory steady-state responses (MASTER): Stimulus and recording parameters. *Audiology, 37,* 59–82.

John, M. S., Dimitrijevic, A., Van Roon, P., & Picton, T. W. (2001). Multiple auditory steady-state responses to AM and FM stimuli. *Audiology and Neurootology, 6,* 12–27.

Kennedy, C., & McCann, D. (2004). Universal neonatal hearing screening moving from evidence to practice. *Archives of Disease in Childhood. Fetal and Neonatal Edition, 89,* 378–383.

Lins, O. G., & Picton, T. W. (1995). Auditory steady-state responses to multiple simultaneous stmuli. *Electroencephalography and Clinical Neurophysiology*, *96*, 420–432.

Moeller, M. P. (2000). Early intervention and language development in children who are deaf and hard of hearing. *Pediatrics*, *106*(3), e43–e60.

Näntänen, R., Gaillard, A. W. K., & Mäntysalo, S. (1978). Early selective-attention effect on evoked potential reinterpretation. *Acta Psychologica*, *42*, 313–329.

Patel, A. D., & Balaban, E. (2004). Human auditory cortical dynamics during perception of long acoustic sequences: Phase tracking of carrier frequency by the auditory steady-state response. *Cerebral Cortex*, *14*, 35–46.

Purcell, D. W., John, M. S., Schneider, B. A., & Picton, T. (2004). Human temporal auditory acuity as assessed by envelope following responses. *Journal of the Acoustical Society of America*, *116* (6), 3581–3593.

Rance, G., Beer, D. E., Cone-Wesson, B., Shepherd R. K., Dowell, R. C., King, A. K., et al. (1999). Clinical findings for a group of infants and young children with auditory neuropathy. *Ear and Hearing*, *20*, 238–252.

Rance, G.. Dowell, R. C., Beer, D. E., Rickards, F. W., & Clark, G. M. (1998). Steady-state evoked potential and behavioural hearing thresholds in a group of children with absent click-evoked auditory brain stem response. *Ear and Hearing*, *19*, 48–61.

Sharma, A., Dorman, M., & Spahr, T. (2002). A sensitive period for the development of the auditory system in children with cochlear implants. *Ear and Hearing*, *23*, 532–539.

Shinn, J. B. (2005). *The auditory steady state response in individuals with neurologic insult of the central auditory nervous system*. Unpublished PhD dissertation, University of Connecticut, Storrs, CT.

Stapells, D. R., Picton, T, W., Durieux-Smith, A., Edwards, C. G., & Moran, L. M. (1990). Thresholds for short-latency auditory-evoked potentials to tones in notched noise in normal-hearing and hearing-impaired subjects. *Audiology*, *29*, 262–274.

Sutton, S., Tueting, P., Zubin, J., & John, E. R. (1965). Evoked potential correlates of stimulus uncertainty. *Science*, *150*, 1187–1188.

Thompson, D. C., McPhillips, H., Davis, R. L., Lieu, T. A., Homer, C. J., & Helfand, M.. (2001). Universal newborn hearing screening. Summary of evidence. *Journal of the American Medical Association*, *286*(16), 2000–2010.

Yoshinago-Itano, C., Sedley, A. L., Coulter, D. K., & Mehl, A. L. (1998). Language of early- and late-identified children with hearing loss. *Pediatrics*, *102*(5), 1161–1171.

CHAPTER 7

Behavioural Threshold Estimation for Auditory Steady-State Response

KATHY VANDER WERFF
TIFFANY JOHNSON
CAROLYN BROWN

Overview

The auditory steady-state response (ASSR) has generated considerable interest over recent years as an objective method for estimation of behavioural thresholds. The primary clinical application proposed for the ASSR has been as a tool used to assist in the diagnosis of hearing loss, particularly the frequency-specific estimation of the audiogram in infants and other populations in whom behavioural testing is difficult or impossible. Objective measures are increasingly relied on in this capacity because the age at which hearing loss is identified and subsequent intervention is initiated has been reduced

as a result of universal newborn hearing screening efforts and early intervention programs. Until recently, the main approach to frequency-specific estimation of behavioural threshold has been to record the auditory brainstem response (ABR) in response to brief tones. With the increased availability of commercial systems, ASSR testing has emerged as an alternative or addition to tone-burst ABR testing for the purpose of behavioural-threshold estimation.

This chapter describes the use of the ASSR for purposes of behavioural-threshold estimation. A brief history of the technique is provided, the literature describing the relationship between ASSR and behavioural thresholds is reviewed, and various approaches to estimating behavioural thresholds from ASSR thresholds are described.

Brief History of the Use of ASSRs for Hearing Threshold Estimation

In the 1980s and early 1990s a number of reports appeared in the literature describing success with recording the ASSR at levels close to behavioural threshold in adults with both normal hearing and hearing loss (e.g., Chambers & Meyer, 1993; Galambos, Makeig, & Talmachoff, 1981; Kuwada, Batra, & Maher, 1986; Picton, Skinner, Champagne, Kellett, & Maiste, 1987). These early reports used modulation (or presentation) rates of approximately 40 Hz. The 40-Hz ASSR has not been widely used clinically because the response is adversely affected by sleep and sedation (Galambos et al., 1981; Picton, Vajsar, Rodriguez, & Campbell, 1987; Plourde, Stapells, & Picton, 1991), and evidence has shown that it is not reliably recorded in infants and young children (Aoyagi et al., 1993; Levi, Folsom, & Dobie, 1993; Maurizi et al., 1990; Stapells, Galambos, Costello, & Makeig, 1988; Suzuki & Kobayashi, 1984). The use of ASSR with tones modulated at rates over 70 Hz for estimating behavioural thresholds was advocated by Cohen, Rickards, and Clark (1991) and demonstrated in newborn infants by Rickards and colleagues (1994). The amplitude of the response at these higher modulation frequencies is smaller than observed for 40-Hz modulation frequencies; however, the response remains stable and detectable when an individual is sleeping or sedated (Aoyagi et al., 1993, 1994a; Cohen et al., 1991). Furthermore, several studies have demonstrated that modulation frequencies in the vicinity of 80 Hz are optimal for detecting responses in sleeping infants and young children (Aoyagi et al., 1993, 1994b; Levi et al., 1993). Although there has been some renewed attention on the 40-Hz ASSR recently (e.g., Riquelme, Kuwada, Filipovic, Hartung, & Leonard, 2006; Tomlin, Rance, Graydon, & Tsialios, 2006; Van Maanen & Stapells, 2005), in this chapter the focus is on results obtained when using modulation frequencies exceeding 70 Hz.

Relationship between ASSR and Behavioural Thresholds Reported in the Literature

Overall, most studies have reported that ASSR thresholds approximate behavioural audiometric thresholds within 5 to 25 dB; however the correlation and the average difference (plus the associated standard deviation) between the two types of thresholds vary according to age, hearing loss, stimulus frequency, and various other test parameters. The following discussion examines the relationship between ASSR and behavioural thresholds in adults and children.

ASSR-Behavioural Threshold Relationship in Adults

Although the ASSR is used primarily to estimate behavioural thresholds for infants and young children who are too young or otherwise unable to be tested accurately using behavioural audiometric procedures, many of the initial studies of the accuracy of ASSR-based threshold estimation have been performed in adult populations. The use of adults makes comparison of ASSR thresholds with behavioural audiometric thresholds relatively simple. In most studies, modulation frequencies in the range of 80 to 90 Hz have been used in order to allow generalization of these results to pediatric populations.

The accuracy of threshold estimation using the ASSR generally has been evaluated by examining correlations between ASSR and behavioural thresholds or by computing mean differences between these thresholds. Excellent correlations between ASSR and behavioural audiometric thresholds have been noted in adults, with most studies reporting Pearson correlation coefficients of 0.85 to 0.95 for the frequencies 1000, 2000, and 4000 Hz (Dimitrijevic, John, Van Roon, Purcell, Adamonis, Ostroff, Nedzelski, & Picton, 2002; Herdman & Stapells, 2003; Herdman & Stapells, 2001a; Hsu, Wu, & Liu, 2003; Van Maanen & Stapells, 2005; Vander Werff & Brown, 2005). Slightly poorer, although still significant, correlations between 500-Hz ASSR and behavioural thresholds have been reported, with correlations ranging from 0.65 to 0.75 in some studies (Herdman & Stapells, 2003; Van Maanen & Stapells, 2005) and 0.85 to 0.87 in others (Dimitrijevic et al., 2002; Hsu et al., 2003; Vander Werff & Brown, 2005).

A number of investigators have evaluated the accuracy of threshold estimation using the ASSR by computing the mean and standard deviations of the difference between ASSR and behavioural thresholds. A comparison of the ASSR-behavioural threshold differences for adults, as reported in the literature, is shown in Figures 7–1 and 7–2 for normal-hearing adults and hearing-impaired adults, respectively. The reader also is referred to reviews by Picton, John, Dimitrijevic, and Purcell (2003) and Herdman and Stapells (2003).

Several trends can be observed by comparing the data across studies. First, a comparison of Figures 7–1 and 7–2 shows a trend for larger differences between ASSR and behavioural thresholds and greater disagreement across studies for normal-hearing adults than for hearing-impaired adults. The mean ASSR thresholds reported by a majority of studies of normal-hearing adults in Figure 7–1 fall between 10 to 25 dB above the behavioural threshold for carrier frequencies ranging from 500 to 4000 Hz. The mean threshold difference exceeded this range in one study (Cone-Wesson, Dowell, Tomlin, Rance, & Ming, 2002) in which a mean ASSR-behavioural threshold difference of 40 dB at 500 Hz was reported, whereas others recorded mean ASSR thresholds within less than 10 dB of behavioural thresholds (Dimitrijevic et al., 2002; Luts & Wouters, 2004). In particular, the greatest variability in studies across the literature is observed for the low stimulus frequencies. Within each study, however, the inter-subject variability in ASSR-behavioural threshold differences has been reported to be relatively small for all stimulus frequencies. Standard deviations for normal-hearing adults have been reported to range from 7 to 15 dB (see bottom panel of Figure 7–1), falling on average around 10 dB across frequencies.

For hearing-impaired adults, as shown in Figure 7–2, the mean ASSR-behavioural threshold difference across studies falls into a somewhat narrower range for all stimulus frequencies. At 1000 Hz and above, this difference has been reported to be as low as 5 dB in some studies (e.g., Dimitrijevic et al., 2002) to as large as 20 dB in others (Hsu et al., 2003; Van Maanen & Stapells, 2005). Five of the seven studies shown in Figure 7–2 obtained mean ASSR-behavioural threshold differences

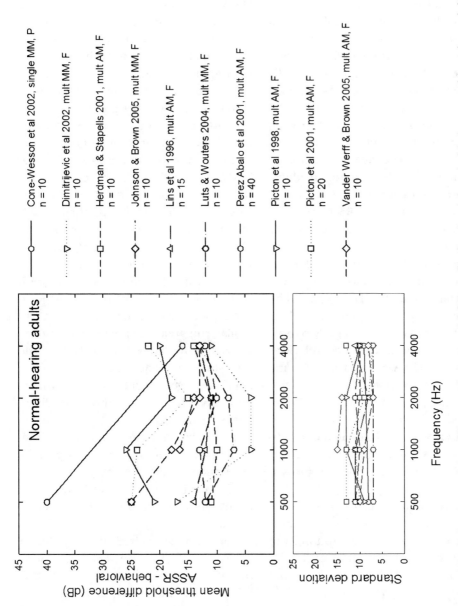

Figure 7–1. Summary of investigations of the difference between ASSR and behavioral thresholds in normal-hearing adults. The figure key indicates the study, stimulus condition (e.g., single versus multiple, AM versus MM), analysis technique (F, F-ratio; P, phase coherence), and number of subjects. *Note:* Results for MM stimuli only reported for Johnson and Brown (2005); means for Luts and Wouters (2004) plotted for the largest number of sweeps reported (48 sweeps).

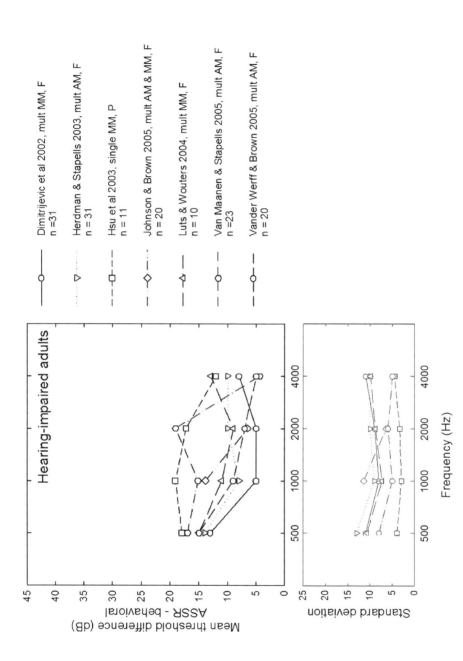

Figure 7–2. Summary of investigations of the difference between ASSR and behavioral thresholds in hearing-impaired adults. The figure key follows the convention used in Figure 7–1. *Note:* Means for Johnson and Brown (2005) reported for AM and MM conditions averaged together; results from Van Maanen and Stapells (2005) reported for 80-Hz stimuli.

of 15 dB or less. Figure 7–2 (bottom panel) also shows a trend for smaller inter-subject variability in hearing-impaired adults than that seen in studies of ASSR in normal-hearing adults, as indicated by standard deviations ranging from 3 to 13 dB. Taken together, the mean and standard deviation data plotted in Figures 7–1 and 7–2 reveal trends in the literature indicating that ASSR thresholds are recorded closer to behavioural thresholds and with less variability in hearing-impaired adults than in normal-hearing adults.

ASSR-Behavioural Threshold Relationship in Children

A number of studies have evaluated the accuracy of threshold estimation using the ASSR in older children, and these findings are described here. As expected, given the more difficult task of obtaining behavioural thresholds in infants, fewer data are available comparing ASSR and behavioural thresholds in infants. Two literature reviews (Picton et al., 2003; John, Brown, Muir, & Picton, 2004) describe ASSR thresholds and response detectability in infants and highlight the across-study variability in methodology and ASSR thresholds for this population. Although these reviews provide useful descriptions of ASSR thresholds in young children, they do not report any behavioural-threshold data, and, as such, do not provide a direct illustration of the relationship between ASSR and behavioural thresholds in infants. In addition, studies reporting results for this population have used differing,methods to obtain ASSR threshold. For example, Lins and colleagues (1996) used multiple simultaneous carrier frequencies and averaged for up to 13 minutes; Cone-Wesson and

Rickards and associates (2002) used a single carrier-frequency stimulus and averaged for 20 to 90 seconds. The effect of many of these methodological factors on ASSR results are discussed later, in the section "Effect of Test Parameters on Auditory Steady-State Response Threshold." Additionally, in the absence of behavioural thresholds, many studies report results of other objective techniques, such as ABR and otoacoustic emissions, or report behavioural threshold results that were obtained some period of time after the ASSR data were measured when establishing normal versus impaired hearing for their subjects. These uncertainties regarding behavioural thresholds at the time ASSR thresholds are measured in infants are largely inescapable; however, these issues should be kept in mind when evaluating the results for this population. Here, we describe the work that has been done in infants and children.

In studies reporting both ASSR and behavioural audiometric thresholds in children, correlations between behavioural and ASSR thresholds generally have been reported to be similar to those previously described in adults, ranging from r = 0.70 to 0.98 (Han, Mo, Liu, Chen, & Huang, 2006; Lins et al., 1996; Luts, Desloovere, Kumar, Vandermeersch, & Wouters, 2004; Luts, Desloovere, & Wouters, 2006; Perez-Abalo, Savio, Torres, Martin, Rodriguez, & Galan, 2001; Rance & Rickards, 2002; Rance, Rickards, Cohen, De Vidi, & Clark, 1995; Rance, Roper, Symons, Moody, Poulis, Dourlay, et al., 2005). Some studies have reported slightly lower correlations at 500 Hz than for higher frequencies (Han et al., 2006; Luts et al., 2006), similar to trends observed in adults. However, recent retrospective studies by Rance and colleagues (Rance & Rickards, 2002; Rance et al.,

2005) that included data from large samples of infants 8 months of age and younger (211 and 556 infants, respectively) found correlations between ASSR and later-obtained behavioural thresholds of 0.96 to 0.98 for all frequencies from 500 to 4000 Hz. These findings are encouraging for the use of the ASSR as a tool for threshold estimation in young infants across frequencies and are the best examples of normative data available to this point. Other studies report poorer correlations between ASSR and behavioural thresholds ranging from 0.58 to 0.76 (Lins et al., 1996; Swanepoel, Hugo, & Roode, 2004); however, the subject pools in these studies were hearing-impaired adolescents with degrees of hearing loss restricted to the severe-to-profound range.

The mean and variability of the difference between ASSR and behavioural thresholds have been examined in several studies of older children and in a few studies of young infants. Figure 7–3 presents a review of studies reporting ASSR-behavioural threshold differences in children from infants to adolescents. The open symbols in the figure show data from studies including infants and children with hearing loss; the filled symbols represent data from a large group of normal-hearing infants in the study by Rance and associates (2005). In this retrospective study, a total of 285 infants younger than 3 months of age underwent ASSR testing and were found to have normal hearing by behavioural testing at 6 to 23 months of age. As can be seen in Figure 7–3, the mean ASSR-behavioural threshold difference for this group of normal-hearing infants was between 22 and 31 dB across frequencies; these are considerably larger differences than those reported by any of the studies including hearing-impaired

infants or children. It should be noted, however, that the standard deviations are among the lowest reported in any of the studies of adults or children, owing to the large sample size.

The difference between ASSR and behavioural thresholds across studies in children with hearing loss (see Figure 7–3) ranges from 1 to 18 dB. However, several of the studies that indicate the largest differences (Lins et al., 1996; Perez-Abalo et al., 2001; Schmulian, Swanepoel, & Hugo, 2005) included older children and adolescents, rather than infants. Larger differences in these older children could perhaps be related to sleep state and higher noise levels in this population. In addition, the studies reporting the smallest differences (approximately 5 dB or less) included primarily or exclusively children with severe-to-profound hearing loss (Rance, Dowell, Rickards, Beer, & Clark, 1998; Stueve & O'Rourke, 2003; Swanepoel et al., 2004). As in to the adult literature, these studies have shown larger differences for infants and children with normal hearing or mild-to-moderate hearing loss compared with those with greater degrees of hearing loss. This may indicate that ASSR is not a reliable indicator of normal versus mild hearing loss in either adults or children. However, although the estimation of thresholds in the normal to mild hearing loss range using the ASSR appears problematic, the technique holds greater value for estimating auditory thresholds for the severely to profoundly hearing-impaired population. ASSR, therefore, may provide an important measure of the amount of residual hearing in children (as well as adults) with absent ABRs at maximum stimulation levels, leading to better informed decisions on rehabilitation with hearing aids and cochlear implants.

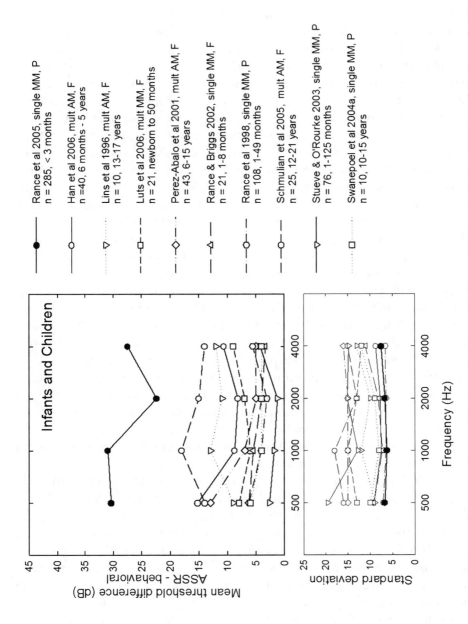

Figure 7–3. Summary of investigations of the difference between ASSR and behavioral thresholds in infants and children. The figure key follows the convention used in Figure 7–1. *Filled symbols* represent results for normal-hearing subjects.

Several studies have in fact documented the presence of ASSR thresholds in the absence of ABR responses in children with severe-to-profound hearing loss (e.g., Cone-Wesson, Dowell, et al., 2002; Rance et al., 1995, 1998; Swanepoel & Hugo, 2004; Vander Werff, Brown, Gienapp, & Schmidt Clay, 2002). The relationship between ASSR and ABR is further reviewed in Chapter 8. It should be noted here that when ASSR testing is used to diagnose severe to profound hearing loss, care should be taken in presenting high-level continuous stimuli. Careful consideration should be made in determining the maximum safe stimulation levels using the ASSR clinically, particularly when presenting multiple frequencies simultaneously. In addition, Gorga and colleagues (2004) have raised concerns that artifact or distortion may be present in recorded responses to high-level stimuli, which could be confused with neural responses. Although manufacturers have taken measures to decrease artifact issues, clinicians should still be cautious in interpreting responses at very high stimulus levels.

Approaches to Establishing Auditory Steady-State Response Thresholds and Estimating Behavioural Audiometric Thresholds from Auditory Steady-State Response Testing

The review presented previously describes the main research findings regarding the relationship between ASSR and behavioural audiometric thresholds. How should cli-

nicians utilize these findings in applying ASSR to clinical practice? This section looks at techniques for establishing ASSR thresholds and use of these thresholds to predict behavioural audiometric thresholds in different populations. The effect of test parameters and other variables that clinicians should consider when implementing ASSR-based threshold estimation also are discussed briefly.

Techniques for Determining Auditory Steady-State Response Thresholds in Clinical Protocols

ASSR thresholds have been determined most frequently using threshold bracketing techniques. Typically responses are recorded at several stimulus intensity levels, starting at an intensity level sufficiently high to elicit a response and then decreasing intensity until a response is no longer identified. *Threshold* is defined as the lowest stimulus level at which a response is detected. With use of the bracketing approach, the threshold for recognizing the physiological ASSR response, as is the case with most auditory evoked potentials, typically exceeds the behavioural threshold for the same stimulus. Determining how close true physiological thresholds are to behavioural thresholds is complicated by the difficulty in detecting the small-amplitude ASSR response due to inadequate signal-to-noise ratio in the electroencephalogram (EEG). One issue in determining physiological threshold, therefore, is how the presence or absence of a response in a background of noise is defined. ASSR analysis is conducted in the frequency domain and relies on statistical comparison of the "signal" amplitude at the stimulus modulation frequency to the "noise" amplitude in immediate neighboring frequency regions. Most research studies, as well as current clinical systems, rely on either phase coherence measures (Jerger, Chmiel, Frost, & Coker, 1986; Stapells, Makeig, & Galambos, 1987) or F-test response statistics (Dobie & Wilson, 1996; Zurek, 1992) to evaluate whether statistical criteria are met in order to determine response presence or absence. The determination of response presence at a given intensity level is, therefore, objective, rather than based on visual waveform identification or other subjective measures, as is typically done with the ABR. However, the accuracy of the determination depends on being able to reduce the noise level sufficiently that ASSR responses close to the true physiological threshold can be detected. That is, in order to determine that a response has not been missed because of excessive background noise, the clinician must consider whether sufficient averaging has taken place and whether the noise level is sufficiently low. One way to ensure that sufficient averaging has occurred is to require that the mean noise level fall below a criterion level before a no-response determination can be made. Although the precise definition of noise varies with the type of device, one example of using such as a criterion is requiring that the noise level fall below 10 to 15 nV for determination of absence of a response (e.g., Dimitrijevic, John, & Picton, 2004; Herdman & Stapells, 2003).

In order to achieve lower mean noise levels, longer periods of averaging are required, particularly at threshold levels. Clinical protocols, which must consider time efficiency as well as accuracy, require decisions such as what noise floor crite-ria to use, how many sweeps to collect, whether to stop as soon as a single significant response is detected or to require a certain number of significant responses, and whether to require a repetition of a response. In addition, the level defined as threshold may depend on whether significant responses are required at all suprathreshold levels. With use of a strict criterion, a response at one stimulus level may be considered a false-positive result if no response is detected at the next higher level (or two levels above, and so on). By contrast, less stringent criteria may label the lowest stimulus level with a significant response as threshold regardless of whether a response is present at any higher stimulus level. Because response presence or absence is based on meeting a statistical criterion, false-positive errors will occur occasionally, and the clinician should be aware of this possibility when developing clinical protocols. These clinical decisions can ultimately influence the threshold level of the ASSR and add variability to the measurement.

In addition to the bracketing technique, methods that use suprathreshold information to define the ASSR threshold have been used (Rodriguez, Picton, Linden, Hamel, & Laframboise, 1986; Vander Werff & Brown, 2005). These studies typically have used regression equations fit to amplitude-intensity or phase-intensity functions to extrapolate threshold from suprathreshold measurements. They are based on the idea that if the amplitude (or phase) of the ASSR changes predictably with level, it is possible to use the responses at higher intensities where responses amplitudes are larger and more easily detected, to predict the threshold level of the response. Additionally, researchers have suggested intensity sweeping methods that slowly but continuously adjust the intensity level up and down, providing response measurements as a function of intensity, and fitting the data points at different intensity levels with mathematical functions to extrapolate threshold (Picton et al., 2003; Rodriguez et al., 1986). A swept intensity technique, therefore, may combine aspects of bracketing and extrapolation methods.

Studies using suprathreshold ASSR measures to estimate threshold have, however, had limited success (Lenarz, Gulzow, Grozinger, & Hoth, 1986; Rodriguez et al., 1986; Vander Werff & Brown, 2005). For example, in the study by Vander Werff and Brown (2005), which used a limited number of suprathreshold amplitude measures to predict behavioural threshold, correlations between estimated and actual behavioural thresholds were poor for most subjects and all stimulus frequencies ($r = 0.10$ to 0.46) except 2000 Hz ($r = 0.79$), despite averaging for up to 15 minutes at each intensity level. The lack of success across studies likely is due to nonlinearity in the relationship between response amplitude and intensity as well as wide individual variability in response amplitudes and growth functions (Lins, Picton, Picton, Champagne, & Durieux-Smith, 1995; Vander Werff & Brown, 2005). In clinical practice, these approaches may not be feasible and may not save time compared to a threshold bracketing procedure.

Effect of Test Parameters on Auditory Steady-State Response Threshold

In evoking the ASSR, a number of test parameters can be manipulated, all of which have the potential to influence the ASSR threshold. For example, the ASSR can be recorded for single-frequency stimulation (much like what is used when recording the tone-burst ABR) or for multiple frequencies presented simultaneously. The ASSR can be recorded using sinusoids that are amplitude-modulated (AM) or both amplitude- and frequency-modulated (AM/FM), known as mixed modulation (MM). There are also differences across studies in the instrumentation used to record the ASSR, amount of averaging, the analysis method and statistical procedure used to detect the response, and the manner in which threshold is defined. Although not all of these parameters have been compared to determine the effect on ASSR threshold, some comparisons have been reported. These are briefly considered next. (The reader is referred to previous chapters for a more thorough review of these issues.)

One basic methodological difference is whether the ASSR is evoked in response to a single modulated tone or in response to a stimulus that consists of multiple carrier tones, each modulated at a slightly different rate. Several groups have compared either the response amplitude or the ASSR threshold recorded using single-frequency stimuli versus multiple simultaneously presented carrier frequencies. For stimulation levels of 60 dB SPL and below, there is no difference in response amplitude or ASSR threshold for the single- and multiple-frequency conditions (Herdman & Stapells, 2001b; John, Lins, Boucher, & Picton, 1998; Lins & Picton, 1995). In addition, Herdman, Picton, and Stapells (2002) reported that ASSRs to moderately intense stimuli (60 dB SPL) reflect activation of an approximately 1-octave-wide cochlear region, whether tones are presented simultaneously or individually. When testing at levels exceeding 60 dB SPL, John and co-workers (1998) reported a significant decrease in response amplitude in the multiple- and single-frequency conditions. Less is known about the influence of multiple- versus single-frequency testing on ASSR thresholds exceeding 60 dB SPL. Additionally, studies using single-frequency stimuli and those using multiple simultaneous stimuli typically have used different recording and analysis procedures, which complicate the comparisons.

A second basic parameter that is varied across studies is the decision to elicit the response to a signal that is sinusoidally amplitude modulated or one that contains both amplitude and frequency modulations. Both AM and MM stimulation have been used for threshold estimation purposes. With use of AM stimuli, the frequency spectrum is narrow, including the carrier frequency plus or minus the modulation frequency. The addition of FM stimulation broadens the stimulus spectrum, thereby stimulating a larger region of the basilar membrane. Several studies have reported larger ASSR amplitudes for MM stimuli compared with AM stimuli when recorded in normal-hearing subjects (Cohen et al., 1991; John, Dimitrijevic, van Roon, & Picton, 2001; John & Picton, 2000). Given this observation of larger amplitude responses with MM stimuli, it is possible that ASSR thresholds for the two stimuli may differ. Johnson and Brown (2005) directly compared ASSR thresholds for AM and MM stimuli in three groups of subjects: subjects with normal hearing, subjects with hearing losses with flat audiometric configurations, and subjects with hearing losses with steeply sloping audiometric configurations. These researchers reported no difference in AM ASSR thresholds compared with MM ASSR thresholds for any

of the three subject groups. This result suggests that the larger amplitude responses observed with MM stimulation in normal-hearing subjects did not change threshold-prediction accuracy.

Trends across the literature for thresholds obtained using AM stimuli compared to MM stimuli can be observed by examining results from the studies in adults reviewed earlier in this chapter (see Figures 7–1 and 7–2). Mean ASSR thresholds across studies were calculated, weighted by sample size, for those studies using either AM or MM multiple-frequency stimuli. As plotted in Figure 7–4, for both normal-hearing and hearing-impaired adults, the weighted-mean ASSR-behavioural threshold difference was 2–7 dB less for MM than for AM stimuli, except at 4000 Hz for hearing-impaired adults, when the thresholds were the same for both types of stimuli. In general, therefore, it appears that mean ASSR thresholds across studies do tend to be slightly closer to behavioural thresholds for MM than for AM stimuli.

Another major factor that varies significantly across studies and may affect the ASSR threshold is the amount of averaging required before a response is determined to be present or absent. This factor also is related to the type of stimuli (single-frequency versus multiple-frequency) and statistical-detection method (phase coherence versus F test) used. Studies using single-frequency stimuli and phase coherence methods generally have used shorter averaging times (e.g., Aoyagi, Suzuki, Yokota, Furuse, Watanabe, & Ito, 1999; Cone-Wesson, Dowell, et al., 2002; Rance et al., 1995, 1998). Response detection times as short as 20 to 90 seconds have been used in some studies (Cone-Wesson, Dowell, et al., 2002; Rance et al., 1995, 1998). Aoyagi and colleagues.

(1999) reported 8 minutes of averaging per intensity level before a no-response judgment was made. By contrast, studies using multiple-frequency stimuli and the F-test procedure typically have used averaging times that exceed 8 minutes before determining that a response is absent (e.g., Dimitrijevic et al., 2002; Johnson & Brown, 2005; Picton et al., 1998; Vander Werff & Brown, 2005).

In general, studies using longer averaging times have reported ASSR thresholds that are closer to behavioural thresholds in normal-hearing subjects than studies using shorter averaging times— compare, for example, the results reported by Dimitrijevic and coworkers (2002) and Cone-Wesson and Dowell and associates (2002) in Figure 7–1. While it appears that the longer averaging times

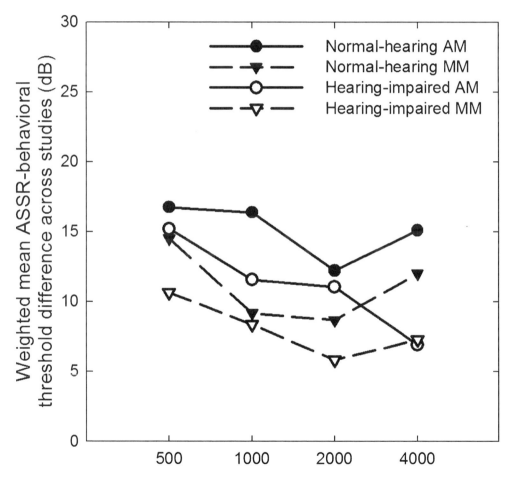

Figure 7–4. Weighted mean (by sample size) of ASSR-behavioral threshold difference for studies of normal-hearing and hearing-impaired adult subjects using AM (*circles*) compared with MM (*triangles*) stimuli. Weighted means were calculated from those studies in Figures 7–1 and 7–2 using multiple-frequency stimuli. *Filled symbols* represent data from normal-hearing subjects; *open symbols* represent data from hearing-impaired subjects.

result in lower thresholds overall, available testing time in clinical situations may impose limits on the test time for each stimulus level. It is encouraging, therefore, that regardless of the length of averaging the difference between ASSR and behavioural thresholds in subjects with hearing loss typically is less than 10 dB (Aoyagi et al., 1999; Cone-Wesson, Dowell, et al., 2002; Dimitrijevic et al., 2002; Johnson & Brown, 2005; Perez-Abalo et al., 2001; Rance, Rickards, Cohen, Burton, & Clark, 1993; Vander Werff & Brown, 2005).

Techniques for Estimating Behavioural Thresholds from ASSR Thresholds

Overall Trends in ASSR-Behavioural Threshold Relationships

In order to use the results of research studies in the clinic to predict audiometric thresholds, it may be valuable to consider overall means and trends across groups in the differences between ASSR and behavioural thresholds. Although limited by the methodological, subject population, and test environment variability across studies, one simple approach to combining results across studies is to calculate a weighted mean based on the sample size of each study (the similarity in standard deviations seen across the various studies, particularly for adults, suggests that this is a valid approach).

Following this approach, Figure 7-5 presents weighted means of the ASSR-behavioural threshold differences for normal-hearing adults, hearing-impaired adults, and hearing-impaired infants and children taken from the studies presented in the previous figures. In general, the difference between mean ASSR and behavioural thresholds is greater in normal-hearing adults than hearing-impaired adults, and greater in adults than in hearing-impaired children. The means for adults shown in Figure 7-5 are higher than those presented in a meta-analysis of seven studies by Herdman and Stapells (2003), who reported mean differences of 10, 6, 7, and 7 dB for 500, 1000, 2000, and 4000 Hz, respectively. The conflicting results for the analysis shown in Figure 7-5 and that of Herdman and Stapells (2003) may be explained by considering that the latter analysis included data for both children and adults and was heavily weighted by the largest study (Rance et al., 1998), which measured ASSR in children with absent ABR (these results are included in the mean for infants and children in Figure 7-5).

Since only one (Rance et al., 2005) of the studies previously reviewed in Figure 7-3 presented data for normal-hearing infants and children, these results are not summarized in Figure 7-5; however, the mean ASSR-behavioural threshold difference for normal-hearing infants and children probably is similar to that seen for normal-hearing adults (see Figure 7-3), although with perhaps greater variability. In Figure 7-5, the small weighted-mean difference observed for hearing-impaired infants and children is influenced by several studies that primarily included children with severe-to-profound hearing loss (Rance et al., 1998; Stueve & O'Rourke, 2003; Swanepoel et al., 2004). ASSR and behavioural threshold comparisons in infants are complicated by maturational issues and variability in how and when behavioural audiometric thresholds are obtained in different studies, which may further influence mean ASSR-behavioural

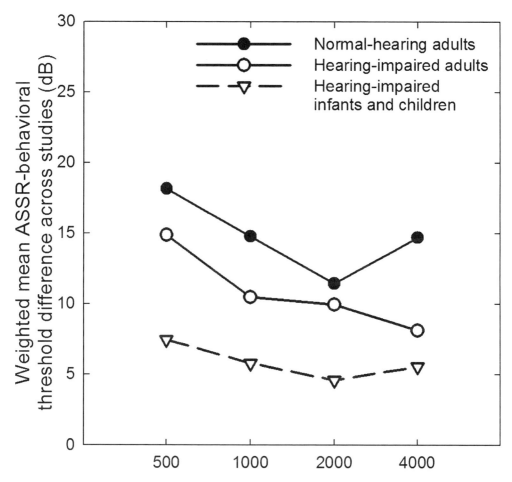

Figure 7–5. Weighted means (by sample size) of ASSR-behavioral threshold difference for studies of normal-hearing and hearing-impaired adults and hearing-impaired infants and children. Weighted means are calculated from the studies shown in Figures 7–1 to 7–3. *Filled* and *open symbols* correspond to data from normal-hearing and hearing-impaired subjects, respectively, whereas *circles* represent data from adults and *triangles* represent data from children.

threshold differences. Studies that have compared ASSR thresholds in subjects of different ages using similar test conditions have found significantly higher ASSR thresholds in young infants compared to older infants and adults (Lins et al., 1996; Rance & Rickards, 2002; Savio, Cardenas, Perez Abalo, Gonzalez, & Valdes, 2001). In a longitudinal study, Rance and Tomlin (2006) found significant develop-

mental changes in ASSR thresholds in normal-hearing neonates over the first 6 weeks of life. Furthermore, behavioural audiometric thresholds typically cannot be obtained until infants are 6 to 12 months of age, and often these thresholds represent "minimum response levels" that are somewhat higher than true behavioural thresholds. This may minimize ASSR-behavioural threshold differences seen in the infant population in some studies. As a result of these variables, the weighted-mean values across studies for infants and children should be viewed with caution; further normative studies are needed to clarify the ASSR-behavioural threshold relationship in this population.

As shown in Figure 7–5, for both adults and children the greatest mean differences between ASSR and behavioural thresholds are observed at 500 Hz. This greater threshold difference, along with poorer correlations and greater variability at 500 Hz, may be due to several factors. Lins and associates (1996) have suggested that elevated ASSR thresholds at 500 Hz may be due to reduced neural synchrony resulting from greater temporal jitter for the 500-Hz region of the basilar membrane. Higher thresholds and greater variability also have been reported for ABRs evoked with low-frequency vs. high-frequency stimuli and have been explained by the same rationale (e.g., Gorga, Kaminski, Beauchaine, & Jesteadt, 1988; Hayes & Jerger, 1982; Munnerley, Greville, Purdy, & Keith, 1991; Stapells, 2000). In addition, ASSR responses at 500 Hz may be reduced because of masking effects from higher-frequency stimuli presented simultaneously (John, Purcell, Dimitrijevic, & Picton, 2002). Background noise levels are higher in the lower frequencies, and because the 500-Hz stimuli typically use the lowest modulation frequencies, the signal-to-noise ratio tends to be slightly poorer for 500 Hz. It also is possible that other stimulus parameters have not been optimized for 500 Hz.

Errors in estimating audiometric thresholds tend to be, as reviewed previously, more common in normal-hearing subjects and in the low frequencies, raising concerns that audiometric configuration may not be well represented using ASSR test-ing. A related concern has been the possibility of underestimating high-frequency behavioural thresholds when low-frequency hearing is normal. Significant underestimation of high-frequency thresholds has been reported when using tone-burst ABRs (Picton, Ouellette, Hamel, & Smith, 1979; Purdy & Abbas, 2002; Stapells, Picton, Durieux-Smith, Edwards, & Moran, 1990). Because of these issues, the effect of audiometric shape has been examined in adults to determine if more errors in threshold estimation using ASSR occur with particular configurations of hearing loss. Several studies have reported general agreement between ASSR threshold and behavioural-threshold configurations (e.g., Dimitrijevic et al., 2002; Perez-Abalo et al., 2001). In particular, it has been shown that the slope of the audiogram in high-frequency sensorineural hearing loss is well represented by ASSR thresholds (Herdman & Stapells, 2003; Johnson & Brown, 2005; Vander Werff & Brown, 2005) with no reported underestimation of threshold even in steeply sloping losses.

Correction versus Regression Techniques

Given the observation that ASSR thresholds typically are recorded at levels that exceed behavioural thresholds, one common practice is to convert or "correct" the ASSR threshold when estimating the behavioural threshold. This typically is done in one of two ways—either by subtracting the average difference between ASSR and behavioural thresholds or by calculating the behavioural threshold using a regression equation derived from the relationship between the two thresholds.

From the data plotted in Figure 7–5, ASSR thresholds are expected to exceed behavioural thresholds by 10 to 12 dB at 2000 Hz in adults. When using a subtraction (or correction factor) approach, 10 to 12 dB would be subtracted from the ASSR threshold to estimate the behavioural threshold at 2000 Hz. It is likely that the correction factor will vary by frequency, because the ASSR-behavioural threshold relationship varies by frequency. The amount of correction at each frequency should be determined using normative values, either obtained locally or by using normative studies and surveys of the literature, such as presented above in Figures 7–1, 7–2, 7–3, and 7–5. Additionally, when using the subtraction approach, the differences in the ASSR-behavioural threshold relationship in normal-hearing versus hearing-impaired subjects should be considered. Because the behavioural threshold will not be known in advance, clinicians may need to consider that a different correction would be applied to a threshold recorded from a normal-hearing subject compared with a hearing-impaired subject. This information may be used to compute the range over which the estimated threshold is likely to occur.

Because the relationship between ASSR and behavioural thresholds has been shown to vary between subjects with normal and impaired hearing (see Figure 7–5) and with the degree of hearing loss (e.g., Rance et al., 1995), a simple correction may not be the most accurate approach to behavioural threshold prediction. As a result of physiological recruitment phenomena, ASSR responses grow more rapidly at levels just above threshold in subjects with cochlear hearing loss than they do in normal-hearing subjects. Because larger-amplitude responses are distinguished more easily from the background EEG activity, ASSR thresholds can be detected at levels closer to behavioural threshold as hearing loss increases. Larger differences between physiological and behavioural thresholds in normal-hearing subjects than in hearing-impaired subjects have been reported in adults (Johnson & Brown, 2005; Lins et al., 1996; Rance et al., 1995; Vander Werff & Brown, 2005) and infants (Rance & Rickards, 2002; Rance et al., 2005). This phenomenon is not unique to ASSR, as larger threshold elevations in normal-hearing subjects also have been found with other physiological measures such as the ABR (Gorga et al., 1988; Johnson & Brown, 2005; Stapells, Picton, & Durieux-Smith, 1994). Owing to the overall smaller amplitude of the ASSR response, however, it may be particularly important to keep the relationship in mind when predicting behavioural thresholds from ASSR.

Whether a regression equation provides more accurate threshold estimation than a simple correction factor depends on the technique used to obtain the ASSR thresholds. Regardless of prediction method, threshold estimation will be more accurate when the background EEG noise is less. The results of a study by Vander Werff and Brown (2005) suggested that predictions based on a simple subtraction method may be as accurate as those based on regression equations when both normal-hearing and hearing-impaired subjects are included in determining the corrections or regressions. However, the biggest errors using the subtraction method occurred for behavioural thresholds in the normal to near-normal hearing range, with the amount of error decreasing for hearing-impaired subjects. Flat and sloping audiometric configurations were predicted equally well by both subtraction and regression methods. The slopes of the regression lines in the Vander Werff and Brown (2005) study, as well as those presented in a study by Dimitrijevic and colleagues (2002), both of which used recording times of 12 to 15 minutes before determining response presence or absence, were close to one. Other studies advocating the use of regression equations for estimation of behavioural thresholds typically have used shorter recording periods (up to 90 seconds) and have shown slopes greater than one (Rance & Rickards, 2002; Rance et al., 1995). By averaging for a longer period of time, the residual noise level is decreased, so responses from normal-hearing subjects can be recorded at intensities closer to threshold. Therefore, as illustrated by Picton and colleagues (2003), the level of the residual noise in the recording has an effect on the slope of the regression equation, and on whether a regression method will be necessary to yield more accurate threshold estimation results. The regression equation also depends on the relative number of data points included for ears with normal hearing or mild hearing loss versus those with severe or profound hearing loss (Luts & Wouters, 2005).

In summary, behavioural thresholds can be predicted from ASSR thresholds by either simple correction or the use of a regression equation. A simple correction may prove just as accurate in cases where the residual noise level is low, which requires a quiet subject and test environment as well as adequate averaging. In the case of shorter averaging times, a regression equation may provide more accurate threshold estimation. The decision of which approach to use depends on the clinical protocol and test parameters used.

Summary and Future Directions

At this time, there remains a lack of established normative data for estimation of behavioural thresholds from ASSR thresholds using the various clinical devices and their differing recording protocols. Rance and colleagues (2005) provide the best sets of data for use with the single-stimulus technique in infants. Additional data are required for the other approaches available in clinical equipment (e.g., multiple frequencies, alternate stimuli), particularly in infants less than 6 months of age. There also is a need for normative data for adults and children with conductive and mixed hearing loss, including data for using bone conduction ASSRs to assess this population. In the meantime, clinicians should be cautious about the use of ASSR thresholds to estimate behavioural thresholds, and they should implement the technique as part of the clinical test battery (e.g., in conjunction with tone-evoked ABR, otoacoustic emissions, or middle ear measures).

Key Points

■ The relationship between auditory steady-state response thresholds and behavioural thresholds has been considered since the 1980s and early 1990s, with a large number of studies describing success at recording the ASSR at levels close to behavioural thresholds (within 5 to 25 dB) in adults and children with both normal hearing and hearing loss.

■ The ASSR-behavioural threshold difference generally has been shown to be greater for normal-hearing persons than for hearing-impaired subjects.

■ ASSR-behavioural threshold relationships have been shown to be different in infants and children than in adults. Maturational factors and difficulty in measuring true behavioural thresholds in young infants may play a role in these age-related trends.

■ The use of either correction factors or regression equations to estimate behavioural thresholds from ASSR thresholds has been supported. The choice of methods may depend on methodological factors and the normative data used for comparison.

■ Further normative data are needed, particularly in the infant population, using the various commercial systems and recording techniques for clinicians to be able to confidently use ASSR thresholds to estimate behavioural thresholds.

References

Aoyagi, M., Kiren, T., Furuse, H., Fuse, T., Suzuki, Y., Yokota, M., ct al. (1994a). Effects of aging on amplitude-modulation following response. *Acta Otolaryngologica Supplementum, 511*, 15–22.

Aoyagi, M., Kiren, T., Furuse, H., Fuse, T., Suzuki, Y., Yokota, M., et al. (1994b). Pure-tone threshold prediction by 80-Hz amplitude-modulation following response. *Acta Otolaryngologica Supplementum, 511*, 7–14.

Aoyagi, M., Kiren, T., Kim, Y., Suzuki, Y., Fuse, T., & Koike, Y. (1993). Optimal modulation frequency for amplitude-modulation following response in young children during sleep. *Hearing Research, 65*(1–2), 253–261.

Aoyagi, M., Suzuki, Y., Yokota, M., Furuse, H., Watanabe, T., & Ito, T. (1999). Reliability of 80-Hz amplitude-modulation following response detected by phase coherence. *Audiology & Neuro-otology, 4*(1), 28–37.

Chambers, R. D., & Meyer, T. A. (1993). Reliability of threshold estimation in hearing-impaired adults using the AMFR. *Journal of the American Academy of Audiology, 4*(1), 22–32.

Cohen, L. T., Rickards, F. W., & Clark, G. M. (1991). A comparison of steady-state evoked potentials to modulated tones in awake and sleeping humans. *Journal of the Acoustical Society of America, 90*(5), 2467–2479.

Cone-Wesson, B., Dowell, R. C., Tomlin, D., Rance, G., & Ming, W. J. (2002). The auditory steady-state response: comparisons with the auditory brainstem response. *Journal of the American Academy of Audiology, 13*(4), 173–187; quiz 225–176.

Cone-Wesson, B., Rickards, F., Poulis, C., Parker, J., Tan, L., & Pollard, J. (2002). The auditory steady-state response: clinical observations and applications in infants and children. *Journal of the American Academy of Audiology, 13*(5), 270–282.

Dimitrijevic, A., John, M. S., & Picton, T. W. (2004). Auditory steady-state responses and word recognition scores in normal-hearing and hearing-impaired adults. *Ear and Hearing, 25*(1), 68–84.

Dimitrijevic, A., John, M. S., Van Roon, P., Purcell, D. W., Adamonis, J., Ostroff, J., et al. (2002). Estimating the audiogram using multiple auditory steady-state responses. *Journal of the American Academy of Audiology, 13*(4), 205–224.

Dobie, R. A., & Wilson, M. J. (1996). A comparison of t test, F test, and coherence methods of detecting steady-state auditory-evoked potentials, distortion-product otoacoustic emissions, or other sinusoids. *Journal of the Acoustical Society of America, 100*(4 Pt 1), 2236–2246.

Galambos, R., Makeig, S., & Talmachoff, P. J. (1981). A 40-Hz auditory potential recorded from the human scalp. *Proceedings of the National Academy of Science of the United States of America*, 78(4), 2643–2647.

Gorga, M. P., Kaminski, J. R., Beauchaine, K. A., & Jesteadt, W. (1988). Auditory brainstem responses to tone bursts in normally hearing subjects. *Journal of Speech and Hearing Research*, 31(1), 87–97.

Gorga, M. P., Neely, S. T., Hoover, B. M., Dierking, D. M., Beauchaine, K. L., & Manning, C. (2004). Determining the upper limits of stimulation for auditory steady-state response measurements. *Ear and Hearing*, 25(3), 302–307.

Han, D., Mo, L., Liu, H., Chen, J., & Huang, L. (2006). Threshold estimation in children using auditory steady-state responses to multiple simultaneous stimuli. *ORL; Journal for Oto-rhino-laryngology and Its Related Specialties*, 68(2), 64–68.

Hayes, D., & Jerger, J. (1982). Auditory brainstem response (ABR) to tone-pips: results in normal and hearing-impaired subjects. *Scandinavian Audiology*, 11(3), 133–142.

Herdman, A. T., Picton, T. W., &Stapells, D. R. (2002). Place specificity of multiple auditory steady-state responses. *Journal of the Acoustical Society of America*, 112(4), 1569–1582.

Herdman, A. T., & Stapells, D. K. (2003). Auditory steady-state response thresholds of adults with sensorineural hearing impairments. *International Journal of Audiology*, 42(5), 237–248.

Herdman, A. T., & Stapells, D. R. (2001a). *Multiple auditory steady-state response thresholds in individuals with sensorineural hearing impairment (preliminary results)*. Paper presented at the 17th Biennial Symposium of the International Evoked Response Audiometry Study Group, University of British Columbia, Vancouver, British Columbia, Canada.

Herdman, A. T., & Stapells, D. R. (2001b). Thresholds determined using the monotic and dichotic multiple auditory steady-state

response technique in normal-hearing subjects. *Scandinavian Audiology*, 30(1), 41–49.

Hsu, W. C., Wu, H. P., & Liu, T. C. (2003). Objective assessment of auditory thresholds in noise-induced hearing loss using steady-state evoked potentials. *Clinical Otolaryngology and Allied Sciences*, 28(3), 195–198.

Jerger, J., Chmiel, R., Frost, J. D., Jr., & Coker, N. (1986). Effect of sleep on the auditory steady state evoked potential. *Ear and Hearing*, 7(4), 240–245.

John, M. S., Brown, D. K., Muir, P. J., & Picton, T. W. (2004). Recording auditory steady-state responses in young infants. *Ear and Hearing*, 25(6), 539–553.

John, M. S., Dimitrijevic, A., van Roon, P., & Picton, T. W. (2001). Multiple auditory steady-state responses to AM and FM stimuli. *Audiology & Neuro-otology*, 6(1), 12–27.

John, M. S., Lins, O. G., Boucher, B. L., & Picton, T. W. (1998). Multiple auditory steady-state responses (MASTER): stimulus and recording parameters. *Audiology*, 37(2), 59–82.

John, M. S., & Picton, T. W. (2000). Human auditory steady-state responses to amplitude-modulated tones: phase and latency measurements. *Hearing Research*, 141(1–2), 57–79.

John, M. S., Purcell, D. W., Dimitrijevic, A., & Picton, T. W. (2002). Advantages and caveats when recording steady-state responses to multiple simultaneous stimuli. *Journal of the American Academy of Audiology*, 13(5), 246–259.

Johnson, T. A., & Brown, C. J. (2005). Threshold prediction using the auditory steady-state response and the tone burst auditory brain stem response: A within-subject comparison. *Ear and Hearing*, 26(6), 559–576.

Kuwada, S., Batra, R., & Maher, V. L. (1986). Scalp potentials of normal and hearing-impaired subjects in response to sinusoidally amplitude-modulated tones. *Hearing Research*, 21(2), 179–192.

Lenarz, T., Gulzow, J., Grozinger, M., & Hoth, S. (1986). Clinical evaluation of 40-Hz middle-latency responses in adults: frequency specific threshold estimation and suprathreshold amplitude characteristics. *ORL; Journal for Oto-rhino-laryngology and Its Related Specialties, 48*(1), 24–32.

Levi, E. C., Folsom, R. C., & Dobie, R. A. (1993). Amplitude-modulation following response (AMFR): Effects of modulation rate, carrier frequency, age, and state. *Hearing Research, 68*(1), 42–52.

Lins, O. G., Picton, P. E., Picton, T. W., Champagne, S. C., & Durieux-Smith, A. (1995). Auditory steady-state responses to tones amplitude-modulated at 80-110 Hz. *Journal of the Acoustical Society of America, 97*(5 Pt 1), 3051–3063.

Lins, O. G., & Picton, T. W. (1995). Auditory steady-state responses to multiple simultaneous stimuli. *Electroencephalography and Clinical Neurophysiology, 96*(5), 420–432.

Lins, O. G., Picton, T. W., Boucher, B. L., Durieux-Smith, A., Champagne, S. C., Moran, L. M., et al. (1996). Frequency-specific audiometry using steady-state responses. *Ear and Hearing, 17*(2), 81–96.

Luts, H., Desloovere, C., Kumar, A., Vandermeersch, E., & Wouters, J. (2004). Objective assessment of frequency-specific hearing thresholds in babies. *International Journal of Pediatric Otorhinolaryngology, 68*(7), 915–926.

Luts, H., Desloovere, C., & Wouters, J. (2006). Clinical application of dichotic multiple-stimulus auditory steady-state responses in high-risk newborns and young children. *Audiology & Neuro-otology, 11*(1), 24–37.

Luts, H., & Wouters, J. (2004). Hearing assessment by recording multiple auditory steady-state responses: the influence of test duration. *International Journal of Audiology, 43*(8), 471–478

Luts, H., & Wouters, J. (2005). Comparison of MASTER and AUDERA for measurement of auditory steady-state responses. *International Journal of Audiology, 44*(4), 244–253.

Maurizi, M., Almadori, G., Paludetti, G., Ottaviani, F., Rosignoli, M., & Luciano, R. (1990). 40-Hz steady-state responses in newborns and in children. *Audiology, 29*(6), 322–328.

Munnerley, G. M., Greville, K. A., Purdy, S. C., & Keith, W. J. (1991). Frequency-specific auditory brainstem responses relationship to behavioural thresholds in cochlear-impaired adults. *Audiology, 30*(1), 25–32.

Perez-Abalo, M. C., Savio, G., Torres, A., Martin, V., Rodriguez, E., & Galan, L. (2001). Steady state responses to multiple amplitude-modulated tones: An optimized method to test frequency-specific thresholds in hearing-impaired children and normal-hearing subjects. *Ear and Hearing, 22*(3), 200–211.

Picton, T. W., Durieux-Smith, A., Champagne, S. C., Whittingham, J., Moran, L. M., Giguere, C., et al. (1998). Objective evaluation of aided thresholds using auditory steady-state responses. *Journal of the American Academy of Audiology, 9*(5), 315–331.

Picton, T. W., John, M. S., Dimitrijevic, A., & Purcell, D. (2003). Human auditory steady-state responses. *International Journal of Audiology, 42*(4), 177–219.

Picton, T. W., Ouellette, J., Hamel, G., & Smith, A. D. (1979). Brainstem evoked potentials to tonepips in notched noise. *Journal of Otolaryngology, 8*(4), 289–314.

Picton, T. W., Skinner, C. R., Champagne, S. C., Kellett, A. J., & Maiste, A. C. (1987). Potentials evoked by the sinusoidal modulation of the amplitude or frequency of a tone. *Journal of the Acoustical Society of America, 82*(1), 165–178.

Picton, T. W., Vajsar, J., Rodriguez, R., & Campbell, K. B. (1987). Reliability estimates for steady-state evoked potentials. *Electroencephalography and Clinical Neurophysiology, 68*(2), 119–131.

Plourde, G., Stapells, D. R., & Picton, T. W. (1991). The human auditory steady-state cvoked potentials. *Acta Otolaryngologica Supplementum, 491*, 153–159; discussion 160.

Purdy, S. C., & Abbas, P. J. (2002). ABR thresholds to tonebursts gated with Blackman and linear windows in adults with high-frequency sensorineural hearing loss. *Ear and Hearing, 23*(4), 358–368.

Rance, G., Dowell, R. C., Rickards, F. W., Beer, D. E., & Clark, G. M. (1998). Steady-state evoked potential and behavioral hearing thresholds in a group of children with absent click-evoked auditory brain stem response. *Ear and Hearing, 19*(1), 48–61.

Rance, G., & Rickards, F. (2002). Prediction of hearing threshold in infants using auditory steady-state evoked potentials. *Journal of the American Academy of Audiology, 13*(5), 236–245.

Rance, G., Rickards, F. W., Cohen, L. T., Burton, M. J., & Clark, G. M. (1993). Steady state evoked potentials: A new tool for the accurate assessment of hearing in cochlear implant candidates. *Advances in Oto-rhino-laryngology, 48*, 44–48.

Rance, G., Rickards, F. W., Cohen, L. T., De Vidi, S., & Clark, G. M. (1995). The automated prediction of hearing thresholds in sleeping subjects using auditory steady-state evoked potentials. *Ear and Hearing, 16*(5), 499–507.

Rance, G., Roper, R., Symons, L., Moody, L. J., Poulis, C., Dourlay, M., & Kelly, T. (2005). Hearing threshold estimation in infants using auditory steady-state responses. *Journal of the American Academy of Audiology, 16*(5), 291–300.

Rance, G., & Tomlin, D. (2006). Maturation of auditory steady-state responses in normal babies. *Ear and Hearing, 27*(1), 20–29.

Rickards, F. W., Tan, L. E., Cohen, L. T., Wilson, O. J., Drew, J. H., & Clark, G. M. (1994). Auditory steady-state evoked potential in newborns. *British Journal of Audiology, 28*(6), 327–337.

Riquelme, R., Kuwada, S., Filipovic, B., Hartung, K., & Leonard, G. (2006). Optimizing the stimuli to evoke the amplitude modulation following response (AMFR) in neonates. *Ear and Hearing, 27*(2), 104–119.

Rodriguez, R., Picton, T., Linden, D., Hamel, G., & Laframboise, G. (1986). Human auditory steady state responses: effects of intensity and frequency. *Ear and Hearing, 7*(5), 300–313.

Savio, G., Cardenas, J., Perez- Abalo, M., Gonzalez, A., & Valdes, J. (2001). The low and high frequency auditory steady state responses mature at different rates. *Audiology & Neuro-otology, 6*(5), 279–287.

Schmulian, D., Swanepoel, D., and Hugo, R. (2005). Predicting pure-tone thresholds with dichotic multiple frequency auditory steady state responses. *Journal of the American Academy of Audiology, 16*(1), 5–17.

Stapells, D. R. (2000). Threshold estimation by the tone-evoked auditory brainstem response: A literature meta-analysis. *Journal of Speech-Language Pathology and Audiology, 24*(2), 74–83.

Stapells, D. R., Galambos, R., Costello, J. A., & Makeig, S. (1988). Inconsistency of auditory middle latency and steady-state responses in infants. *Electroencephalography and Clinical Neurophysiology, 71*(4), 289–295.

Stapells, D. R., Makeig, S., & Galambos, R. (1987). Auditory steady-state responses: Threshold prediction using phase coherence. *Electroencephalography and Clinical Neurophysiology, 67*(3), 260–270.

Stapells, D. R., Picton, T. W., & Durieux-Smith, A. (1994). Electrophysiologic measures of frequency-specific auditory function. In J. T. Jacobson (Ed.), *Principles and applications in auditory evoked potentials* (pp. 251–283). New York: Allyn & Bacon.

Stapells, D. R., Picton, T. W., Durieux-Smith, A., Edwards, C. G., & Moran, L. M. (1990). Thresholds for short-latency auditory-evoked potentials to tones in notched noise in normal-hearing and hearing-impaired subjects. *Audiology, 29*(5), 262–274.

Stueve, M. P., & O'Rourke, C. (2003). Estimation of hearing loss in children: comparison of auditory steady-state response, auditory brainstem response, and behavioral test methods. *American Journal of Audiology, 12*(2), 125–136.

Suzuki, T., & Kobayashi, K. (1984). An evaluation of 40-Hz event-related potentials in young children. *Audiology, 23*(6), 599–604.

Swanepoel, D., & Hugo, R. (2004). Estimations of auditory sensitivity for young cochlear implant candidates using the ASSR: Preliminary results. *International Journal of Audiology*, *43*(7), 377–382.

Swanepoel, D., Hugo, R., & Roode, R. (2004). Auditory steady-state responses for children with severe to profound hearing loss. *Archives of Otolaryngology Head and Neck Surgery*, *130*(5), 531–535.

Tomlin, D., Rance, G., Graydon, K., & Tsialios, I. (2006). A comparison of 40 Hz auditory steady-state response (ASSR) and cortical auditory evoked potential (CAEP) thresholds in awake adult subjects. *International Journal of Audiology*, *45*(10), 580–588.

Van Maanen, A., & Stapells, D. R. (2005). Comparison of multiple auditory steady-state responses (80 versus 40 Hz) and slow cortical potentials for threshold estimation in hearing-impaired adults. *International Journal of Audiology*, *44*(11), 613–624.

Vander Werff, K. R., & Brown, C. J. (2005). Effect of audiometric configuration on threshold and suprathreshold auditory steady-state responses. *Ear and Hearing*, *26*(3), 310–326.

Vander Werff, K. R., Brown, C. J., Gienapp, B. A., Schmidt Clay, K. M. (2002). Comparison of auditory steady-state response and auditory brainstem response thresholds in children. *Journal of the American Academy of Audiology*, *13*(5), 227–235.

Zurek, P. M. (1992). Detectability of transient and sinusoidal otoacoustic emissions. *Ear and Hearing*, *13*(5), 307–310.

CHAPTER 8

The 80-Hz Auditory Steady-State Response Compared with Other Auditory Evoked Potentials

DAVID R. STAPELLS

Introduction

As clearly indicated in other chapters of this book, there is much interest in audiologic applications of the auditory steady-state response (ASSR) to stimuli modulated with rates between 70 and 110 Hz (the "80-Hz ASSR"), especially for threshold estimation in infants and young children with hearing loss. This heightened interest is well justified. Nevertheless, in certain circumstances, other auditory evoked potential (AEP) measures may be more appropriate. Furthermore, some

comparisons of the 80-Hz ASSR with other AEPs may not have been made under equivalent circumstances and are thus still unresolved, especially related to the tone-evoked auditory brainstem response ("tone-ABR"). Finally, as a "brainstem" response, the 80-Hz ASSR is limited in what it can tell us about auditory processing—obtaining measures from anatomically and hierarchically higher areas of the auditory system may prove informative for normal and disordered functions. This chapter considers the 80-Hz ASSR relative to the tone-ABR, the 40-Hz ASSR, and the slow cortical potential (SCP).

Basic Principles

Keeping Apples with Apples: Compare only Thresholds For Techniques Using Frequency-Specific Stimuli

The recent literature is replete with studies that compare thresholds for the 80-Hz ASSR (to frequency-specific tonal stimuli) with those for the click-evoked ABR. Comparing clicks, a completely non–frequency-specific stimulus (typically with equal energy from less than 0.1 kHz to approximately 6 to 8 kHz), with narrow-band, sinusoidally amplitude-modulated (AM) tones is equivalent to comparing apples and oranges. Those frequencies that dominate a particular subject's click-ABR cannot be determined with certainty; this is especially true when hearing loss is present. This chapter, therefore, considers only results for frequency-specific measures.

There is More Than One "ASSR"

A reading of the ASSR literature since 1996 may lead to the erroneous impression that there is only one "ASSR." However, the ASSR is not a unitary response. Use of different modulation rates, if the difference is large enough, results in responses dominated by different regions of the brain. Moreover, because they reflect overlapped responses, the ASSRs typically reflect contributions from a wide area of the auditory system. For example, the 80-Hz ASSR is primarily brainstem in origin but contains some cortical contribution; the 40-Hz ASSR has both brainstem and cortical generators, with the cortex dominating in awake adults; responses to slow rates (less than 20 Hz) are likely to be dominated by cortical sources but must contain brainstem contributions (Herdman et al., 2002). As described in this chapter, the ASSRs to different rates often have quite different properties (and different uses), so ASSRs cannot be considered as a single response.

Comparisons of the 80-Hz Auditory Steady-State Response and Tone-Evoked Auditory Brainstem Response

Considering the clear relevance of the 80-Hz ASSR to infant audiometry, there are surprisingly few comparisons of tone-ABR and 80-Hz ASSR thresholds in the same individuals, and especially in infants with hearing loss. Such studies are faced with two major differences between these techniques: (1) The ASSR is detected objectively by a computer using frequency-based measures, whereas the tone-ABR is detected by a clinician observing the visual replication of responses and thus is subjective in nature; and (2) ASSR stimuli are typically continuous and calibrated in dB HL, whereas tone-ABR stimuli are brief in duration and calibrated in "nHL." In the latter situation concerning calibrations, such differences may potentially be overcome by (1) determining differences in acoustic terms, such as *peak-to-peak equivalent* (ppe) SPL, and, (2) when assessing listeners with impaired hearing, by using predictive formulae and correlation coefficients determined using the relevant metric (i.e., nHL and HL).

In normal adults, whether 80-Hz ASSR thresholds are better than tone-ABR thresholds when both are considered in ppe SPL is still uncertain, although recent studies suggest they are better. Cone-Wesson and colleagues (Cone-Wesson, Dowell, Tomlin, Rance, & Ming, 2002) report single-stimulus 80-Hz ASSR thresholds of 52 and 23 dB SPL for 500 and 4000 Hz, respectively. Tone-ABR thresholds were lower (better): 33 and 20 dB ppe SPL for 500 and 2000 Hz. More recently, however, Johnson and Brown (2005) present results that suggest, in dB ppeSPL, 80-Hz ASSR thresholds in normal adults are better than tone-ABR thresholds by about 24, 22, and 18 dB at 1000, 1500, and 2000 Hz. Van der Reijden, Mens, and Snik (2006) similarly provide results suggesting that the 80-Hz ASSR shows lower thresholds in dB ppe SPL than tone-ABR.

Comparisons of the 80-Hz ASSR and tone-ABR thresholds in normal infants are still relatively scarce. Recently, Rance, Tomlin, and Rickards (2006) reported that infants' 500- and 4000-Hz single-stimulus 80-Hz ASSR thresholds are higher than their tone-ABR thresholds at birth and nearly identical (within 4 dB) at age 6 weeks, as shown in Table 8–1. Importantly, Rance and colleagues note that the ASSR thresholds show twice the variability of ABR thresholds (standard deviations of about 11 dB versus about 4 dB). In my own laboratory, in a study in which ASSRs to equivalent response noise levels were recorded (using the Fsp noise measure), older infants were found to show nearly identical thresholds (in dB ppe SPL) for the two measures (2000 Hz: ASSR, 29 dB ppe SPL; ABR, 30 dB ppe SPL) (Herdman & Stapells, unpublished data). Also, similar to the findings of Rance and colleagues, the infant ASSR thresholds showed greater variability than that observed for the tone-ABR thresholds.

Thus, in normal-hearing subjects, there appears to be a difference in the relationship between tone-ABR and 80-Hz ASSR thresholds in adults compared with infants, with ASSR thresholds (in dB SPL) better than ABR thresholds in adults, but

Table 8–1. Tone-ABR and 80-Hz ASSR thresholds (in dB SPL) for young infants

	500 Hz		4000 Hz	
	ABR	ASSR	ABR	ASSR
Newborn (age 0 weeks)				
MEAN	53.0	57.1	41.8	50.6
SD	4.3	10.7	4.2	10.6
Infant (age 6 weeks)				
MEAN	52.4	52.4	41.2	44.8
SD	6.5	6.0	5.1	8.5

SD = standard deviation.
Data from Rance, Tomlin, & Rickards, 2006.

worse than or equal to ABR thresholds in young infants (and with greater variability). The reasons for this discrepancy are not clear but may be related to maturational factors (such as infants' ability to follow very fast stimuli) or to procedural issues (e.g., recording durations, signal-to-noise measures). Further research is warranted.

Comparisons of tone-ABR and 80-Hz ASSR thresholds in subjects, adult or infant, with hearing loss are also relatively scarce. Aoyagi and coworkers (1999) compared tone-ABR and 80-Hz single-stimulus ASSR estimates of threshold in hearing-impaired children and reported similarly good correlations between 1000-Hz tone-ABR and behavioural thresholds (r = .83) and between ASSR and behavioural thresholds (r = .86). Vander Werff, Brown, Gienapp, and Schmidt Clay (2002) reported a correlation of 0.86 between tone-ABR and 80-Hz single-stimulus ASSR thresholds in children with significant hearing loss. More recently, Johnson and Brown (2005) compared tone-ABR and 80-Hz ASSR thresholds in adults with flat or steeply sloping audiograms and reported that both methods predict behavioural thresholds equally well. These investigators' results show that the tone-ABR threshold (in nHL) was closer than the ASSR (in HL) to pure-tone behavioural threshold (in dB HL); however, if their thresholds are converted to dB SPL, the opposite would be concluded, with ASSR thresholds being closer to pure-tone behavioural thresholds (in dB SPL).

One comparison between the ABR and the 80-Hz ASSR that has received much attention is that of thresholds for individuals with profound sensorineural hearing loss. Specifically, numerous papers have reported that the ASSR was present when the ABR (usually to clicks) was absent to maximum-intensity stimuli. There are a sufficient number of instances of this finding to suggest that it is a real phenomenon (e.g., Firszt, Gaggl, Runge-Samuelson, Burg, & Wackym, 2004; Rance, Dowell, Rickards, Beer, & Clark, 1998; Roberson, O'Rourke, & Stidham, 2003; Stueve & O'Rourke, 2003; Vander Werff et al., 2002). Several methodological issues, however, make these comparisons complicated: (1) In some cases, artifactual ASSRs may have been obtained as a result of A/D processing errors (Gorga et al., 2004; Picton & John, 2004; Small & Stapells, 2004); (2) in other cases, the ASSRs obtained may reflect physiologic but nonauditory responses (possibly vestibular) (Small & Stapells, 2004); (3) calibration of stimuli for the two responses is quite different (especially for the ABR, where each study may have used a different SPL for "0 dB nHL"); and, finally (4) in no case has the level at the specific carrier frequency been made equivalent between ABR and ASSR tests (e.g., a click spreads its energy across a wide band of frequencies; a 100-dB ppe SPL click will have 30 to 40 dB less energy at 500 Hz than a 100-dB ppe SPL 500-Hz AM tone). Thus, further research and careful thought are required to elucidate any differences between the ABR and ASSR in estimating thresholds in profound hearing loss.

In conclusion, when both tone-ABR and 80-Hz ASSR thresholds are obtained in the same subjects, the limited data to date indicate that both predict behavioural hearing threshold equally well in subjects with hearing loss. When considered in dB SPL, ASSR thresholds are 10 to 20 dB lower (better) than tone-ABR thresholds, at least in adults. This relationship may be different in infants, in whom higher, more variable ASSR thresholds are seen. It must be noted, however, that the data are very limited, owing to the small number of subjects tested and to considerable differences in methodology (e.g., single versus multiple ASSR, varied recording durations). Clearly, further research is required. Although the literature for the 80-Hz ASSR is growing rapidly, significant gaps in data remain, especially concerning the response in young infants. Data for 80-Hz ASSR prediction of behavioural threshold in infants with sensorineural hearing loss are limited primarily to single-stimulus ASSR (e.g., Rance et al., 2005) with only few similar data for the multiple-ASSR technique (Han, Mo, Liu, Chen, & Huang, 2006; Luts, Desloovere, & Wouters, 2006). No ASSR data exist for children with conductive or mixed hearing loss. The tone-ABR, therefore, with its long clinical history and research base, remains an essential component in the diagnostic test battery for infants with hearing loss (Stapells, Herdman, Small, Dimitrijevic, & Hatton, 2005).

Comparisons of the 80-Hz and the 40-Hz Auditory Steady-State Responses

The current high level of interest by audiologists in the 80-Hz ASSR is reminiscent of the first time ASSRs stimulated great interest for threshold estimation purposes: In 1981, Galambos and colleagues published their paper on the "40-Hz Event-Related Potential" demonstrating that ASSR to tones repeated at 40/s could be used to accurately assess threshold (Galambos, Makeig, & Talmachoff, 1981). So great was the interest in the 1980s that one equipment manufacturer developed the "first automatic and objective infant audiometer" based on Fourier

analyses of the infant 40-Hz ASSR. The outcome of this 40-Hz audiometer bears sober reflection in these days of excitement and new equipment for the 80-Hz ASSR: Even as this machine was marketed, several researchers demonstrated that the 40-Hz ASSR was not reliably recorded in sleeping infants (Stapells, Galambos, Costello, & Makeig, 1988; Suzuki & Kobayashi, 1984). By the 1990s, interest in the 40-Hz ASSR in audiology had all but disappeared.

Currently, the slow cortical potential (SCP) testing is considered the gold standard diagnostic method for verification of behavioural pure-tone thresholds to rule out nonorganic hearing loss in adult medicolegal/compensation cases (Alberti, Hyde, & Riko, 1987; Bonvier, 2002; Hyde, 1997; Hyde, Alberti, Matsumoto, & Li, 1986; Kaf, Durrant, Sabo, et al., 2006; Kaf, Sabo, Durrant, & Rubinstein, 2006; Stapells, 2002; Van Maanen & Stapells, 2005). Although accurate (see later on), SCP testing typically involves clinician-based response detection and is thus subject to the detrimental effects of inexperience and bias. Although the 40-Hz ASSR proved not to be useful for threshold estimation in infants, good reasons exist to consider this response for the assessment of adults for medicolegal and compensation purposes. The research of the 1980s had clearly shown that the largest and most easily recorded ASSR in adults was the response to stimuli modulated in the 35- to 45-Hz range (the "40-Hz ASSR") (Galambos et al., 1981; Stapells, Linden, Suffield, Hamel, & Picton, 1984; Stapells, Makeig, & Galambos, 1987). Moreover, this response provided excellent and objective predictions of behavioural threshold (e.g., Dobie & Wilson, 1998; Galambos et al., 1981; Kileny & Shea, 1986; Sammeth & Barry, 1985; Stapells et al., 1984; Stapells et al., 1987; Van der Reijden et al., 2006; Van Maanen & Stapells, 2005). A recent study has shown that the multiple-stimulus technique could be used with the 40-Hz ASSR (Van Maanen & Stapells, 2005).

Recently, researchers have begun to reconsider the 40-Hz ASSR for threshold testing of alert adults. In three recent independent studies, the 40-Hz ASSR has been shown to be a better measure of behavioural thresholds than the 80-Hz ASSR. Studying adults with sensorineural hearing loss, data from Van Maanen and Stapells (2005), presented in Figure 8–1,

show that thresholds for the multiple 40-Hz ASSR were significantly closer to pure-tone behavioural threshold than multiple 80-Hz ASSR thresholds, although both provided accurate estimates (i.e., both showed similar correlations between ASSR threshold and pure-tone behavioural threshold). Importantly, as Table 8–2 shows, the mean time to obtain a four-frequency audiogram (in 1 ear) was nearly twice that for 80-Hz ASSR (36 minutes) compared with the 40-Hz ASSR (21 minutes). Further, many subjects could not complete the 80-Hz ASSR testing because they were too physiologi-

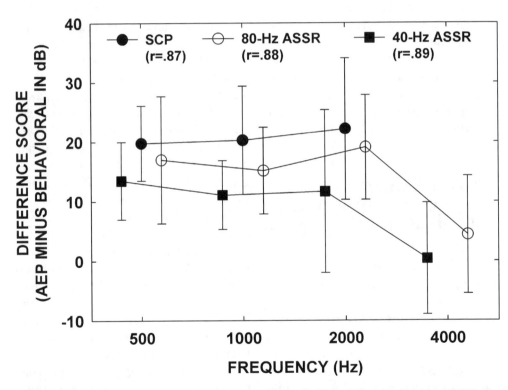

Figure 8–1. Estimation of pure-tone behavioural threshold by the 80-Hz ASSR, the 40-Hz ASSR, and the transient slow cortical potential (SCP) in adult subjects with sensorineural hearing loss. Shown are the difference scores (in dB), calculated as evoked potential threshold (in dB HL) minus behavioural threshold. Also shown are the Pearson correlation coefficients between the evoked potential thresholds and the pure-tone behavioural thresholds (pooled across frequency). SCP thresholds were not obtained for 4000 Hz. (Data from Van Maanen & Stapells, 2005.)

Table 8–2. Estimated time for four pure-tone thresholds

	80-Hz ASSR	40-Hz ASSR	Slow Cortical Potential
Mean time (minutes)	36.0	20.6	14.9
SD	18.5	9.5	1.0
% Within 15 minutes	13%	43%	56%
% Within 30 minutes	43%	89%	100%

SD = standard deviation.
Data from Van Maanen & Stapells, 2005.

cally "noisy" (Van Maanen & Stapells, 2005). Petitot and coworkers compared multiple-stimulus 40-Hz and 80-Hz ASSR thresholds in normal-hearing adults and showed 40-Hz ASSR thresholds to be significantly lower (better) by about 8 to 10 dB (Petitot, Collet, & Durrant, 2005). Recently, Van der Reijden and associates (2006) showed similar results in a group of adults with normal hearing: Compared with the 80-Hz ASSR, the 40-Hz ASSR thresholds were 8 dB better at 500 Hz and 2 dB better at 2000 Hz.

Thus, for assessing adult thresholds using the ASSR, the 40-Hz ASSR is preferable to the 80-Hz ASSR. As the 40-Hz ASSR decreases in amplitude with sleep (for a review, see the work of Picton, John, Dimitrijevic, & Purcell [2003]), adults should be tested while awake. As noted earlier, infants do not show reliable 40-Hz ASSRs. It is not clear at what age the 40-Hz ASSR is mature. Aoyagi and colleagues (1994) reported a general increase in detectability of the 40-Hz ASSR from age 6 months to 15 years of age. More recently, results obtained by Pethe and colleagues suggest that the optimal modulation rate range (based on response signal to noise ratio) for the

ASSR changes from 80 Hz to 40 Hz at about 13 years of age (Pethe, Muhler, Siewert, & von Specht, 2004).

Comparisons of the Auditory Steady-State Responses and Slow Cortical Potential

If the SCP is currently the "gold standard" evoked-potential test for the assessment of medicolegal/compensation cases (in adults), how well do ASSRs compare with the SCP? Recently, Kaf and colleagues compared 2000-Hz threshold estimates for the SCP and 80-Hz ASSR in noise masked normal adults and found high correlations between thresholds for the two measures (Kaf, Durrant, et al., 2006; Kaf, Sabo, Durrant, & Rubinstein, 2006). These investigators did not, however, assess the speed of the two tests. This was a primary question of recent research by Van Maanen and Stapells (2005). As indicated earlier (see Figure 8–1), although the 80-Hz ASSR indeed provided reasonably accurate predictions of pure-tone behavioural threshold in adults with sensorineural hearing loss, these estimates took 75% more time than the 40-Hz ASSR (see Table 8–2). Compared with the SCP, although threshold estimation accuracy was similar, the 80-Hz ASSR test took 240% longer (Van Maanen & Stapells) (see Table 8–2). On the basis of these results, the SCP would clearly be favored over the 80-Hz ASSR for assessment of adults.

Comparison of 40-Hz ASSR and SCP techniques for estimation of awake adults' thresholds raises a more interesting question. In a 2005 study of adults with sensorineural hearing loss, the evoked potential minus pure-tone behavioural threshold differences were significantly higher (by 6 to 10 dB) for the SCP than for the 40-ASSR (Van Maanen and Stapells, 2005) (see Figure 8–1). Although these SCP difference scores are somewhat higher than has been shown in the literature (e.g., Tomlin, Rance, Graydon, & Tsialios, 2006; Tsui, Wong, & Wong, 2002), both measures showed similarly high correlations between pure-tone behavioural threshold and evoked potential threshold (all in dB HL), indicating that they would both give good estimates of behavioural threshold. Tomlin and colleagues also showed good correlations between 40-Hz ASSR, SCP, and pure-tone behavioural thresholds in normal-hearing and hearing-impaired adult subjects (Tomlin et al., 2006). In contrast with Van Maanen and Stapells (2005), their SCP results show smaller difference scores. They also note that the 40-Hz ASSR thresholds showed greater variability. They concluded that the SCP may be the better evoked potential threshold technique for adults.

More recently, Yeung and Wong reported significantly lower (better) difference scores for SCP compared with 40-Hz ASSR, with SCP showing a greater number of cases within 10 dB of pure-tone behavioural audiometry than the 40-Hz ASSR (Yeung & Wong, 2007). One other measure argues in favor of the SCP: it appears to be faster. The SCP estimate (mean, 15 minutes) of the audiogram was found to be faster than the 40-Hz ASSR (mean, 21 minutes), although the difference did not quite reach significance (see Table 8–2) (Van Maanen & Stapells, 2005).

In conclusion, the SCP may still be the better evoked potential test for adults undergoing medicolegal/compensation assessments. However, as the SCP is typically detected using visual judgements, clinicians must have experience and skill with assessment of these transient responses. Given the objectivity of response detection of the 40-Hz ASSR, especially in the context of medicolegal/compensation issues, this response must still be considered a strong candidate for adult testing.

Higher-Level Processing and the Auditory Steady-State Response: The Slow Cortical (Less than 20 Hz) ASSR

Amid all of the excitement about the 80-Hz ASSR, it must be remembered that this response represents processing at a fairly low level of the auditory system. As noted previously, the 80-Hz ASSR is primarily brainstem in origin (e.g., Herdman et al., 2002)—indeed, it may be very similar to wave V of the ABR (Stapells et al., 2005). As such, it does not reflect many complex processes. For example, the 80-Hz ASSR does not seem to assess binaural processing: It does not demonstrate the *binaural masking level difference* (BMLD) (Wong & Stapells, 2004) and shows little or no binaural interaction component (Lins, Picton, Picton, Champagne, & Durieux-Smith, 1995; Ponton, Hatton, & Stapells, 2007). In contrast with the 80-Hz ASSR, the ASSRs to stimuli modulated or repeated at rates less than 20 Hz—the slow cortical ASSR—do reflect more complex processes. For example, the 7-Hz (or 13-Hz) ASSR does demonstrate the BMLD (Wong & Stapells, 2004). Interestingly, although primarily cortical in origin, the 40-Hz ASSR does not demonstrate the BMLD (Galambos and Makeig [1992]; Ishida and Stapells [2007].) Similarly, Dajani and Picton recently investigated binaural perception by recording the slow cortical ASSRs to changes in interaural correlation of stimuli occurring at a rate of 4 Hz (Dajani & Picton, 2006). Armstrong and Stapells recently demonstrated that adding multiple simultaneous stimuli (either multiple monaural or binaural) shows effects on ASSR amplitudes that are completely different for the slow cortical 14-Hz ASSR than for the 40- and 80-Hz ASSRs (Armstrong & Stapells, 2007). These interaction patterns may prove useful in assessing complex auditory processing and its disorders. For example, Stefanatos and colleagues have shown correlations between slow cortical ASSRs and developmental dysphasia (Stefanatos, Green, & Ratcliff, 1989). In conclusion, although much research is still required, clinicians are likely to see future clinical application of the slow cortical (below 20 Hz) ASSR.

Conclusions

Although optimism about clinical application of the 80-Hz ASSR is certainly warranted, clinicians must consider the intended application (and patient group). The 80-Hz ASSR currently is best suited for the assessment of hearing in young infants. Nevertheless, owing to gaps in the evidence base, 80-Hz ASSR results in infants with hearing loss currently must be confirmed and expanded on by air- and bone-conducted tone-evoked ABR thresholds. For assessment of adults, such as with medicolegal/compensation assessment, the 40-Hz ASSR is preferable to the 80-Hz ASSR for evoked potential threshold verification of behavioural thresholds. The transient SCP, however, is the current "gold standard" method and may be better than the 40-Hz ASSR. Finally, assessment of higher-order auditory processing may require recordings of ASSRs to slower rate modulations; the slow cortical (less than 20 Hz) ASSR appears to be a candidate.

Acknowledgments. Research projects with Maxine Armstrong, Anthony Herdman, Elais Ponton, and Anna Van Maanen contributed to some of the findings reported in this chapter. Their assistance is gratefully acknowledged. This research was supported by the Canadian Institutes of Health Research and the Natural Sciences and Engineering Research Council of Canada.

References

Alberti, P. W., Hyde, M. L., & Riko, K. (1987). Exaggerated hearing loss in compensation claimants. *Journal of Otolaryngology*, *16*(6), 362–366.

Aoyagi, M., Kiren, T., Furuse, H., Fuse, T., Suzuki, Y., Yokota, M., et al. (1994). Effects of aging on amplitude-modulation following response. *Acta Otolaryngologica Supplementum*, *511*, 15–22.

Aoyagi, M., Suzuki, Y., Yokota, M., Furruse, H., Watanabe, T., & Ito, T. (1999). Reliability of 80-Hz amplitude modulation-following response detected by phase coherence. *Audiology and Neuro-otology, 4*, 28–37.

Armstrong, M., & Stapells, D. R. (2007, June 10–14). *Frequency-channel interactions in brainstem and cortical auditory steady-state responses (ASSRs)*. Paper presented at the 20th Biennial Symposium of the International Evoked Response Audiometry Study Group, Bled, Slovenia.

Bonvier, R. (2002). Slow auditory evoked potentials: The end of malingering in audiology. *International Tinnitus Journal, 8*, 58–61.

Cone-Wesson, B., Dowell, R. C., Tomlin, D., Rance, G., & Ming, W. J. (2002). The auditory steady-state response: comparisons with the auditory brainstem response. *Journal of the American Academy of Audiology, 13*(4), 173–187.

Dajani, H., & Picton, T. (2006). Human auditory steady-state responses to changes in interaural correlation. *Hearing Research, 219*, 85–100.

Dobie, R. A., & Wilson, M. J. (1998). Low-level steady-state auditory evoked potentials: Effects of rate and sedation on detectability. *Journal of the Accoustical Society of America, 104*(6), 3482–3488.

Firszt, J. B., Gaggl, W., Runge-Samuelson, C. L., Burg, L. S., & Wackym, P. A. (2004). Auditory sensitivity in children using the auditory steady-state response. *Archives of Otolaryngology–Head & Neck Surgery, 130*(5), 536–540.

Galambos, R., & Makeig, S. (1992). Physiological studies of central masking in man. II: Tonepips SSRs and the masking level difference. *Journal of the Acoustical Society of America, 92*, 2691–2697.

Galambos, R., Makeig, S., & Talmachoff, P. (1981). A 40-Hz auditory potential recorded from the human scalp. *Proceedings of the National Academy of Science of the United States of America, 78*(4), 2643–2647.

Gorga, M. P., Neely, S. T., Hoover, B. M., Dierking, D. M., Beauchaine, K. L., & Manning, C. (2004). Determining the upper limits of stimulation for auditory steady-state response measurements. *Ear and Hearing, 25*(3), 302–307.

Han, D., Mo, M., Liu, H., Chen, J., & Huang, L. (2006). Threshold estimation in children using auditory steady-state responses to multiple simultaneous stimuli. *O-R-L, 68*, 64–68.

Herdman, A., Lins, O., Van Roon, P., Stapells, D., Scherg, M., & Picton, T. (2002). Intracerebral sources of human auditory steady-state responses. *Brain Topography, 15*, 69–86.

Hyde, M. (1997). The N1 response and its applications. *Audiology and Neuro-otology, 2*, 281–307.

Hyde, M., Alberti, P., Matsumoto, N., & Li, Y. L. (1986). Auditory evoked potentials in audiometric assessment of compensation and medicolegal patients. *Annals of Otology, Rhinology and Laryngology, 95*, 514–519.

Ishida, I. M., & Stapells, D. R. (2007, June 10–14). *Does the 40-Hz ASSR show the binaural masking level difference?* Paper presented at the 20th Biennial Symposium of the International Evoked Response Audiometry Study Group, Bled, Slovenia.

Johnson, T. A., & Brown, T. A. (2005). Threshold prediction using the auditory steady-state response and the tone burst auditory brain stem response: A within-subject comparison. *Ear and Hearing, 26*, 559–576.

Kaf, W. A., Durrant, J. D., Sabo, D. L., Boston, J. R., Taubman, L. B., & Kovacyk, K. (2006). Validity and accuracy of electric response audiometry using the auditory steady-state response: Evaluation in an empirical design. *International Journal of Audiology, 45*, 211–223.

Kaf, W. A., Sabo, D. L., Durrant, J. D., & Rubinstein, E. (2006). Reliability of electric response audiometry using 80 Hz auditory steady-state responses. *International Journal of Audiology, 45*, 477–486.

Kileny, P., & Shea, S. L. (1986). Middle-latency and 40-Hz auditory evoked responses in normal-hearing subjects: Click and 500-Hz thresholds. *Journal of Speech and Hearing Research, 29,* 20–28.

Lins, O. G., Picton, P. E., Picton, T. W., Champagne, S. C., & Durieux-Smith, A. (1995). Auditory steady-state responses to tones amplitude-modulated at 80–110 Hz. *Journal of the Acoustical Society of America, 97,* 3051–3063.

Luts, H., Desloovere, C., & Wouters, J. (2006). Clinical application of dichotic multiple-stimulus auditory steady-state responses in high-risk newborns and children. *Audiology and Neuro-otology, 11,* 24–37.

Pethe, J., Muhler, R., Siewert, K., & von Specht, H. (2004). Near-threshold recordings of ampitude modulation following responses (AMFR) in children of different ages. *International Journal of Audiology, 43,* 339–345.

Petitot, C., Collet, L., & Durrant, J. D. (2005). Auditory steady-state responses (ASSR): effects of modulation and carrier frequencies. *International Journal of Audiology, 44,* 567–573.

Picton, T., John, M., Dimitrijevic, A., & Purcell, D. (2003). Human auditory steady-state responses. *International Journal of Audiology, 42,* 177–219.

Picton, T. W., & John, M. S. (2004). Avoiding electromagnetic artifacts when recording auditory steady-state responses. *Journal of the American Academy of Audiology, 15*(8), 541–554.

Ponton, E., Hatton, J. & Stapells, D. R. (2007, June 10–14). *ASSR measures of binaural processing: Effect of dichotic modulation rate separation on brainstem (80 Hz) and cortical (40 Hz) ASSRs.* Paper presented at the 20th Biennial Symposium of the International Evoked Response Audiometry Study Group, Bled, Slovenia.

Rance, G., Dowell, R. C., Rickards, F. W., Beer, D. E., & Clark, G. M. (1998). Steady-state evoked potential and behavioral hearing thresholds in a group of children with absent click-evoked auditory brain stem response. *Ear and Hearing, 19*(1), 48–61.

Rance, G. R. R., Symons, L., Moody, L.-J., Poulis, C., Dourlay, M., et al. (2005). Hearing threshold estimation in infants using auditory steady-state responses. *Journal of the American Academy of Audiology, 16,* 291–300.

Rance, G., Tomlin, D., & Rickards, F. (2006). Comparison of auditory steady-state responses and tone-burst auditory brainstem responses in normal babies. *Ear and Hearing, 27,* 751–762.

Roberson, J. B., Jr., O'Rourke, C., & Stidham, K. R. (2003). Auditory steady-state response testing in children: Evaluation of a new technology. *Otolaryngology–Head and Neck Surgery, 129*(1), 107–113.

Sammeth, C. A., & Barry, S. J. (1985). The 40-Hz event-related potential as a measure of audiotry sensitivity in normals. *Scandinavian Audiology, 14,* 51–55.

Small, S. A., & Stapells, D. R. (2004). Artifactual responses when recording auditory steady-state responses. *Ear and Hearing, 25*(6), 611–623.

Stapells, D. R. (2002). Cortical event-related potentials to auditory stimuli. In J. Katz (Ed.), *Handbook of clinical audiology* (5th ed., pp. 378–406). Baltimore: Lippincott Williams & Wilkins.

Stapells, D. R., Galambos, R., Costello, J. A., & Makeig, S. (1988). Inconsistency of auditory middle latency and steady-state responses in infants. *Electroencephalography and Clinical Neurophysiology, 71,* 289–295.

Stapells, D. R., Herdman, A., Small, S. A., Dimitrijevic, A., & Hatton, J. (2005). Current status of the auditory steady-state responses for estimating an infant's audiogram. In R. Seewald & J. Bamford (Eds.), *A sound foundation through early amplification 2004* (pp. 43–59). Basel: Phonak AG.

Stapells, D. R., Linden, D., Suffield, J. B., Hamel, G., & Picton, T. W. (1984). Human auditory steady state potentials. *Ear and Hearing, 5*(2), 105–113.

Stapells, D. R., Makeig, S., & Galambos, R. (1987). Auditory steady-state responses: threshold prediction using phase coherence. *Electroencephalography and Clinical Neurophysiology, 67,* 260-270.

Stefanatos, G. A., Green, G. G., & Ratcliff, G. G. (1989). Neurophysiological evidence of auditory channel anomalies in developmental dysphasia. *Archives of Neurology, 46,* 871-875.

Stueve, M. P., & O'Rourke, C. (2003). Estimation of hearing loss in children: Comparison of auditory steady-state response, auditory brainstem response, and behavioral test methods. *American Journal of Audiology, 12*(2), 125-136.

Suzuki, T., & Kobayashi, K. (1984). An evaluation of 40-Hz event-related potentials in young children. *Audiology, 23,* 599-604.

Tomlin, D., Rance, G., Graydon, K., & Tsialios, I. (2006). A comparison of 40 Hz auditory steady-state response (ASSR) and cortical auditory evoked potential (CAEP) thresholds in awake adult subjects. *International Journal of Audiology, 45,* 580-588.

Tsui, B., Wong, L. L., & Wong, E. C. (2002). Accuracy of cortical evoked response audiometry in the identification of nonorganic hearing loss. *International Journal of Audiology, 41,* 330-333.

Van der Reijden, C. S., Mens, L. H. M., & Snik, A. F. M. (2006). Frequency-specific objective audiometry: Tone-evoked brainstem responses and steady-state responses to 40 Hz and 90 Hz amplitude modulated stimuli. *International Journal of Audiology, 45,* 40-45.

Van Maanen, A., & Stapells, D. R. (2005). Comparison of multiple auditory steady-state responses (80 vs 40 Hz) and slow cortical potentials for threshold estimation in hearing-impaired adults. *International Journal of Audiology, 44,* 613-624.

Vander Werff, K. R., Brown, C. J., Gienapp, B. A., & Schmidt Clay, K. M. (2002). Comparison of auditory steady-state response and auditory brainstem response thresholds in children. *Journal of the American Academy of Audiology, 13*(5), 227-235.

Wong, W. Y., & Stapells, D. R. (2004). Brain stem and cortical mechanisms underlying the binaural masking level difference in humans: an auditory steady-state response study. *Ear and Hearing, 25*(1), 57-67.

Yeung, K. N. K., & Wong, L. L. N. (2007). Prediction of hearing thresholds: Comparison of cortical evoked response audiometry and auditory steady state response audiometry techniques. *International Journal of Audiology, 46,* 17-25.

CHAPTER 9

Auditory Steady-State Responses in Neonates and Infants

GARY RANCE

Introduction

As the developmental course of the auditory pathway is not consistent along its length (Goodin, Squires, Henderson, & Starr, 1978; Ponton, Egermont, Kwong, & Don, 2000), the reliability of auditory steady-state response (ASSR) measurement in children is highly dependent on the neural generators involved and, hence, on the stimulus presentation rate. The ASSR elicited by signals at 40 Hz (the "40-Hz response"), which in awake adult subjects can be detected at levels close to hearing threshold (Boettcher, Poth, Mills, & Dubno, 2001; Tomlin, Rance, Graydon, & Tsialios, 2006; Van Maanen

& Stapells, 2005), is not consistently recordable in young children (Levi, Folsom, & Dubie, 1993; 1995; Maurizi et al., 1990; Stapells, Galambos, Costello, & Makeig, 1988). There are two main reasons for this. The first relates to the practicalities of pediatric testing. Obtaining recordings with acceptably low levels of electroencephalogram (EEG) noise in youngsters requires that they be in either natural or sedated sleep. Unfortunately, in both sleeping adults and children, the amplitude of the 40-Hz response is reduced to less than 50% of that obtained in awake subjects (Cohen, Rickards, & Clark, 1991; Levi et al., 1993; Pethe, von Specht, Muhler, & Hocke, 2001; Petitot, Collet, & Durrant, 2005; Plourde &

Picton, 1990), so response thresholds are significantly higher (Galambos, Makeig, & Talmachoff, 1981; Klein, 1983; Picton, Vajsar, Rodriguez, & Campbell, 1987). Picton and colleagues (1987), for example, recorded ASSRs to 500-Hz tones in adult subjects (tested awake and asleep) and found that responses generally were less reliable, and detection thresholds were on average 11 dB higher, during sleep. This subject state effect is not surprising, because transient auditory evoked potentials with similar latencies to those of the 40-Hz ASSR (approximately 30 ms) are also affected by sleep and sedation (Osterhammel, Shallop, & Terkildsen, 1985).

The second major limitation on the recording of the 40-Hz ASSR in children is that the response is immature not only in infancy but also through the first decade of life. While the developmental course of this response is yet to be fully determined, Aoyagi and colleagues (1994) did show a general increase in detectability in subjects 6 months to 15 years of age, and Pethe, Muhler, Siewert, and von Specht (2004) found amplitude increases throughout childhood, with the response not reaching adult proportions until around the age of 14 years.

The amplitude of the infant ASSR decreases with increasing presentation rate (as does the adult response), but unlike adults, young children do not show an enhancement for modulation frequencies around 40 Hz (Aoyagi et al., 1994; Levi et al., 1993; Riquelme, Kuwada, Filipovic, Hartung, & Leonard, 2006; Suzuki & Kobayashi, 1984). The infant ASSR at 40 Hz, for example, is around half the size of the response at 10 Hz, whereas the adult ASSR is about 50% larger.[1] The lack of amplitude enhancement at 40 Hz in children suggests that the auditory cortex (the approximate region of origin for this response) is immature and unable to support the ASSR at high rates. Comparable results have been demonstrated in transient auditory evoked potentials of similar latency. Jerger, Chmiel, Glaze, and Frost (1987), for example, also found that middle latency responses (MLRs) could only be recognized in young children for stimuli at very low (less than 2 Hz) presentation rates.

Unlike the 40-Hz response, ASSRs to stimuli presented at rates of approximately 70 to 100 Hz can be recorded in children of all ages including newborns (Aoyagi et al., 1993; Cone-Wesson, Parker, Swiderski, & Rickards, 2002; John, Brown, Muir, & Picton (2004); Levi et al., 1993; Lins & Picton, 1995; Luts, Desloovere, & Wouters, 2006; Rance, Tomlin, & Rickards, 2006; Rance et al., 2005; Rickards et al., 1994; Savio, Cardenas, Perez-Abalo, Gonzalez, & Valdes, 2001). These "high-rate" ASSRs, which show equivalent latencies around 10 ms, are better suited to pediatric application in that they are appear to be unaffected by response state (Cohen et al.,1991; Linden, Campbell, Hamel, & Picton, 1985; Levi et al., 1993; Rance, Rickards, Cohen, De Vidi, & Clark, 1995) and less affected by developmental factors, at least in children younger than 12 months of age at assessment. Recent findings, however, have pointed to some maturational changes in the first year of life, and it is these developments (and their clinical implications) that are the focus of this chapter.

---

[1]This does not necessarily mean that response detectability in babies is greater for frequencies around 10 Hz, because background EEG levels typically are higher in this region (Riquelme et al., 2006).

Auditory Steady-State Response Development in Normal Babies

Maturation of high-rate ASSRs occurs through the neonatal and infant periods. Response latency delays have been reported in neonates (Cone-Wesson, Parker, et al., 2002; Rickards et al., 1994), and more importantly, a number of recent studies have shown that ASSR amplitudes are significantly lower (relative to adults and older children) for normal infants in the first year of life.

The Neonatal Auditory Steady-State Response

The amplitude of the high-rate (greater than 70 Hz) ASSR in the neonatal period is highly variable across subjects and is generally considerably smaller than that observed in older subjects (John et al., 2004; Luts et al., 2006). Table 9–1 shows average response amplitudes obtained across a range of carrier frequencies for babies tested within 3 days of birth in

the study by John and associates, and at an average corrected age of 12 days in the investigation by Luts and colleagues (2006).

The test stimuli used in these two studies were slightly different—in the former, tonal stimuli with an exponential envelope, and in the latter, sinusoidally modulated mixed amplitude- and frequency-modulated (AM/FM) tones.[2] Both investigations, however, revealed average response levels of only 10 to 20 nV for stimuli at 50 dB SPL. These response amplitudes are significantly lower than those obtained using identical test methodologies in normally hearing adult subjects. John, Dimitrijevic, and Picton (2002), for example, found adult responses approximately twice that of the newborn level (approximately 35 nV); Luts and associates (2006) found response amplitudes approximately three to four times higher in their group of adult controls (Table 9–1). Figure 9–1 demonstrates this response amplitude difference, showing the averaged amplitude spectrum obtained (in this case to stimuli at 30 dB SPL) for groups of infant and adult subjects (Luts et al., 2006).

Table 9–1. Average neonatal ASSR amplitudes (nV) obtained for simultaneous stimuli at the audiometric octave frequencies at a presentation level of 50 dB SPL

Study	500 Hz	1000 Hz	2000 Hz	4000 Hz
John et al., 2004 (newborns)	17.5 ± 13.7	20.6 ± 11.2	22.4 ± 9.3	15.3 ± 5.6
Luts et al., 2006 (newborns)	9 ± 6	12 ± 7	11 ± 5	8 ± 5
Luts et al., 2006 (adults)	32 ± 15	51 ± 18	45 ± 15	22 ± 11

---

[2]A discussion of the types of stimuli used to elicit the ASSR in babies can be found in Chapters 2 and 3.

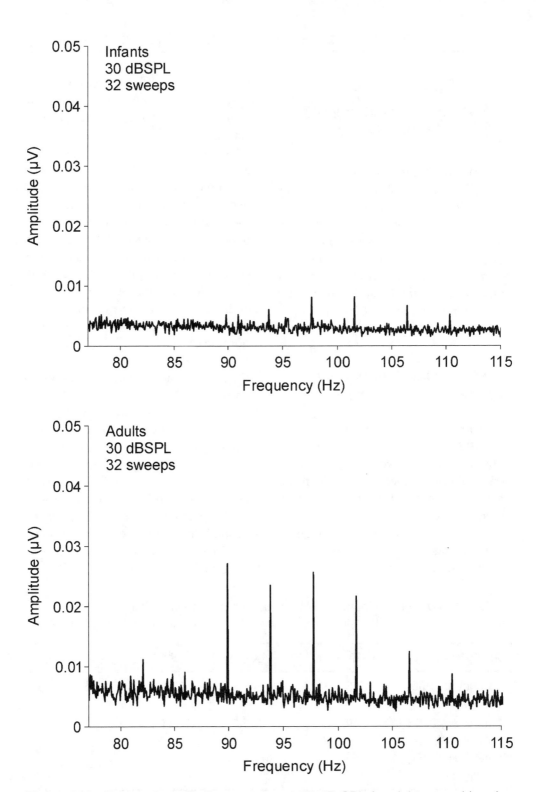

Figure 9–1. Averaged amplitude spectrum at 30 dB SPL for eight normal-hearing infants and adults (both ears). (Figure 3 from Luts et al. [2006]. *Audiology & Neuro-otology, 11*, 24–37. Copyright 2006 Karger. Reproduced with permission.)

Amplitude Development in Infancy

The point at which the ASSR in babies reaches adult dimensions is yet to be determined. Lins and associates (1996) measured responses to simultaneously presented AM tones in a group of babies (ages 1 to 10 months at assessment) and in a cohort of normal-hearing adult subjects and found that infant response amplitudes in this range were still only one-third to one-half adult size.

Subsequent studies have suggested that the bulk of the amplitude change occurs in the neonatal period (John et al., 2004; Savio et al., 2001). In their study, Savio and coworkers measured ASSR amplitudes to simultaneously presented AM tones at 70 dB SPL in three groups of children ages 0 to 29 days, 1 to 6 months, and 7 to 13 months at assessment. Clear age effects were observed, and responses in the neonatal cohort were significantly smaller than those of the children in both older groups. No difference was obtained between these older subject groups, indicating that most amplitude increase occurs in the first weeks of life. John and his associates also found significant neonatal amplitude changes. In this case, responses obtained to AM/FM stimuli at 50 dB SPL from full-term babies younger than 3 days at assessment were approximately 22% smaller than those of children aged 3 to 15 weeks.

Both of the foregoing studies found that responses to low-frequency stimuli showed lower amplitudes (relative to the other test frequencies) and a longer developmental course. Mean ASSR amplitudes at 500 Hz in the data from the study by John and associates (2004), for example, were not significantly different in the neonatal and infant test cohorts, whereas responses to higher-frequency stimuli did show a developmental effect. This finding is inconsistent with electrophysiological and behavioural data, which has tended to show greater responsivity to low-frequency stimuli in normal-hearing infants (Hepper & Shahidullah, 1994; Teas, Klein, & Kramer, 1982; Yamada, Ashikawa, Kodern, & Yamane, 1983).

Detection of Auditory Steady-State Responses in the Neonatal and Infant Period

Identification of the ASSR (and other evoked potentials) requires that the response be extracted from within the EEG. As such, detection is determined by both the amplitude of the response and the amplitude of the background EEG noise (the signal/noise ratio). Various factors that affect this ratio have been investigated, and optimal test parameters (in adult subjects at least) have been reasonably well established (Picton, John, Dimitrijevic, & Purcell, 2003; Picton, Dimitrijevic, Perez-Abalo, & Van Roon, 2005). EEG noise levels, for example, are strongly influenced by factors such subject state of arousal, EEG frequency range, and test duration. Signal amplitude can be affected by a range of stimulus and recording parameters including stimulus type, modulation rate, carrier frequency, and electrode configuration. These issues are reviewed in detail in the studies by Picton and colleagues (2003, 2005) and elsewhere in this book.

Each of these factors still apply to the assessment of babies but, as discussed in the previous section, the ASSR in the neonatal/early infant period is still developing. This immaturity raises the possibility that different test parameters may be appropriate for this age range. As such, a number of researchers have considered the stimulus characteristics that maximize the ASSR signal-to-noise ratio in newborns. Rickards and associates (1994), in their study of full-term neonates, measured the effect of modulation frequency (MF) on the response. An "efficiency" metric was used to determine optimal MFs for AM/FM tones with central frequencies at 500, 1500, and 4000 Hz that were modulated at rates between 40 and 190 Hz. As can be seen in Figure 9–2, optimal modulation rates varied with carrier tone, but were all within the range of 70 to 100 Hz. More recently, Riquelme and colleagues (2006) measured ASSRs to "transposed" tones modulated at rates between 25 and 88 Hz in a group of newborn subjects. These authors showed a

result pattern similar to that in the study by Rickards and coworkers (1994), obtaining optimal S/N ratios for MFs at the high end of their test range (65–88 Hz). Significantly, Riquelme and associates (2006) actually found that response amplitudes were greater to stimuli at low modulation rates (25–37 Hz) but that detection efficiencies in this range were comparatively low because background EEG noise levels were also higher in this region.

Direct comparison of ASSR signal-to-noise ratios in adult and infant subjects (at these optimal test frequencies) is complicated by the fact that the subjects typically are in different response states. Various researchers have measured noise levels in these subject groups, but where assessment of babies requires that the child be asleep or sedated, adult subjects are typically "relaxed" rather than asleep during testing. That being the case, background EEG levels in the frequency

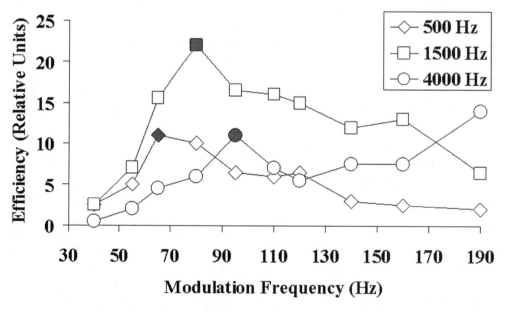

Figure 9–2. ASSR detection efficiency plotted against modulation frequency. Optimal modulation rate for each carrier tone in the range 70 to 100 Hz is represented by the filled data point. (From Rickards et al., 1994.)

range of 70 to 100 Hz in sleeping infants tend to be equivalent to or lower than those in older subjects. Luts and coworkers (2006), for example, found an average noise level of 5.1 nV in a group of adults and only 3.0 nV in a cohort of sleeping neonates after 10 minutes of recording. The relatively low noise level in babies has definite advantages for response detection but does not entirely compensate for the low-response amplitudes seen in early infancy (Luts et al., 2006). As such, it is not surprising to find that detection of the ASSR to low-level stimuli is more difficult in normal-hearing youngsters than in older subjects.

The Auditory Steady-State Response Threshold in Babies

ASSR threshold levels in normal babies tend to be higher than those in older subjects. Findings reported for normal-hearing adults (to high-modulation-rate [70 to 100 Hz] stimuli) have varied across studies but have broadly shown minimum response levels around 20 to 30 dB HL for low-frequency tones and 15 to 20 dB HL for mid- to- high-frequency signals (Aoyagi et al., 1994; Cone-Wesson, Parker, et al., 2002; Herdman & Stapells, 2001; Lins et al., 1996; Lins & Picton, 1995; Picton et al., 1998; Picton et al., 2005). ASSR thresholds in neonates and infants, on the other hand, have typically been around 10 dB higher, with most investigations showing average threshold levels of around 35 to 45 dB HL for low carrier frequencies and 25 to 40 dB HL for mid-to-high frequencies (Cone-Wesson, Rickards, et al., 2002; Levi et al., 1995; Lins et al, 1996; Luts et al., 2006; Perez-Abalo et al., 2007; Rance & Rickards, 2002; Rance & Tomlin, 2006; Rance

et al; 2005; Rickards et al., 1994; Savio et al., 2001). Table 9–2 shows a summary of the threshold values obtained in studies involving normal babies in the first year of life. Threshold levels are expressed in dB HL and have been converted in some cases from dB SPL values using the earphones and calibration materials described in each study.

Direct comparison of ASSR threshold findings across studies is complicated by methodological differences. As discussed previously, detection of low-level responses is strongly affected by factors influencing both the signal amplitude and the level of the EEG noise floor. Comparison of adult and infant findings, however, is possible in the (few) investigations that have measured ASSRs using similar test conditions for both subject groups. Lins and associates (1996) established ASSR thresholds to 500- 1000- 2000- and 4000-Hz AM tones in a cohort of normal-hearing adults and a group of infants aged 1 to 10 months at assessment. Response threshold levels in these subjects showed a significant group difference for the 500-Hz carrier and typically were 10 to 15 dB higher in the babies for each of the test frequencies. Similar results also have been obtained in our own laboratory where ASSR thresholds in a cohort of children (most of whom were less than 3 months of age) were approximately 10 to 15 dB higher than those previously measured in older children and adults (Rance & Rickards, 2002). More recently, Luts and colleagues (2006) used identical test protocols to assess a group of adult subjects and a group of infants (with a mean corrected age of 12 days) and found that response thresholds in the babies were on average 11 dB higher for stimuli across the audiometric range.

Table 9–2. ASSR threshold levels in (presumed) normally hearing neonates and infants. Mean and standard deviation values (in dB HL) are shown

Study	Subject Age	Stimulus Type	Test Time(s)	500 Hz	1000 Hz	2000 Hz	4000 Hz
Infants							
Lins et al. (1996)	1–10 mo.	Multiple AM	180–780	33 ± 13	22 ± 10	17 ± 8	21 ± 10
Savio et al.* (2001)	7–12 mo.	Multiple AM	180–480	46 ± 9	44 ± 10	37 ± 8	33 ± 9
Cone–Wesson, Rickards, et al. (2002)	1–79 mo.	Single AM/FM	22–90	39 ± 8	34 ± 10	26 ± 10	39 ± 12
Rance & Rickards[†] (2002)	1–8 mo.	Single AM/FM	22–90	43 ± 12	42 ± 10	35 ± 8	34 ± 10
Rance et al. (2005)	1–3 mo.	Single AM/FM	22–90	32 ± 7	32 ± 7	24 ± 6	28 ± 7
Rance & Tomlin (2006)	6 weeks	Single AM/FM	22–90	40 ± 7			33 ± 8
Neonates							
Rickards et al. (1994)	1–7 days	Single AM/FM	30–210	41 ± 10	*1500 Hz:* 24 ± 9		35 ± 11
Levi et al. (1995)	1 mo.	Single AM	100	36 ± 11	42 ± 11	34 ± 15	
Savio et al.* (2001)	0–1 mo.	Multiple AM	180–480	57 ± 11	55 ± 12	51 ± 12	48 ± 13
Luts et al. (2006)	<3 mo. (12 days)	Multiple AM/FM	600	37 ± 10	35 ± 10	32 ± 10	36 ± 9
Rance & Tomlin (2006)	3–7 days	Single AM/FM	22–90	46 ± 11			
Perez–Abalo et al. (2007)	<1 mo.	Multiple AM	180–480	43 ± 7		36 ± 6	38 ± 11

[†]Only subjects with hearing thresholds of up to 15 dB HL from this dataset have been included.

*Data in this study were obtained in the presence of high levels of environmental noise, which the authors considered may have affected the results.

168

In summary, it has become clear that ASSR threshold levels in (presumed) normal-hearing children obtained in the neonatal and infant periods are consistently higher than those of older subjects. The point at which the response reaches maturity in normally developing babies is currently under investigation.

Auditory Steady-State Response Threshold Changes in Infancy

The course of ASSR threshold development in babies is yet to be firmly established. Savio and coworkers (2001) compared a group of normal infants tested in the neonatal period and a second cohort assessed between the ages of 7 and 12 months and found significant threshold decreases with increasing age. Mean threshold differences between the groups in this study were 7, 10, 12, and 14 dB for the 500-, 1000-, 2000- and 4000-Hz test frequencies, respectively. These findings broadly suggested maturational changes somewhere in the first year of life.

A more detailed investigation of ASSR threshold changes occurring in the first 6 weeks of life (the age range in which children typically are referred for clinical diagnostic testing) was presented by Rance and Tomlin (2006). This longitudinal study tracked ASSR thresholds in healthy, full-term babies from the neonatal period (3 to 6 days at initial assessment) to 6 weeks of age. Consistent within-subject decreases across this period of around 5 dB were observed at both test frequencies (500 Hz and 4000 Hz). Figure 9–3 shows the threshold data obtained at the four collection points for all of the subjects in this study. Results

for two children are highlighted to show within-subject changes over time.

In addition to showing response changes through the first weeks of life, the data collected by Rance and Tomlin (2006) also demonstrated that ASSR threshold maturation was not yet complete at 6 weeks of age in normally developing babies. Mean threshold values obtained at the final data collection point (39.7 dB for the 500-Hz tone and 32.1 dB for the 4000-Hz tone) in this study were still approximately 10 dB higher than typical adult levels.

Unpublished follow-up data from the Rance and Tomlin cohort (2006) did suggest that ASSR threshold development was complete (for high-frequency stimuli at least) by the end of the first year of life. ASSR thresholds at the 4 kHz-test frequency obtained at 12 months of age in these babies had decreased significantly to near-adult levels. Mean threshold levels for this group had reduced from 33 dB HL at 6 weeks of age to 22 dB HL at 52 weeks. Results at the 500-Hz test frequency, however, were still relatively immature, showing a mean threshold of 35 dB HL at 52 weeks (a decrease of only 5 dB) (see Figure 9–4 for details). This frequency difference is consistent with studies of ASSR amplitude development that have shown a longer maturational course for low-frequency responses (John et al., 2004; Savio et al., 2001).

Developmental Mechanisms Affecting Auditory Steady-State Response Thresholds in Infancy

ASSR amplitude increases and threshold decreases in the first year of life are likely to be largely the result of neural development in the auditory pathway rather than

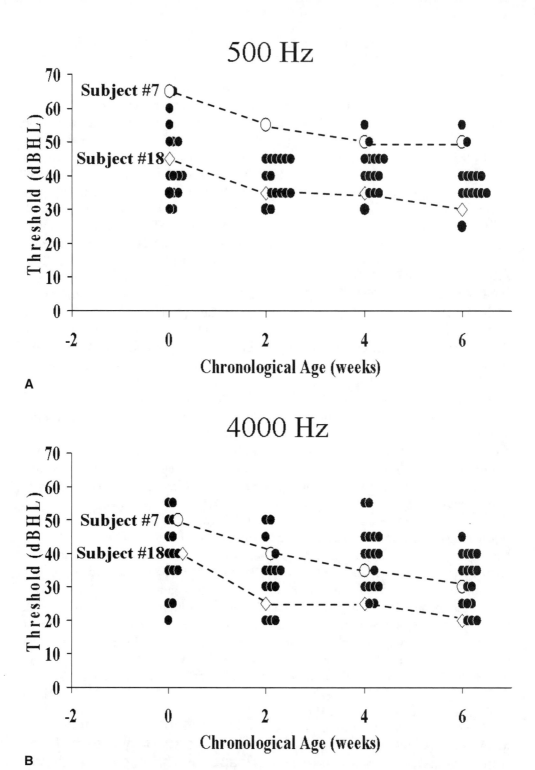

Figure 9–3. A, ASSR thresholds obtained for 500-Hz stimuli. Findings for two subjects are highlighted: Subject #7 is represented by the *open circles*; Subject #18, by *open diamonds*. **B**, ASSR thresholds obtained for 4-kHz stimuli. Findings for two subjects are highlighted: Subject #7 is represented by the *open circles*; Subject #18, by *open diamonds*.

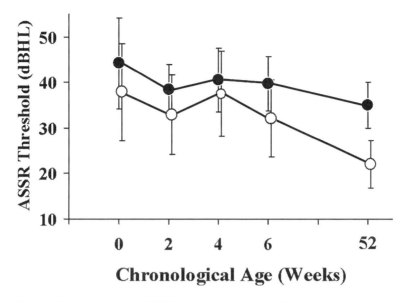

Figure 9–4. Average ASSR threshold levels for a cohort of normally hearing subjects tested through the first year of life. The *error bars* represent mean ± 1 standard deviation.

maturation of peripheral mechanisms. Ear canal changes (particularly through the neonatal and early infant periods) can affect the level of the stimuli reaching the cochlea. Rance and Tomlin (2006), for example, measured ear canal SPLs for AM/FM tones and found that sound levels at the tympanic membrane decreased by approximately 6 dB (for a consistent input) across the first 6 weeks of life. Such decreases would, however, work against the observed changes to ASSR amplitude and threshold, as ear canal stimulus levels (for a given coupler calibrated signal) effectively decrease over time.[3]

Development of the middle ear system also is unlikely to account for the observed ASSR maturational effects. Although it is possible that subtle variations in power transfer through the developing middle ear may influence signal levels at the cochlea, the scale of this effect is unlikely to alter ASSR findings significantly (Keefe & Levi, 1996; Sininger, Abdala, & Cone-Wesson, 1997). Inner ear development is also unlikely to produce measurable changes in ASSR amplitude or detection because the cochlea is both anatomically and physiologically mature in full-term newborns (Abdala, Sininger, Ekelid, & Zeng, 1996; Eggermont, Ponton, Coupland, & Winkelaar, 1991; Johnsen, Bagi, & Elberling, 1983; Smurzynski et al., 1993).

Unlike the inner ear, the auditory neural pathway is not completely developed in the full-term neonate. The auditory

---

[3]Rance and Tomlin (2006) in fact found that within-subject ASSR thresholds calculated using actual ear canal sound levels decreased by on average 11.1 dB for a 500-Hz tone and 10.1 dB for a 4-kHz tone over the Week 0 to 6.recording period.

brainstem response (ABR) shows both amplitude and morphological changes that occur through infancy and up to 2 to 3 years of age (Salamy, 1984), and later evoked potentials from the auditory midbrain and cortex have developmental courses that may not be complete until adolescence (Goodin et al., 1978; Ponton et al., 2000). Furthermore, elevated ABR thresholds have been reported for both click and tone-burst stimuli throughout the neonatal and early infant periods (Adelman, Levi, Lindner, & Sohmer, 1990; Schulman-Galambos & Galambos, 1979; Sininger et al., 1997; Stapells, Gravell, & Martin, 1995). Sininger and colleagues (1997), for example, used an in situ calibration system to equate ear canal SPLs across subjects and found click-evoked ABR thresholds in a group of neonates to be approximately 17 dB higher than those of adult controls, and tone burst–ABR thresholds that were 3 to 24 dB higher (depending on test frequency). As such, it is not surprising that ASSRs should also show developmental changes through the first months of life.

Auditory Steady-State Responses and Tone Burst–Evoked Auditory Brainstem Responses in Neonates and Young Infants

ASSRs and tone burst–evoked ABRs (TB-ABRs) have emerged as the two most promising "objective" measures of auditory function in children too immature to undergo conditioned audiometric testing. A number of investigators have compared threshold levels for these auditory evoked potentials in adult subjects

(Cone-Wesson, Dowell, et al., 2002; Johnson & Brown, 2005; Swanpoel, Hugo, & Roode, 2004) and in children 3 months of age and older at assessment (Aoyagi et al., 1999; Stueve & O'Rourke, 2003; Vander Werff, Brown, Gienapp, & Schmidt Clay, 2002). Results have varied across studies, but overall, TB-ABR threshold levels typically have been obtained at lower presentation levels (about 3 to 10 dB lower) in subjects with normal hearing and those with sensorineural hearing loss.

Direct comparison of response thresholds, does however, need to take into account the fact that the stimuli for the two techniques are calibrated differently. Stimulus levels for ASSR testing are usually presented in dB HL as behavioural detection thresholds for the continuous modulated tones used to elicit the response are typically within 1 to 2 dB of American National Standards Institute reference levels for pure tones (0 dB HL) (ANSI, 1996). By contrast, stimulus levels for tone-burst stimuli are typically referred to as dB nHL, reflecting the fact that their brevity results in detection thresholds that are elevated compared with pure tone levels. As such, actual peak equivalent SPL values may be 5 to 15 dB higher for tone bursts at 0 dB nHL than for modulated tones at 0 dB HL.

ASSR thresholds are significantly higher than TB-ABR levels in normally developing newborns. Where ASSRs can typically only be recorded to stimuli 30 to 40 dB HL or above, TB-ABRs can be reliably detected in normal babies at levels as low as 5 to 15 dB nHL (Klein, 1984; Sininger et al., 1997). A study by Rance and associates (2006) compared ASSR and TB-ABR findings in a group of infants and found that within each subject, ASSR thresholds were on average 4.8 dB higher at the

500-Hz frequency and 19.3 dB higher at the 4000-Hz frequency. Within-subject differences for each data collection point are shown in Figure 9–5.

A number of factors may contribute to the finding that threshold differences between ASSRs and TB-ABRs are more pronounced in early infancy. The first is that the two responses may have different developmental courses. While the infant ABR does mature in the first years of life, changes in response threshold appear to be less dramatic than for the ASSR. Rance and coworkers (2006), for example, found that ASSR threshold levels typically decreased (within each subject) by 5 dB more than ABR thresholds over the 6-week test period. As such, differences between tests appear to decrease (somewhat) over time (see Figure 9–5).

Another likely contributor to the clear threshold difference between techniques in infancy is the relative size of the responses. The amplitude of the ASSR in normally developing babies is significantly less than that of the TB-ABR. For example, John and associates (2004) and Luts and colleagues. (2006) reported mean neonatal ASSR amplitudes of approximately 10 to 20nV for a range of carrier tones presented at 50 dB SPL (see Table 9–1). Sininger and coworkers. (1997) in contrast, measured TB-ABR amplitudes of approximately 250 nV for a 500-Hz tone burst signal at equivalent presentation levels.

The obvious question arising from these findings is why ASSR amplitudes are so much smaller than TB-ABR amplitudes. Certainly these two responses have a number of similarities. TB-ABR

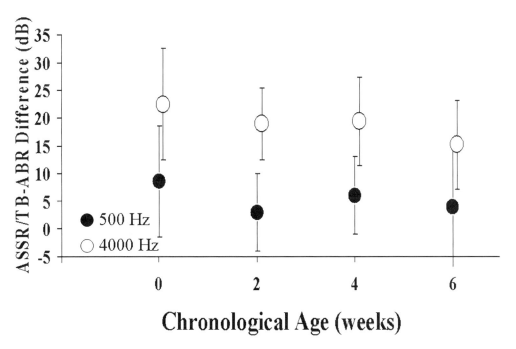

Figure 9–5. Within-subject difference levels (ASSR threshold minus TB-ABR threshold) for a group of normal babies tested through the first 6 weeks of life. The *error bars* represent mean ± 1 standard deviation.

latencies in babies are broadly equivalent to those of the high-rate ASSRs (Cone-Wesson, Parker, et al., 2002; Rickards et al., 1994), and the two are similar in their imperviousness to changes in response state (Cohen et al., 1991; Osterhammel et al., 1985). Furthermore, the two responses also are alike in their pattern of responsiveness to stimuli at different frequencies, both showing relatively higher detection thresholds to low-frequency stimuli (Rance et al., 2006). However, these shared characteristics do not confirm that the tests have common generators, and it may be that the amplitude difference between tests reflects different sources within the auditory pathway (see Chapter 4 for details).

Another possible explanation for the pronounced amplitude difference between tests in neonates and infants may be related to a reduced ability to process stimuli at high presentation rates. In subjects with mature auditory pathways, stimulus presentation rates of up to 50 per second tend to have no clinically significant effects on the ABR (Burkhard, Shi, & Hecox, 1990; Sininger & Don, 1989). Stimulus rates beyond this value, however, result in dramatic response latency increase, amplitude decrease, and hence, threshold elevation. The effects of presentation rate on the developing auditory brainstem are yet to be fully investigated, but obvious changes in click-ABR latency have been reported in neonates for rates as low as 10 Hz (Lasky, 1984; Lasky & Rupert, 1982), suggesting a higher sensitivity to rapidly repeating signals. As such, ABR presentation rates in infant testing typically are restricted to less than 40 Hz. ASSR assessment, by contrast, requires modulation frequencies in the range of 70 to 100 Hz to elicit reliable responses in sleeping children,

and it may be that stimulus peaks occurring at such high rates exceed refractory periods within the immature auditory systems in normal babies and result in comparatively low response amplitudes.

Another potential contributor to the apparent ASSR/ABR sensitivity difference in infants (and older subjects as well) relates to the way in which test stimuli are calibrated. As mentioned previously, both the tone bursts used for ABR assessment and the modulated tones used for ASSR testing are referenced to behavioural detection thresholds (typically using cohorts of normal-hearing adults). However, the different temporal characteristics of these stimuli (tone bursts being much shorter) mean that the actual SPL values at behavioural threshold for these stimuli are quite different. As such, the peak equivalent SPL (dB peSPL) for tone bursts (at 0 dB nHL) are significantly higher than those of modulated tones (at 0 dB HL). For example, peSPL levels for tone-burst stimuli used in the study by Rance and associates. (2006) were 3.5 dB higher at 500 Hz and 12.6 dB higher at 4 kHz than dB peSPL values for the modulated tones at these frequencies. So how might this affect ASSR and TB-ABR threshold levels? It may be that the underlying physiologic processes that generate these electrophysiological responses are dependent on the peak values of the acoustic waveform, rather than on perceptual detection levels. If this is the case, then comparison of detection levels for the two tests needs to be made using the same unit (dB peSPL). Interestingly, studies involving normal infants that have expressed ASSR and TB-ABRs in this way have shown similar response thresholds (Rance et al., 2006, Stapells, Herdman, Small, Dimitrijevic, & Hatton, 2005).

Hearing Level Prediction Using Auditory Steady-State Responses in Normal Babies

Maturation of the ASSR in the neonatal and infant periods poses two particular challenges with regard to prediction of hearing level. The first relates to response sensation level, and the second concerns response variability. Hearing levels are most commonly predicted from evoked potentials using mean threshold difference levels or sensation levels. That is, when the evoked potential threshold exceeds the hearing level by an amount that is consistent across subjects and test occasions, the most likely hearing level can be predicted for an individual from the ASSR threshold by subtracting the typical response sensation or difference level.[4] (This issue is discussed in detail in Chapter 7). For older children and adult subjects, the ASSR-behavioural threshold correlation has been empirically established. In normally developing babies however, this relationship is not well defined, and it is clear that ASSR levels change significantly over an as-yet ill-defined time course. As such, there is a clear need to determine typical response levels for babies of different ages and developmental stages.

A second factor limiting the accuracy of threshold estimation in the infant period is the variability of ASSR thresholds. It does not matter, for example, if the ASSR threshold (for a given set of test conditions) is 20, 30, or even 40 dB above hearing level, provided it occurs at the same level each time a child is tested. The sensation level can be subtracted once the typical level is known, but the

confidence with which a prediction can be made is determined by the range of possible hearing levels that can correspond to a particular ASSR threshold (Picton et al., 2005; Rance et al., 1995).

ASSR threshold variance in babies is higher than for older subjects. This is particularly the case in the neonatal period when response thresholds in groups of normal babies can vary by more than 30 dB (Luts et al., 2006; Rance & Tomlin, 2006; Rickards et al., 1994; Savio et al., 2001). Each of the studies measuring ASSR thresholds in neonates, for example, has shown standard deviations greater than 10 dB across a range of carrier frequencies (see Table 9–2). Part of this variability may be due to ear canal differences between subjects. For example, in a study by Rance and Tomlin (2006), when ASSR thresholds were recalculated using actual SPLs (measured at the eardrum), the spread of response detection levels was significantly reduced.

In essence though, the problem of high ASSR threshold variance in normal babies is due to low response amplitude (John et al., 2004; Luts et al., 2006). As ASSRs are smaller and more variable (John et al., 2004) in neonates and infants, small fluctuations in either the level of the ASSR or the ambient EEG noise result in significant fluctuations in detection threshold.

Auditory Steady-State Responses in Hearing-Impaired Babies

ASSRs can be consistently recorded at low sensation levels in adults and older

---

[4]Regression formulae describing the ASSR/behavioral threshold relationship can also be used in situations where factors such as degree of hearing loss affect this relationship.

children with sensorineural hearing loss (Aoyagi et al., 1999; Johnson & Brown, 2005; Rance & Rickards, 2002; Rance et al., 1995, 2005; Stueve & O'Rourke, 2003; Swanepoel et al., 2004; Vander Werff et al., 2002). Accordingly, the technique has been used in these populations to predict both the degree and the configuration of the behavioural audiogram (see Chapter 7 for details). In fact, the behavioural-ASSR threshold relationship in cochlear hearing-impaired subjects is stronger than has been observed for normal-hearing subjects. Recent studies by Vander Werff and Brown (2005) and Picton and colleagues (2005), for example, have compared groups of adults with normal hearing and groups with sensorineural loss and found smaller ASSR-behavioural difference levels and reduced response variability in hearing-impaired cases. The likely explanation for this result is a "recruitment-like" phenomenon (Rance et al., 1995). Recruitment is an abnormally rapid growth in perceived loudness that is often reported by subjects with sensorineural hearing loss. The physiological correlate of this perceptual effect of cochlear damage is an abnormally rapid increase in the size of the ASSR (once the signal has exceeded the subject's hearing level). Both Vander Werff and Brown (2005) and Picton and coworkers (2005) demonstrated this effect, showing steeper ASSR amplitude growth functions in their hearing-impaired subjects. The results of this rapid amplitude growth are that responses can be recorded close to hearing threshold, and that the transition between stimulus levels that produce a measurable potential and those that do not is more pronounced. This in turn results in relatively low ASSR threshold variability.

The effect of sensorineural hearing loss on the ASSR in the newborn period is yet be fully explored, but preliminary data suggest that responses can also be reliably obtained at low sensation levels in this subject group. That is, the response amplitude advantages afforded by the recruitment-like effect appear to override the maturational factors observed in normal-hearing babies. For example, Luts and associates (2006) found mean ASSR threshold sensation levels of around 5 to 10 dB (depending on carrier frequency) in a group of 20 hearing-impaired infants tested in the first few months of life, where threshold sensation levels in babies with (presumed) normal hearing in this study were approximately 30 to 40 dB.

ASSR threshold data from a larger group of babies with sensorineural hearing loss was presented by Rance and colleagues (2005). Figure 9–6 shows a subset of the findings from this cohort, only including results for those children ($n = 121$) who underwent assessment at 6 weeks of age or younger (corrected). As can be seen in this distribution, ASSRs in these children were consistently recordable at low-sensation levels. Furthermore, the relatively low spread of the data suggests that ASSR thresholds obtained in the early infant period can reliably reflect the behavioural audiogram particularly in ears with significant sensorineural hearing loss.

Auditory Steady-State Responses in Premature Babies

As discussed previously in this chapter, the ASSR is still developing in healthy, full-term neonates. Not surprisingly, attempts to record the response in premature babies (before their due date) have also shown clear maturational changes. Luts and associates (2006) measured ASSR

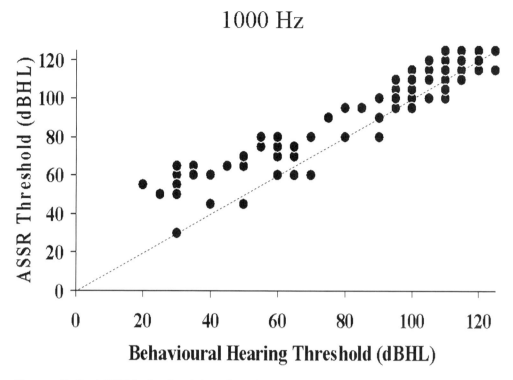

Figure 9–6. ASSR-behavioral hearing threshold comparisons at the 1-kHz test frequency for 121 children with sensorineural-type hearing loss. Evoked potential assessments were carried out between the ages of 2 and 6 weeks (corrected age). Behavioral thresholds were obtained when the child was mature enough to provide reliable conditioned audiometric results (7 to 12 months of age).

signal-to-noise ratios in normal-hearing premature babies assessed between 36 and 40 weeks postconceptual age and in term-born babies tested between 41 and 50 weeks postconceptual age. These investigators found that for stimuli presented at 50 dB SPL, ASSR signal-to-noise ratios typically were approximately 40% lower in the "younger" children. Similarly, Cone-Wesson, Parker, and coworkers (2002) measured ASSRs at moderately high screening levels (66 dB SPL for a 500-Hz carrier and 56 dB SPL for a 2-kHz carrier) and found higher "pass" rates in full-term babies assessed during the first week of life compared with pre-

mature children born at 23 to 34 weeks of gestation and tested at around 31 weeks.

These findings clearly suggest that clinical ASSR testing of premature babies should at least be postponed until they have passed their due date. Whether the auditory pathways of these babies develop to the level of their full-term peers by 40 weeks postconceptual age is unclear. Riquelme and associates (2006) found no significant difference in the proportion of ASSR runs reaching response criterion for a group of full-term babies in the first week of life and a cohort of neonatal intensive care unit (NICU) graduates tested at a similar age (i.e., assessment in the premature infants was undertaken when they had reached a postconceptual age of 39 weeks). However, ABR results obtained in premature babies suggest that response development can lag behind that of healthy, full-term children (Salamy et al., 1984), and it may be that ASSR findings in this group will show similar delays.

Clinical Application of ASSR-Based Hearing Estimation Techniques in Newborns

The advent of newborn hearing screening has meant that children are now routinely referred for diagnostic hearing testing in the first weeks of life. Assessment techniques based on the ASSR are in many respects well suited to this task. ASSR testing offers an objective, frequency-specific method that can provide information detailed enough to form a basis for intervention in young children with significant sensorineural hearing loss (Rance & Briggs, 2002). Unfortunately, low-response amplitude and high-threshold variability in normal babies limits our ability to differentiate between ears with normal acuity and those with mild-degree hearing loss. This is a crucial clinical issue because a high proportion of babies (approximately 75%) referred through newborn hearing screening subsequently show normal or near-normal hearing (Kennedy et al., 2000). As recent

evidence suggests that even mild sensorineural hearing loss can affect long-term developmental outcomes (Bess, Dodd-Murphy, & Parler, 1998) it is important that diagnostic procedures can identify affected babies.

Improving the clinical applicability of ASSR testing in the first weeks of life requires a better understanding of the course of response development in neonates and young infants with normal hearing. Age-related norms for ASSR thresholds (obtained using optimized test procedures) need to be established for this population. Furthermore, normative data also are required for newborn babies with sensorineural hearing loss, particularly those with lesser degrees of impairment in whom recruitment-like effects may not be sufficient to override developmental changes in the first weeks of life.

Conductive hearing loss and its effect on ASSR findings in neonates is also a major clinical issue as most babies presenting with impairment in this period suffer middle-ear rather than cochlear pathology. ASSR thresholds to air-conducted stimuli in affected children are likely to show similar sensation levels (re. cochlear hearing thresholds) to those seen in subjects with normal acuity. This of course assumes that stimulus presentation level (which needs to be higher to overcome the air-bone gap in these cases) is not a factor.[5] Further consideration of the ways in which ASSR findings to air-conducted and also bone-conducted stimuli can be used to supplement the

---

[5]As response sensation levels in normal neonates are large, it is possible to obtain quite high ASSR threshold levels in ears with middle-ear pathology. For example in a child with normal cochlear reserve and a conductive hearing loss of 50 dB at a frequency of 500 Hz, the likely ASSR threshold will be approximately 90 dB HL (40 dB HL mean ASSR threshold + 50 dB HL conductive overlay).

existing infant assessment battery is required generally, but in particular in relation to babies with conductive hearing loss. ASSR testing to stimuli presented via bone conduction is discussed in detail in Chapter 11, and case examples showing ways in which ASSR findings can be used in differential diagnosis are presented in Chapter 14.

In addition to establishing expected ASSR sensation levels in young babies, confident prediction of hearing levels requires that response variability is minimized. Current data suggest that in this population, a broad range of hearing levels can correspond to a particular ASSR threshold. This necessarily reduces the confidence with which hearing level predictions can be made.

In addition to optimizing test parameters, a number of clinical factors may affect the reliability of findings in this group. First, selecting an appropriate time to carry out the assessment may be important. There are a number of valid reasons for undertaking diagnostic assessment as early as possible, such as initiating the intervention process (if required), reducing parental anxiety, and accessing the child when periods of natural sleep are frequent. On the other hand, as discussed throughout this chapter, auditory pathway development limits the reliability of the response in the first weeks of life. An optimal test age is yet to be firmly established, but all of the studies conducted thus far have concluded that ASSR assessment in the neonatal period (particularly week 1 for full-term babies) should be avoided (John et al., 2004; Luts et al., 2006; Rance & Tomlin, 2006).

Reducing signal-level variability may help to improve the reliability of ASSR threshold measures in newborns. Insert transducers are commonly used in the clinical assessment of babies because these devices are less likely to collapse a soft ear canal than are standard headphones (Hosford-Dunn et al., 1983). However, inserts are more likely to accentuate the effects of ear canal-size on the presentation level because the enclosed volume (between the end of the insert and the eardrum) is relatively smaller than when circumural transducers are used. For example, in a recent study (Rance et al., 2006) that employed insert phones and measured signal levels at the eardrum, SPLs (for a consistent transducer output measured in a 2-cc coupler) varied by up to 10 dB across subjects assessed at the some postconceptual age. Furthermore, within-subject comparisons obtained when the insert phone was removed and replaced through the course of a test session also showed significant fluctuations, despite the fact that the tester was an experienced clinician following a strict protocol. Therefore, employing transducers that minimize differences in presentation level between subjects, such as the "Ear-Muffin" or "Ear-Coupler," or designing evoked potential systems that can measure ear canal sound levels may reduce ASSR variability in young patients.

ASSR testing, using current approaches at least, may not be the most accurate hearing assessment option for all children in the neonatal period. Tone-burst ABR testing appears to offer more reliable results in newborns with normal acuity (Rance et al., 2006). ASSR testing on the other hand, with its potential for greater frequency specificity and higher stimulus presentation levels, has advantages for babies with significant sensorineural hearing loss (Rance & Briggs, 2002;

Rance et al., 1995). As such, clinicians should consider (particularly when undertaking diagnostic assessment in very young children) using ASSR-based techniques in concert with other components in the electrophysiological, electroacoustic, and behavioural hearing test batteries.[6]

Summary and Research Directions

Over the past few years it has become clear that maturational factors do affect the ASSR in the first months of life. Responses from normal-hearing babies tend to have longer equivalent latencies and significantly lower amplitudes than those obtained from adults and older children. As a result, detection thresholds are higher and more variable, particularly in the neonatal period.

The key to improving hearing level prediction in neonates and young infants lies in the optimization of the ASSR signal-to-noise ratio. Background EEG levels are affected by a number of test parameters in subjects of all ages, but an obvious area for investigation in babies concerns the test duration. While it is clear that increasing the recording period in the laboratory (where EEG levels in cooperative subjects are relatively stable over time) results in lower noise floors, establishing a balance between long run times and the clinical constraints imposed by infant sleep patterns is an area in need of further investigation. Other aspects of test efficiency such as the use of multiple simultaneous stimuli and binaural testing

(which are discussed elsewhere in this book) are yet to be thoroughly explored in infant populations.

Improving ASSR amplitude in babies through the optimization of test parameters should be another research focus for the immediate future. Manipulation of the stimuli used to elicit the response in this population is one approach that has been recently considered by a number of research groups. ASSRs can be evoked by a range of noise and tonal stimuli (see Chapter 2 for details). Sinusoidally AM tones have been most vigorously investigated for clinical application because they are relatively precise in terms of their frequency content and have been shown to reflect the configuration of the behavioural audiogram in adults and older children (Johnson & Brown, 2005; Rance et al., 1995). Recent work by John and associates (2004) and Riquelme and colleagues (2006) has experimented with different stimulus envelope shapes (notably steeper on/off slopes) and has shown significant response amplitude advantages (over AM tones) in infant subjects. As always, in this area there is a trade-off between response precision and stimulus frequency specificity, but these (and other) technical developments may find clinical application in the future.

In conclusion, ASSR assessment does appear to have a place in the infant test battery. The technique is well suited as a diagnostic measure for those children with significant sensorineural hearing loss who have failed neonatal hearing screening. There is, however, more progress to be made before the response can be reliably used to differentiate between those

---

[6]The inability of the ASSR technique to differentiate between peripheral (cochlear) hearing losses and those related to neural transmission disorders such as auditory neuropathy/dyssynchrony is another good reason to combine ABR and ASSR measures in the diagnostic clinic.

children with normal hearing and those with mild hearing loss in the first weeks of life.

References

Abdala, C., Sininger, Y. S., Ekelid, M., & Zeng, F. G. (1996). Distortion product otoacoustic emission suppression tuning curves in human adults and neonates. *Hearing Research*, *98*, 38–53.

Adelman, C., Levi, H., Lindner, N., & Sohmer, H. (1990). Neonatal auditory brainstem-response threshold and latency: 1 hour to 5 months. *Electroencephalography and Clinical Neurophysiology*, *77*, 77–80.

Aoyagi, M., Kiren, T., Kim, Y., Suzuki, Y., Fuse, T. & Koike, Y. (1993). Optimal modulation frequency for amplitude-modulation following response in young children during sleep. *Hearing Research*, *65*, 253–261.

Aoyagi, M., Kiren, T., Furuse, H., Fuse, T., Suzuki, Y., Yokota, S., et al. (1994). Puretone threshold prediction by 80-Hz amplitude-modulation following response. *Acta Oto-laryngologica. Supplementum*, *511*, 7–14.

Aoyagi, M., Suzuki, Y., Yokota, M., Furuse, H., Watanabe, T., & Ito, T. (1999). Reliability of 80-Hz amplitude-modulation-following response detected by phase coherence. *Audiology & Neuro otology*, *4*, 28–37.

ANSI. (1996). *ANSI S3.6-1996, specifications for audiometers*. New York: American Institute of Physics.

Bess, F. H., Dodd-Murphy, J., & Parker, R. A. (1998). Infants with minimal sensorineural hearing loss: Prevalence, educational performance and functional status. *Ear and Hearing*, *19*, 339–354.

Boettcher, F. A., Poth, E. A., Mills, J. H., & Dubno, J. R. (2001). The amplitude-modulation following response in young and aged human subjects. *Hearing Research*, *153*, 32–42.

Burkhard, R., Shi, Y., & Hecox, K. (1990). A comparison of maximum length sequences for the derivation of brainstem auditory-evoked responses at rapid rates of stimulation. *Journal of the Acoustical Society of America*, *87*, 1656–1664.

Cohen, L. T., Rickards, F. W., & Clark, G. M. (1991). A comparison of steady-state evoked potentials to modulated tones in awake and sleeping humans. *Journal of the Acoustical Society of America*, *90*, 2467–2479.

Cone-Wesson, B., Parker, J., Swiderski, N., & Rickards, F. (2002). The auditory steady-state response: Full-term and premature neonates. *Journal of the American Academy of Audiology*, *13*, 260–269.

Cone-Wesson, B., Dowell, R. C., Tomlin, D., Rance, G., & Ming, W. J. (2002). The auditory steady-state response: Comparisons with auditory brainstem response. *Journal of the American Academy of Audiology*, *13*, 173–187.

Cone-Wesson, B., Rickards, F. W., Poulis, C., Parker, J., Tan, L., & Pollard, J. (2002). The auditory steady-state response. III. Clinical applications in infants and children. *Journal of the American Academy of Audiology*, *13*, 270–282.

Eggermont, J. J., Ponton, C. W., Coupland, S. G., & Winkelaar, R. (1991). Maturation of traveling-wave delay in the human cochlea. *Journal of the Acoustical Society of America*, *90*, 288–298.

Galambos, R., Makeig, S., & Talmachoff, P. J. (1981). A 40-Hz potential recorded from the human scalp. *Proceedings of the National Academy of Sciences of the United States of America*, *78*, 2643–2647.

Goodin, D., Squires, K., Henderson, B., & Starr, A. (1978). Age-related variations in evoked potentials to auditory stimuli in normal human subjects. *Electroencephalography and Clinical Neurophysiology*, *44*, 337–358.

Hepper, P.G., & Shahidullah, B. S. (1994). Development of fetal hearing. *Archives of Disease in Childhood*, *71*, 81–87.

Herdman, A. T., & Stapells, D. R. (2001). Thresholds determined using the monotic and diotic multiple auditory steady-state response technique in normal-hearing subjects. *Scandinavian Audiology, 30,* 41–49.

Hosford-Dunne, H., Runge, C.A., Hillel, A. & Johnson, S.J. (1983). Auditory brain stem response testing in infants with collapsed ear canals. *Ear Hear, 4,* 258–260.

Jerger, J., Chmiel, R., Glaze, D., & Frost, J. D., Jr. (1987). Rate and filter dependence of the middle latency response in infants. *Audiology, 26,* 269–283.

John, M. S., Brown, D. K., Muir, P. J., & Picton, T. W. (2004). Recording steady-state responses in young infants. *Ear and Hearing, 25,* 539–553.

John, M. S., Dimitrijevic, A. & Picton, T. W. (2002). Auditory steady-state responses to exponential modulation envelopes. *Ear and Hearing, 23,* 106–117.

Johnsen, N. J., Bagi, P., & Elberling, C. (1983). Evoked acoustic emissions from the human ear. III. Findings in neonates. *Scandavian Audiology, 12,* 17–24.

Johnson, T. A., & Brown, C. J. (2005). Threshold prediction using the auditory steady-state response and the tone burst auditory brain stem response; a within subject comparison. *Ear and Hearing, 26,* 559–576.

Keefe, D. H., & Levi, E. (1996). Maturation of the middle and external ears: Acoustic power-based responses and reflectance tympanometry. *Ear and Hearing, 17,* 361–373.

Kennedy, C. R., Kimm, L., Thornton, A. R. D., & Davis, A. (2000). False positives in universal neonatal screening for permanent childhood hearing impairment. *Lancet, 356,* 1903–1904.

Klein, A. J. (1983). Properties of brain-stem response slow-wave component. I. Latency, amplitude and threshold sensitivity. *Archives of Otololaryngology–Head & Neck Surgery, 109,* 6–12.

Klein, A. J. (1984). Frequency and age-dependent auditory evoked potential

thresholds in infants. *Hearing Research, 16,* 291–297.

Lasky, R. E. (1984). A developmental study on the effect of stimulus rate on the auditory evoked brain-stem response. *Electroencephalography and Clinical Neurophysiology, 59,* 411–419.

Lasky, R. E., & Rupert, A. (1982). Temporal masking of auditory evoked brainstem responses in human newborns and adults. *Hearing Research, 6,* 315–334.

Levi, E. C., Folsom, R. C., & Dobie, R. A. (1993). Amplitude-modulation following response (AMFR): Effects of modulation rate, carrier frequency, age and state. *Hearing Research, 5,* 366–370.

Levi, E. C., Folsom, R. C., & Dobie, R. A (1995). Coherence analysis of envelope-following responses (EFRs) and frequency-following responses (FFRs) in infants and adults. *Hearing Research, 89,* 21–27.

Linden, R. D., Campbell, K. B., Hamel, G., & Picton, T. W. (1985). Human auditory steady-state potentials during sleep. *Ear and Hearing, 6,* 167–174.

Lins, O. G., & Picton, T. W. (1995). Auditory steady-state responses to multiple simultaneous stmuli. *Electroencephalography and Clinical Neurophysiology, 96,* 420–432.

Lins, O. G., Picton, T. W., Boucher, B. L., Durieux-Smith, A., Champagne, S. C., Moran, L. M., et al. (1996). Frequency-specific audiometry using steady-state responses. *Ear and Hearing, 2,* 81–96.

Luts, H., Desloovere, C., Kumar, A., Vandermeersch, E., & Wouters, J. (2004). Objective assessment of frequency-specific hearing in babies. *International Journal of Pediatric Otorhinolaryngology, 68,* 915–926.

Luts, H., Desloovere, C., & Wouters, J. (2006). Clinical application of dichotic multiple-stimulus auditory steady-state responses in high-risk newborns and young children. *Audiology & Neuro-otology, 11,* 24–37.

Maurizi, M., Almadori, G., Paludetti, G., Ottaviani, F., Rosignoli, M., & Luciano, R. (1990). 40-Hz steady-state in newborns and in children. *Audiology, 29,* 322–328.

Osterhammel, P. A., Shallop, J. K., & Terkildsen, K. (1985). The effect of sleep on the auditory brainstem response (ABR) and the middle latency response (MLR). *Scandinavian Audiology, 14,* 47–50.

Petitot, C., Collet, L., & Durrant, J. D. (2005). Auditory steady-state responses (ASSR): Effects of modulation and carrier frequencies. *International Journal of Audiology, 44,* 567–573.

Pethe, J., von Specht, H., Muhler, R., & Hocke, T. (2001). Amplitude modulation following responses in awake and sleeping humans—a comparison for 40 Hz and 80 Hz modulation frequency. *Scandinavian Audiology. Supplementum, 52,* 152–155.

Pethe, J., Muhler, R., Siewert, K., & von Specht, H. (2004). Near-threshold recordings of amplitude modulation following responses (AMFR) in children of all ages. *International Journal of Audiology, 43,* 339–345.

Perez-Abalo, M. C., Mijares, E., Savio, G., Santos, E., Herrera, D., & Lage, A. (in press). Automated c-ABR and MSSR neonatal screening: Relative efficiency as measured by ROC methodology. *International Journal of Audiology.*

Picton, T. W., Vajsar, J., Rodriguez, R., & Campbell, K. B. (1987). Reliability estimates for steady state evoked potentials. *Electroencephalography and Clinical Neurophysiology, 68,* 119–131.

Picton, T. W., Dimitrijevic, A., Perez-Abalo, M. C., & Van Roon, P. (2005). Estimating audiometric thresholds using auditory steady-state responses. *Journal of the American Academy of Audiology, 16,* 140–156.

Picton, T. W., Durieux-Smith, A., Champagne, S. C., Whittingham, J. A., Moran, L. M., et al. (1998). Objective evaluation of aided thresholds using auditory steady-state responses. *Journal of the American Academy of Audiology, 9,* 315–331.

Picton, T. W., John, M. S., Dimitrijevic, A., & Purcell, D. (2003). Human auditory steady-state responses. *International Journal of Audiology, 42,* 177–219.

Plourde, G., & Picton, T. W. (1990). Human auditory steady-state responses during general anaesthesia. *Anesthesia and Analgesia, 82,* 75–83.

Ponton, C. W., Egermont, J. J., Kwong, B., & Don, M. (2000). Maturation of human central auditory system activity: Evidence from multi-channel evoked potentials. *Clinical Neurophysiology, 111*(2), 220–236.

Rance, G., & Rickards, F. W. (2002). Prediction of hearing threshold in infants using auditory steady-state evoked potentials. *Journal of the American Academy of Audiology, 13,* 236–245.

Rance, G., & Briggs, R. J. S. (2002). Assessment of hearing level in infants with significant hearing loss: The Melbourne experience with steady-state evoked potential threshold testing. *Annals of Otology, Rhinology, & Laryngology, 111*(5), 22–28.

Rance, G., Rickards, F. W., Cohen, L. T., De Vidi, S., & Clark, G. M. (1995). The automated prediction of hearing thresholds in sleeping subjects using auditory steady-state evoked potentials. *Ear and Hearing, 16,* 499–507.

Rance, G., Roper, R., Symonds, L., Moody, L. J., Poulis, C., Dourlay, M., et al. (2005). Hearing threshold estimation in infants using auditory steady state responses. *Journal of the American Academy of Audiology, 16,* 293–302.

Rance, G., & Tomlin, D. (2006). Maturation of auditory steady-state responses in normal babies. *Ear and Hearing, 27,* 20–29.

Rance, G., Tomlin, D., & Rickards, F. W. (2006). Comparison of auditory steady-state responses and tone-burst auditory brainstem responses in normal babies. *Ear and Hearing, 27,* 751–762.

Rickards, F. W., Tan, L. E., Cohen, L. T., Wilson, O. J., Drew, J. H., & Clark, G. M. (1994). Auditory steady-state evoked potentials in newborns. *British Journal of Audiology, 28,* 327–337.

Riquelme, R., Kuwada, S., Filipovic, B., Hartung, K., & Leonard, G. (2006). Optimizing the stimuli to evoke the amplitude modulation following response (AMFR) in neonates. *Ear and Hearing, 27*, 104–119.

Salamy, A. (1984). Maturation of the auditory brainstem response from birth through early childhood. *Journal of Clinical Neurophysiology, 1*, 293–329.

Savio, G., Cardenas, J., Perez-Abalo, M., Gonzalez, A., & Valdes, J. (2001). The low and high frequency auditory steady-state responses mature at different rates. *Audiology & Neuro-otology, 6*, 279–287.

Schulman-Galambos, C., & Galambos, R. (1979). Brain stem evoked response audiometry in newborn hearing screening. *Archives of Otololaryngology–Head & Neck Surgery, 105*, 86–90.

Sininger, Y. S., Abdala, C., & Cone-Wesson, B. (1997). Auditory threshold sensitivity of the human neonate as measured by the auditory brainstem response. *Hearing Research, 104*, 27–38.

Sininger, Y. S., & Don, M. (1989). Effects of click rate and electrode orientation on threshold detectability of the auditory brainstem response. *Journal of Speech and Hearing Research, 32*, 880–886.

Smurzynski, J., Jung, M. D., Lafreniere, D., Kim, D. O., Kamath, M. V., Rowe, J. C., et al. (1993). Distortion-product and click-evoked otoacoustic emissions of preterm and full-term infants. *Ear and Hearing, 14*, 258–274.

Stapells, D. R., Galambos, R., Costello, J. A., & Makeig, S. (1988). Inconsistency of auditory middle latency and steady-state responses in infants. *Electroencephalography and Clinical Neurophysiology, 71*, 289–295.

Stapells, D. R, Herdman, A., Small, S. A., Dimitrijevic, A., & Hatton, J. (2005). Current status of the auditory steady-state responses for estimating an infant's audiogram. In R. C. Seewald & I. Bamford (Eds.), *A sound foundation through early amplification* (pp. 43–59). Basel: Phonak AG.

Stapells, D. R., Gravel, J. S., & Martin, B. A. (1995). Thresholds for auditory brain stem responses to tones in notched noise from

infants and young children with normal hearing or sensorineural hearing loss. *Ear and Hearing, 16*, 361–371.

Suzuki, T., & Kobayashi, K. (1984). An evaluation of 40-Hz event-related potentials in young children. *Audiology, 23*, 599–604.

Stueve, M. P., & O'Rourke, C. (2003). Estimation of hearing loss in children: Comparison of auditory steady-state response, auditory brainstem response, and behavioral test methods. *American Journal of Audiology, 12*(2), 125–136.

Swanepoel, D., Hugo, R., & Roode, R. (2004). Auditory steady-state response for children with severe to profound hearing loss. *Archives of Otololaryngology–Head & Neck Surgery, 130*(5), 531–535.

Teas, D. C., Klein, A. J., & Kramer, S. K. (1982). An analysis of auditory brainstem responses in infants. *Hearing Research, 7*, 19–54.

Tomlin, D., Rance, G., Graydon, K., & Tsialios, I. (2006). A comparison of 40 Hz ASSR and CAEP thresholds in awake adult subjects. *International Journal of Audiology, 45*, 580–588.

Van Maanen, A., & Stapells, D. R. (2005). Comparison of multiple auditory steady-state responses (80 versus 40 Hz) and slow cortical potentials for threshold estimation in hearing impaired adults. *International Journal of Audiology, 44*, 613–624.

Vander Werff, K. R. and Brown, C. J. (2005). Effect of audiometric configuration on threshold and suprathreshold auditory steady-state responses. *Ear Hear, 26*(3), 310–326.

Vander Werff, K. R., Brown, C. J., Gienapp, B. A., & Schmidt Clay, K. M. (2002). Comparison of auditory steady-state response and auditory brainstem response thresholds in children. *Journal of the American Academy of Audiology, 13*, 227–235.

Yamada, O., Ashikawa, H., Kodera, K., & Yamane, H. (1983). Frequency selective auditory brainstem response in newborns and infants. *Archives of Otology—Head & Neck Surgery, 109*, 79–82.

CHAPTER 10

Auditory Steady-State Responses and Hearing Screening

GUILLERMO SAVIO
MARIA CECILIA PEREZ-ABALO

Overview

The rapid growth of universal newborn hearing screening (UNHS) programs worldwide has had an enormous impact on the practice in pediatric audiology and on the impetus of research in electrical response audiometry (ERA). To evaluate all infants at birth, efficient screening devices (usually automated) are necessary. Although a variety of such equipment is available at present, continuous technological improvements are still needed to further enhance the performance of such devices. A second important step, once the child is identified as being at risk for a hearing loss, is to make the diagno-sis and initiate appropriate intervention before 6 months of age (Joint Committee on Infant Hearing, 2000). Because behavioural audiometric techniques cannot provide accurate information in such young infants, physiological methods (frequency-specific audiometry) have become essential for exact determination of the degree, type, and configuration of the hearing loss. As well, the initial treatment for hearing impairment involves fitting of hearing aids or perhaps a more permanent decision for cochlear implantation, which also will require precise objective methodology.

The recent advent of techniques using auditory steady-state responses (ASSRs) to stimuli presented using repetition (or modulation) rates in the 70- to 110-Hz range (the "80-Hz ASSR") has raised considerable interest among audiologists for potential applications in the assessment (and treatment) of hearing-impaired infants and children. Moreover, other potential applications of ASSR within the context of screening can be envisioned as well. This chapter considers the possible benefits and potential difficulties associated with using ASSR assessment for UNHS.

Introduction

Some general features of the 80-Hz ASSR technique are inherently advantageous for infant screening:

■ At stimulation rates between 70 and 110 Hz, the ASSR is generated mostly in the brainstem; therefore, it is not affected by sleep or sedation (Lins, Picton, Picton, Champagne, & Durieux-Smith, 1995; Picton, John, Dimitrijevic, & Purcell, 2003).

■ The ASSR can be elicited by multiple simultaneously presented stimuli. This allows the determination of various frequency-specific thresholds (in both ears) at the same time, with consequent reduction in testing time (Lins & Picton, 1995).

■ Responses are best represented in the frequency domain (using fast Fourier transform analysis) and can be effectively identified (by automatic detection) using different statistics (Dobie & Wilson, 1989; Valdes et al., 1997; Victor & Mast, 1991).

■ Over the last several years, some clinical findings have been accumu-

lated that seem to substantiate the potential applicability of ASSR within a screening context (Cone-Wesson, Parker, Swiderski, & Rickards, 2002; Savio, Perez-Abalo, Gaya, Hernandez, & Mijares, 2006).

This chapter reviews the advantages and caveats of using the 80-Hz ASSR in screening both for early detection of hearing losses and for subsequent assessment (i.e., characterization of residual hearing). In addition, relevant issues regarding testing time, ease of automation, and the need for further technology improvements also are analyzed.

Auditory Steady-State Responses in Normal-Hearing Infants

An important consideration with use of ASSR testing within a screening context is accuracy in the prediction of normal hearing sensitivity in babies. Many studies have concluded that the 80-Hz ASSR can be reliably recorded in infants (see Table 9–2, Chapter 9) down to intensities reasonably close to the sensitivity thresholds in normal-hearing adults (John, Brown, Muir, & Picton, 2004; Lins et al., 1996; Luts, Desloovere, & Wouters, 2006; Rance & Rickards, 2002; Rance et al., 2005; Rance & Tomlin, 2006; Rickards et al., 1994; Savio, Cardenas, Perez-Abalo, Gonzalez, & Valdes, 2001). However, recent concerns have arisen regarding the stability of ASSR in neonates and very young infants (Luts et al., 2006; Rance & Tomlin, 2006; Rance, Tomlin, & Rickards, 2006). Some current results (reviewed in Chapter 9) indicate that in the first 6 weeks of life, the ASSR threshold levels can differ from those observed in older infants and adults, probably reflecting developmental changes. In addition, there is much variability in the reported data across studies of work with infants (John et al., 2004).

All of these "dissenting findings" seem to imply that the ASSR technique is not quite ready for use within screening contexts, or that it should be used with caution, applied more as a complement to than as a substitute for tone-evoked auditory brainstem responses (ABRs) (Stapells, Herdman Small, Dimitrijevic, & Hatton, 2005). However, many complicating factors should be considered that would limit this data interpretation. Considerable differences exist in experimental (stimulation and recording) procedures, testing time, recording environments, sample size, and age range across infant studies. Another important issue is the lack of agreement on the optimal duration of ASSR testing. A trade-off between test duration and test accuracy has been recognized. More prolonged recording times have been recommended as an alternative for identifying the near-threshold responses (which are much smaller and variable in infants than in adults) (John et al., 2004; Luts et al., 2006; Picton et al., 2003; Rance et al., 2006; Savio et al., 2001). This would decrease the time efficiency of the ASSR test so that it may become impracticable for screening purposes. Some experimental results recently published suggest that ASSR testing can be further optimized using more efficient stimuli or analysis methods that will enhance the signal-to-noise ratio (Cebulla, Sturzebecher, & Elberling, 2006; John, Dimitrijevic, & Picton, 2002; Picton, John, Dimitrijevic, & Purcell, 2003; Sturzebecher, Cebulla, Elberling, & Berger, 2006). Nevertheless, these new methods

await further clinical validation in both normal-hearing and hearing-impaired infant populations.

Applicability of Auditory Steady-State Response Testing as a Screening Tool

UNHS most commonly uses automated otoacoustic emission (OAE) for testing well babies in the nursery and automated click-evoked ABR ("click-ABR") for testing those at risk (as in the neonatal intensive care unit). Also, a second confirmation test (usually with click-ABR) is scheduled for all infants who fail at the first screen before discharge from the maternity ward. In an elegantly designed long-term follow-up study, Norton, Gorga, and Widen (2000) used receiver operating characteristic (ROC) curve methodology to evaluate the performance of different variants of OAE and automated ABR devices in screening a large sample of infants ($n = 4911$) for hearing loss. These investigators found that any of these automated devices performed with reasonable efficiency, correctly identifying approximately 80% of all cases of congenital hearing loss, with a 20% false-positive rate. Also, no significant differences were found in comparing the efficiency of OAE or automated ABR equipment. Therefore, although the efficiency of the present practice and methods used for early detection of hearing loss is adequate, it still needs to be improved further.

The ASSR may offer some potential advantages over click-ABR and OAE for screening. Like the click-ABR, the ASSR can be affected by auditory pathway disorders otherwise missed with OAE (Rance et al., 1999; Tapia & Savio, 2005). As well, it may be useful for identifying mid- to low-frequency hearing losses that typically are missed with use of click-ABR (Durieux-Smith, Picton, Bernard, Mac-Murray, & Goodman, 1991). Some promising data already have been published on the use of ASSR in infant screening (Cone-Wesson, Parker, et al., 2002, Savio et al., 2006). Cone-Wesson and Parker and colleagues (2002) tested 82 newborn recruited (as part of an UNHS program) from the neonatal intensive care unit and well-baby nursery at the Los Angeles County + University of Southern California Medical Center. All neonates had passed a click-ABR and OAE screening test. The "pass" rates for ASSR trials (250 to 4000 Hz) in the presumably normal-hearing neonates were higher than 90% for all amplitude-modulated tones and reached 100% for 2000 Hz tones. This study, however, was not designed for determining the actual diagnostic efficiency of the ASSR as a screening tool. First, no infants who failed the screening test were evaluated. Second, the "gold standard" diagnostic test was use of another physiological measure (OAE and click-ABR) and not (as recommended) an independent test such as behavioural audiometry (Norton et al., 2000).

In a recently published long-term follow-up study on the diagnostic efficiency of ASSR for targeted screening, Savio and coworkers (2006) used conventional pure-tone behavioural audiometry (determined when the child was 3 to 4 years old) as the "gold standard" diagnostic method. In this study, a large sample of high-risk babies ($n = 508$) were screened at 3 months of age using multiple 80-Hz ASSR to amplitude-modulated tones (500 and 2000 Hz) and a standard click-ABR test. Pass-fail criteria were set for both screening methods at 40 dB nHL (equivalent to 75 dB peak SPL for the click and 62 dB SPL RMS for multiple-frequency stimuli). Although both click-ABR and ASSR screening methods demonstrated equally good performance (sensitivity 100% and specificity 92%), the sensitivity of click ABR may have been lower (94%). One child failed the multiple-ASSR screen (at 500 Hz) and passed the click-ABR test. At confirmation audiometry (1 month later), this child showed elevated ASSR thresholds at 500 and 1000 Hz with normal values at the higher frequencies (2000 and 4000 Hz) and a clear click-ABR at 30 dB nHL. Although these data could not be included in the analysis of diagnostic efficiency (because the child was lost to follow-up), the findings suggest that the ASSR also may have a potential value to identify low-frequency hearing loss. Further studies, however, are needed in this area.

On the other hand, possible limitations may be anticipated for ASSR screening within the context of UNHS protocols. As discussed previously, the ASSR thresholds are not yet mature and thus are more variable in neonates (Rance et al., 2006). It could be hypothesized on this basis that the accuracy of ASSR screening may be lower at these early stages of development. Findings from a recent study using an ASSR algorithm specifically designed for screening purposes (with adaptive stopping criteria) in neonates seem to suggest the contrary (Perez-Abalo et al., 2007). In this study, 35 normal-hearing neonates were tested (7 to 18 days after birth) with multiple ASSR to 500- and 2000-Hz amplitude-modulated tones presented at a fixed intensity of 40 dB nHL. Recordings with and without stimulation were obtained in each case. The ASSR screening efficiency was as high (100% sensitivity and 96% specificity) in the neonates as that previously found in older infants (Savio et al., 2006). However, the diagnostic accuracy of the ASSR screening test may be somewhat overestimated. Because no follow-up information is available yet on these infants, another electrophysiological technique (standard click-ABR) had to be used as the definitive test for determining normal-hearing status. Thus, to determine the actual effectiveness of an ASSR screening test within a UNHS context, further investigations are needed providing long-term follow-up data with an independent hearing assessment.

Assessment of Hearing-Impaired Infants with Auditory Steady-State Response Testing

The need for some form of objective audiometry to characterize the residual hearing before the age of 6 months has been recognized by a number of researchers (Hayes, 2003; Mencher, Davis, DeVoe, Beresford, & Bamford, 2001; Norton et al., 2000; Savio et al., 2006). Current guidelines still recommend the use of transient auditory evoked potentials recorded in response to brief acoustic stimuli (tone-evoked ABR) for frequency-specific audiometric testing to guide the initial fitting of amplification in infants younger than 6 months of age (Joint Committee on Infant Hearing, 2000; Stapells et al., 2005). A large body of research and many successful clinical studies published since the late 1970s (Stapells, 2000) support the ability of tone-evoked ABR to estimate behavioural thresholds in normal-hearing and hearing-impaired

infants. In practice, however, only a minority of UNHS programs nowadays routinely obtain ABR thresholds using tonal stimuli for such purposes (Stapells, 2000). Among several possible reasons for this problem, some limitations of tone-evoked ABR are recognized, stemming from the relative complexity of threshold determination (by visual inspection), which will require more skill from the clinician, the nature of the brief stimuli used in relation with the severity and configuration of the hearing loss, and the need for prolonged recording sessions (because only one ear and frequency can be tested at a time). For more details on tone-evoked ABR, see Chapter 8.

Nevertheless, the ASSR can be a more feasible alternative for objective estimation of the audiogram in these young infants. Despite the relatively recent advent of ASSR commercial equipment and its more widespread use, some compelling evidence has been rapidly accumulating, suggesting that the technique can be used as an effective measure of frequency-specific hearing thresholds in hearing-impaired infants or young children suspected to have hearing loss (Cone Wesson, Dowell, Tomlin, Rance, & Ming, 2002; Firszt, Gaggl, Runge-Samuelson, Burg, & Wackym, 2004; Luts, Desloovere, Kumar, Vandermeersch, & Wouters, 2004; Perez-Abalo et al., 2001; Rance & Rickards, 2002; Stueve & O'Rourke, 2003; Swanepoel, Hugo, & Roode, 2004; Vander Werff, Brown, Gienapp, & Schmidt Clay, 2002).

Most of the aforementioned studies conclude favorably on the value of ASSR technique to provide audiometric information that is essential in the management of children with moderate-to-severe or profound hearing loss. Consensus is lacking, however, on how well the ASSR technique can predict hearing losses in the mild-to-moderate range; additional data in this area are needed as well. Further investigations are required.

Some long-term follow-up data in infants screening are available showing that early ASSR audiometry can predict accurately the behavioural audiometric results (Cone-Wesson, Rickards, et al., 2002; Luts et al., 2006; Savio et al., 2006). Cone-Wesson and Rickards and their colleagues (2002) successfully used the 80-Hz ASSR (to single modulated tones) for the assessment of hearing sensitivity in a hospital-based pediatric audiology clinic that was part of a UNHS program. A high correlation was found between physiological ASSR thresholds at 1000, 2000, and 4000 Hz and the click-ABR thresholds in children referred for diagnostic testing with both ASSR and click-ABR at 3 to 6 months of age. Savio and coworkers (2006) also evaluated how well ASSR audiometry performed at early stages of development (4- to 5-month old infants) could predict the behavioural pure-tone audiogram obtained when the children were 3 to 4 years of age. These researchers found significantly higher correlation coefficients between the physiological and the behavioural pure-tone average (PTA) for the multiple ASSR than for the single-click-ABR threshold in both normal hearing and hearing impaired infants (ASSR: $r = 0.97$; click-ABR: $r = 0.88$) (Figure 10–1).

Moreover, the differences between subjective and objective audiograms (measured by the Z scores) were significantly smaller for multiple ASSRs at 500, 1000, and 2000 Hz than for click-ABR (Figure 10–2). This implies that the multiple-ASSR technique can predict more closely the configuration of the audiogram using frequencies below 4000 Hz in both groups (normal-hearing and hearing-impaired children).

These results have been recently confirmed and expanded to newborns by Luts and associates (2006). Using ASSR testing, these investigators evaluated a sample of newborns at risk for hearing loss ($n = 53$) previously detected by neonatal screening and also found a strong overall correlation ($r = 0.87$) between the ASSR thresholds (at audiometric frequencies from 500 to 4000 Hz) and those obtained subsequently (7 months later) using visual reinforcement audiometry.

All of these results taken together strongly suggest that ASSR testing may be considered a reasonably accurate method for characterizing residual hearing in infants with hearing impairment early detected by means of a screening protocol, providing valuable information for diagnosis and intervention. Table 10–1 summarizes the main findings for 80-Hz ASSR in the screening context.

Testing Time Requirements

Timing is an important issue in the screening context. The goal of UNHS is to screen all babies in natural sleep before discharge from the maternity hospital. For this purpose, the screening test needs to be safe, simple, and quick to administer. Furthermore, and of most importance, the technology used need to be adapted to the neonatal environment. This is not yet the case with ASSR technology but might well be in the near future. Much variability exists in reported durations of ASSR recording in infants, ranging from very quick tests (at a fixed, near-threshold intensity), completed in 20 to 90 s (Cone-Wesson, Parker, et al.,

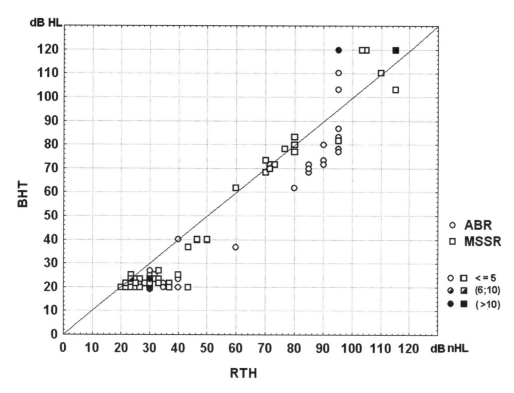

Figure 10–1. The overlaid scatterplots illustrate the correspondence between the overall physiological and behavioral hearing estimates (PTA) calculated for each technique (click-ABR and MSSR). Only the results for those babies (*n* = 96 ears) who were evaluated audiometrically with both techniques at 4 to 5 months of age, and returned 3 years later for the final (behavioral) follow-up assessment, were plotted. Each data point represents, for the MSSR and behavioral audiometry studies, an average threshold calculated across audiometric frequencies (500 to 4000 Hz), whereas for the click-ABR, the physiological threshold was directly computed as the PTA. In those cases with no measurable response at the maximum stimulus intensity, the physiological thresholds were arbitrarily assigned at 5 dB above the limits of the equipment for each technique. *Circles* represent click-ABR data; and *squares* MSSR data. The number of overlaid data points in each symbol is specified by the legend at the *lower right*. *Open symbols* represent between 1 and 5 data points, *half-filled symbols* between 6 and 10 data points, and *filled symbols* more than 10 data points. Note that there are more overlaid data points in the diagonal, or close to it, for the MSSR than for click-ABR. PTA, pure tone average (500 to 4000 Hz); RTH, average response threshold; BTH, average behavioural threshold; MSSR, multiple auditory steady-state responses. (From Savio, G., Perez Abalo, M. C., Gaya, J., Hernandez, O., & Mijares, E. (2006). Test accuracy and prognostic validity of multiple auditory steady state responses for targeted hearing screening. *International Journal of Audiology, 45*(2), 115. Copyright 2006 Taylor & Francis. Reproduced with permission.)

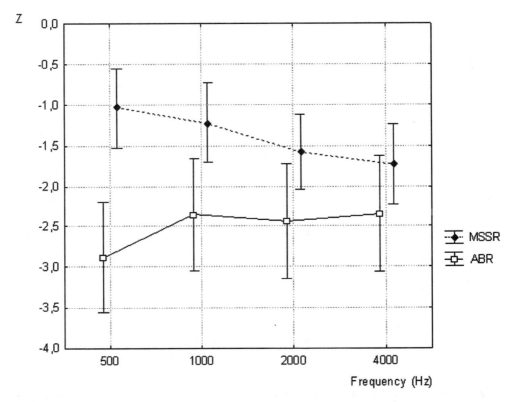

Figure 10–2. The interaction between the accuracy of the technique (as measured by the standardized distance between the objective and the subjective audiograms) and the audiometric frequency is shown graphically. The *y-axis* represents Z values (vector across frequencies). The *x-axis* corresponds to the different audiometric frequencies. The *filled circles* represent the MSSR technique; the *open squares* correspond to the click-ABR technique. *Vertical bars* denote the 0.95 confidence intervals. MSSR, multiple auditory steady-state responses; Z, standardized distance between the objective and the subjective audiograms. By using the Z vector, the differences in scale (or magnitude effect) between physiological and behavioral technique can be corrected. (From Savio, G., Perez Abalo, M. C., Gaya, J., Hernandez, O., & Mijares, E. (2006). Test accuracy and prognostic validity of multiple auditory steady state responses for targeted hearing screening. *International Journal of Audiology, 45*(2), 115. Copyright 2006 Taylor & Francis. Reproduced with permission.)

2002), up to more prolonged recording times of 12 minutes per run (John et al., 2004), which would be unfeasible for screening. Also, and probably related, some reliability problems have been found in testing neonates in the first few days after birth (John et al., 2004; Luts et al., 2006; Rance et al., 2006). An important consideration in this context is the lack of appropriate stopping criteria for ASSR testing, particularly in the absence of a significant response. Averaging typically is stopped when either a stable significant response is detected (with any of the available statistical methods) or a maximum number of sweeps have been reached.

Table 10–1. Accuracy and prognostic validity of auditory steady-state response (ASSR) screening

Study	N	Age	Stimulus	Accuracy		Prognostic Validity (Correlation Coefficient) by Frequency*			
				Sensitivity	Specificity	500 Hz	1000 Hz	2000 Hz	4000 Hz
Cone-Wesson, Parker et al., 2002	82	<1 mo	Single AM	NA	~92%	NA			
Luts et al., 2006	30	<3 mo	Multiple AM/FM	NA	NA	0.82	0.84	0.89	0.91
Savio et al., 2006	508	3 mo	Multiple AM	100%	92%	0.88	0.93	0.98	0.95
Perez Abalo et al., 2007	35	<1 mo	Multiple AM	100%	96%	NA			

*ASSR-behavioral thresholds.

This latter criterion does not always ensure that a small near-threshold signal can be resolved from the more variable residual noise. This issue highlights the importance of basing averaging stopping criteria on signal-to-noise ratio estimates, rather than on a fixed number of sweeps.

Such an approach was successfully used in the laboratory recently. In a previous study by Savio and coworkers (2007), a multiple-ASSR (500 and 2000 Hz) technique, with average test durations of 319 ($\pm$ 150) seconds, was used to screen 3-month-old infants, with high diagnostic accuracy. In a subsequent study, Perez-Abalo and colleagues (2007) tested a sample of 35 newborns (7 to 18 days old) in natural sleep, using a new automated software algorithm specifically designed for screening purposes and a portable AUDIX system. Because this software includes more flexible stopping criteria (adjusted on the basis of signal size, background noise, and the significance of the Hotelling T2 statistic), it ensured a more stable signal-to-noise ratio, avoiding excessive or insufficient averaged sweeps. Under such conditions, the multiple-ASSR (500 and 2000 Hz) screening test could be completed in about half the time (mean duration 156 $\pm$ 96 seconds), with similarly high sensitivity and specificity rates (100% and 96%, respectively).

Ease of Automation

Regardless of the technique used for screening (ABR, OAE, or ASSR) in any automatic device, the presence of artifacts or noisy recordings may be incorrectly judged as a threshold response. This could be due to, among other factors, the inefficiency of the automatic procedures built into the equipment to recognize the signals from the noise. The ASSR is a quasi-sinusoidal response. This simplifies the quantitative description of the response (represented in the frequency domain with only two parameters: amplitude and phase). Several statistical methods are available for detecting the ASSR based on only phase information (Aoyagi, Fuse, Suzuki, Kim, & Koike, 1993; Jerger, Chmiel, Frost, & Coker, 1986), or on both parameters (amplitude and phase), such as the Hotelling T2 (Picton, Vajsar, Rodriguez, & Campbell, 1987; Valdes et al., 1997), the circular T2 (Victor & Mast, 1991), the F test, or test for hidden periodicity (Lins & Picton, 1995), and the magnitude of squared coherence (MSC) (Dobie & Wilson, 1989).

The advantages with automatic detection of ASSR over other transient responses such as click-ABR were recently demonstrated (using ROC methodology) by Savio and coworkers. (2007). In each case, ROC curves were computed with a sample of 222 recordings (with and without response) obtained in 3-month-old high-risk infants. For automatic detection of the click-ABR, the standard deviation ratio (SDR) and the linear correlation coefficient between two replicates (CCR) were calculated as described by Picton, Linden, Hamel, and Maru (1983). On the other hand, for the multiple ASSR, two frequency domain statistics, the Hotelling T2 (HT2) and the circular T2 (CT2), were computed. Significantly higher areas under the ROC curve were found for the multiple ASSR statistics (HT2: 0.91 to 0.95; CT2: 0.90 to 0.91 at 500 and 2000 Hz, respectively) than for the click-ABR statistics (CCR: 0.60; SDR: 0.87). These results, shown graphically in Figure 10–3, are promising and could serve as an additional foundation for a future design of an automatic ASSR screening device.

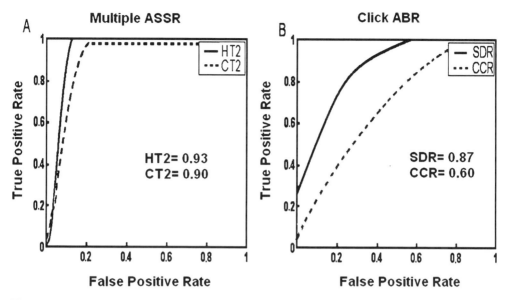

Figure 10–3. Receiver operating characteristic (ROC) curves for the statistics used in the automatic detection of multiple ASSR and click-ABR. In each graphic, the *y-axis* corresponds to the true-positive rate and the *x-axis* to the false-positive rate, both of which are represented as proportions. In **A** the ROC curves (overlaid) of the statistics HT2 and CT2 used for automatic detection of multiple ASSR (500 and 2000 Hz, both frequencies averaged). In **B** the ROC curves for the statistics SDR and CCR used for automatic detection of click-ABR. The values of the area-under-the-ROC-curves (for the different statistics) are also shown in the figure. SDR, standard deviation ratio; CCR, correlation coefficient; CT2, circular T2; HT2, Hotelling T2. (From Savio, G., Mijares, E., Perez Abalo, M. C., Vega, M., Lage, A., & Hernandez, D. (2007). Efficiency of the automatic detection of multiple auditory steady state responses measured with ROC methodology. *Revista de Logopedia, Foniatría y Audiología Española, 27*(1), 18. Copyright 2007 AELFA y Grupo Ars XXI de Comunicación, S.L. Reproduced with permission.)

Auditory Steady-State Response Technology

Because the advent of commercial equipment for recording ASSR is relatively recent, this technology will need to be further improved for its use in neonatal screening or to adapt more easily to a pediatric audiology clinical context. Most ASSR commercial equipment systems have been developed from previous research systems allowing much flexibility in the selection of experimental parameters (Stapells et al., 2005). Also, too much detailed and relatively complex information, such as the power spectrum of the signal, phase, amplitude, statistical values, and its probability, is shown. Thus, an appropriate use of ASSR techniques requires expertise to correctly define the recording and stimulation parameters, and to interpret the results. The importance of these requirements is further highlighted by the "artifactual" or spurious ASSRs to high-intensity stimuli reported in deaf persons (Jeng, Brown, Johnson, & Vander Werff, 2004; Small & Stapells,

2004). These findings initially raised some doubts about whether the ASSR technique is ready to be used in clinical practice and probably delayed a wider introduction. It subsequently was demonstrated that these artifacts were due to electromagnetic aliasing and can be avoided by using specific recording and stimulation parameters (Picton & John, 2004).

This suggests, then, that the ASSR technology needs some improvement and redesigning before it can be ready for screening. Software systems need to be simplified and more user-friendly. Automated algorithms should be used so that it can be operated by less skilled personnel such as volunteers or nurses. The equipment (hardware) also needs to be more appropriate for testing neonates (in their crib) while asleep, without interference from a noisy environment. Also, the experimental procedures (recording and stimulation) should be standardized, with selection of those that are more appropriate in carefully designed and controlled clinical studies (preferably using different equipment).

Key Points

Over the past decade, a considerable body of research has been published that supports the clinical usefulness of ASSR to predict hearing sensitivity in normal-hearing and hearing-impaired infants (Firszt et al., 2004; John et al., 2004; Luts et al., 2004; Rance et al., 2005; Savio et al., 2006; Stueve & O'Rourke, 2003; Swanepoel et al., 2004). Nowadays, the accumulated ASSR data in infants are more comprehensive (in tested frequencies) and represent a population of considerable size (n = approximately 1200) when compared with data previously reported for tone-evoked ABR. Also, the ASSR offers significant advantages over transient response for automation and for testing multiple thresholds (and both ears) at the same time in a relatively short period (less than 1 hour). Taken together, these results strongly suggest that the technique already may have an important role in the assessment of those infants earlier identified as hearing-impaired by UNHS, supplementing the clinical testing battery to allow a precise diagnosis of the auditory status. To facilitate more widespread and appropriate use of ASSR in screening contexts, however, the recording and stimulation protocols need to be standardized. More adequate stopping criteria based on quantitative estimates of the signal-to-noise ratio, rather than number of sweeps (which varies widely across studies), are required. Finally, although the time efficiency of frequency-specific audiometry with multiple ASSR represents a significant improvement over that for tone-evoked ABR (which is the currently recommended method for use in the assessment stage), it would have to be significantly improved for initial detection of hearing loss. New stimuli and optimized analysis and artifact rejection methods could be a valid alternative, provided that these are more extensively tested. The available ASSR technology (hardware and software) needs to be improved and better adapted for testing neonates in a screening context.

References

Aoyagi, M., Fuse, T., Suzuki, T., Kim, Y., & Koike, Y. (1993). An application of phase spectral analysis to amplitude-modulation following response. *Acta Oto-laryngologica Supplementum, 511*, 82–88.

Cebulla, M., Stürzebecher, E., & Erberling, C. (2006). Objective detection of auditory steady-state responses: Comparison of one-sample and q-sample tests. *Journal of the American Academy of Audiology, 17*, 93–103.

Cone-Wesson, B., Dowell, R., Tomlin, D., Rance, G., & Ming, W. J. (2002). The auditory steady state response: Comparisons with the auditory brainstem response. *Journal of the American Academy of Audiology, 13*, 173–187.

Cone-Wesson, B., Parker, J., Swiderski, N., & Rickards, F. (2002). The auditory steady-state response: Full-term and premature neonates. *Journal of the American Academy of Audiology, 13*, 260–269.

Cone-Wesson, B., Rickards, F., Poulis, C., Parker, J., Tan, L., & Pollard, J. (2002). The auditory steady-state response: Clinical observations and applications in infants and children. *Journal of the American Academy of Audiology, 13*, 270–282.

Dobie, R .A., & Wilson, M. J. (1989). Analysis of auditory evoked potentials by magnitude-squared coherence. *Ear and Hearing, 10*, 2–13.

Durieux-Smith, A., Picton. T. W., Bernard, P., MacMurray, B., & Goodman, J. T. (1991). Prognostic validity of brain-stem electrical response audiometry in infants of neonatal intensive care unit. *Audiology, 30*, 249–265.

Firszt, J. B., Gaggl, W., Runge-Samuelson, C. L., Burg, L. S., & Wackym, P. A. (2004). Auditory sensitivity in children using the auditory steady state response. *Archives of Otolaryngology–Head & Neck Surgery, 130*, 536–540.

Jerger, J., Chmiel, R., Frost, J. D., & Coker, N. (1986). Effect of sleep on the auditory steady state evoked potential. *Ear and Hearing, 7*, 240–245.

Jeng, F. C., Brown, C., Johnson, T. A., & Vander Werff, K. R. (2004). Estimating air-bone gaps using auditory steady state responses. *Journal of the American Academy of Audiology, 15*, 67–78.

John, M. S., Dimitrijevic, A., & Picton, T. W. (2002). Auditory steady-state responses to exponential modulation envelopes. *Ear and Hearing, 23*, 106–117.

John, M. S., Brown, D. K., Muir, P. J., & Picton, T. W. (2004). Recording auditory steady state responses in young infants. *Ear and Hearing, 25*, 539–553.

Joint Committee on Infant Hearing. (2000). Year 2000 position statement: Principles and guidelines for early hearing detection and intervention programs. *Pediatrics, 106*.

Hayes, D. (2003). Screening methods: Current status. *Mental Retardation and Developmental Disabilities Research Reviews, 9*, 65–72.

Lins, O. G. , Picton, P. E. , Picton, T. W., Champagne, S. C. , & Deurieux-Smith, A. (1995). Auditory steady-state response to tones amplitude-modulated at 80 to 110 Hz. *Journal of the Acoustical Society of America, 97*, 3051–3063.

Lins, O. G., & Picton, T. W. (1995). Auditory steady-state response to multiple simultaneous stimuli. *Electroencephalography and Clinical Neurophysiology, 96*, 420–432.

Lins, O. G., Picton, T. W., Boucher, B. L., Durieux-Smith, A., Champagne, S. C., Moran, L.M., et al. (1996). Frequency-specific audiometry using steady-state response. *Ear and Hearing, 17*, 81–96.

Luts, H., Desloovere, C., Kumar, A., Vandermeersch, E., & Wouters, J. (2004). Objective assessment of frequency-specific hearing thresholds in babies. *International Journal of Pediatric Otorhinolaryngology, 68*, 915–926.

Luts, H., Desloovere, C., & Wouters, J. (2006). Clinical application of dichotic multiple stimulus auditory steady state responses in high risk newborns and young children. *Audiology and Neuro-otology, 11*, 24–37.

Mencher, G., Davis, A., DeVoe, S., Beresford, D., & Bamford, J. (2001) Universal neonatal hearing screening: Past, present, and future. *American Journal of Audiology, 10*, 3–12.

Norton, S. J., Gorga, M. P., & Widen, J. E. (2000). Identification of neonatal hearing impairment: Evaluation of transient evoked otoacustic emission, distortion product otoacustic emission, and auditory brain stem response test performance. *Ear and Hearing, 21,* 508-528.

Pérez-Abalo, M. C., Savio, G., Torres, A., Martin, V., Rodríguez, E., & Galán, L. (2001). Steady state responses to multiple amplitude modulated tones: An optimized method to test frequency specific thresholds in hearing impaired children and normal subjects. *Ear and Hearing, 22,* 200-211.

Pérez-Abalo, M. C., Mijares, E., Savio, G., Santos, E., Herrera, D.,& Lage, A. (2007). *Automated c-ABR and MSSR neonatal screening: Relative efficiency as measured by ROC methodology.* Manuscript in preparation.

Picton, T. W., Linden, R. D., Hamel, G., & Maru, J. T. (1983). Aspects of averaging. *Seminars in Hearing, 4,* 324-340.

Picton, T. W., Vajsar, J., Rodriguez, R., & Campbell, K. B. (1987). Reliability estimates for steady-state evoked potentials. *Electroencephalography and Clinical Neurophysiology, 68,* 119-131.

Picton, T. W., John, M. S., Dimitrijevic, A., & Purcell, D. (2003). Human auditory steady state responses. *International Journal of Audiology, 42,* 177-219.

Picton T. W., & John, M. S. (2004). Avoiding electromagnetic artifacts when recording auditory steady state responses. *Journal of the American Academy of Audiology, 15,* 541-554.

Rance, G., Beer, D. E., Cone-Wesson, B., Shepherd, R. K., Dowell, R. C., King, A. M., et al. (1999). Clinical findings for a group of infants and young children with auditory neuropathy. *Ear and Hearing, 20,* 238-252.

Rance, G., & Rickards, F. (2002). Prediction of hearing threshold in infants using auditory steady-state evoked potentials. *Journal of the American Academy of Audiology, 13,* 236-245.

Rance, G., Roper, R., Symons, L., Moody, L. J., Poulis, C., Dourlay, M., et al. (2005). Hearing threshold estimation in infants using auditory steady-state responses. *Journal of the American Academy of Audiology, 16,* 291-300.

Rance, G., & Tomlin, D. (2006). Maturation of auditory steady state responses in normal babies. *Ear and Hearing, 27,* 20-29.

Rance, G., Tomlin, D., & Rickards, F. W. (2006). Comparison of auditory steady state responses and tone burst auditory brain stem responses in normal babies. *Ear and Hearing, 27,* 751-762.

Rickards, F. W., Tan, L. E., Cohen, L. T., Wilson, O. J., Drew, J. H., & Clark, G. M. (1994). Auditory steady state evoked potentials in newborns. *British Journal of Audiology, 28,* 327-337.

Savio, G., Cardenas, J., Perez-Abalo, M. C., Gonzalez, A., & Valdes, J. (2001). The low and high frequency auditory steady state responses mature at different rates. *Audiology and Neuro-otology, 6,* 279-287.

Savio, G., Perez-Abalo, M. C., Gaya, J., Hernandez, O., & Mijares, E. (2006). Test accuracy and prognostic validity of multiple auditory steady state responses for targeted hearing screening. *International Journal of Audiology, 45,* 109-120.

Savio, G., Mijares, E., Perez-Abalo, M.C., Vega, M., Lage, A., & Hernández D. (2007). Efficiency of the automatic detection of multiple auditory steady state responses measured with ROC methodology. *Revista de Logopedia, Foniatría y Audiología Española, 27,* 12-23.

Small, S.A., & Stapells, D. R. (2004). Artifactual responses when recording auditory steady state responses. *Ear and Hearing, 25,* 611-623.

Stapells, D. R. (2000). Threshold estimation by the tone-evoked auditory brainstem response: A literature meta-analysis. *Journal of Speech-Language Pathology and Audiology, 24,* 74-83.

Stapells, D. R., Herdman, A., Small, S. A., Dimitrijevic, A., & Hatton, J. (2005). Current status of auditory steady-state responses for estimating the infant's audiogram. In R. C. Seewald & J. Bamford (Eds.), *A sound foundation through early amplification* (pp. 43-59). Basel: Phonac AG.

Stueve, M., & O'Rourke, C. (2003). Estimation of hearing loss in children: Comparison of auditory steady-state response, auditory brainstem response and behavioral test methods. *American Journal of Audiology*, *12*, 125–136.

Stürzebecher, E., Cebulla, M., Erberling, C., & Berger, T. (2006). New efficient stimuli for evoking frequency-specific auditory steady-state responses. *Journal of the American Academy of Audiology*, *17*, 448–461.

Swanepoel, D., Hugo, R., & Roode, R. (2004). Auditory steady-state responses for children with severe to profound hearing loss. *Archives of Otolaryngology—Head & Neck Surgery*, *130*, 531–535.

Tapia, M. C., & Savio, G. (2005). Auditory steady state responses in the study of two patients with auditory neuropathy.

Acta Otorrinolaringólogica Española, *56*, 240–245.

Valdes, J. L., Pérez-Abalo, M. C., Martín, V., Savio, G., Sierra, C., & Rodríguez, E. (1997). Comparison of statistical indicators for the automatic detection of 80 Hz auditory steady state response. *Ear and Hearing*, *18*, 420–429.

Vander Werff, K. R., Brown, C. J., Gienapp, B. A., & Schmidt Clay, K. M. (2002). Comparison of auditory steady-state response and auditory brainstem response thresholds in children. *Journal of the American Academy of Audiology*, *13*, 227–235.

Victor, J. D., & Mast, J. (1991). A new statistic for steady-state evoked potentials. *Electroencephalography and Clinical Neurophysiology*, *78*, 378–388.

CHAPTER 11

Bone Conduction Auditory Steady-State Responses

SUSAN SMALL
DAVID STAPELLS

Introduction

Normal hearing sensitivity during the first few years of life is essential for normal speech and language development. Internationally, there is a major focus in hearing health care on implementation of universal newborn hearing screening to identify infants who are at risk for hearing loss before the age of 3 months, in order to diagnose hearing loss and begin intervention by 6 months of age (Joint Committee on Infant Hearing, 2000). To initiate early intervention and to maximize speech and language development, accurate and reliable audiometric information is needed to diagnose the type and configuration of hearing loss in early infancy. Typically, air and bone con-

duction thresholds to frequency-specific stimuli in the speech frequency range are obtained. In order to achieve this goal, accurate and efficient techniques that are appropriate for very young infants are needed to assess frequency-specific hearing thresholds. The 80-Hz auditory steady-state response (ASSR) to multiple simultaneously presented stimuli is a technique that is well suited to this task and is well on the way to becoming a standard clinical tool for assessing infants.

Accurate bone conduction thresholds are particularly important in assessing infants and young children who have unilateral or bilateral otits media or atresia (Jahrsdoerfer, Yeakley, Hal, Robbins, & Gray, 1985; Stapells & Ruben, 1989). The early diagnosis of a conductive or mixed hearing loss is necessary in order to plan medical intervention and aural rehabilitation. To make use of the ASSR as a diagnostic tool, it is imperative that air and bone conduction ASSR threshold data in normal-hearing and hearing-impaired infants of different ages are available to interpret both "normal" and "elevated" thresholds.

This chapter reviews current knowledge about bone conduction ASSRs in infant and adults with normal and impaired hearing and describes how this knowledge can be applied clinically. Also included is a look at the gaps in understanding of bone conduction ASSRs and the limitations that they impose on their clinical use.

Bone Conduction Auditory Steady-State Responses in Individuals with Normal Hearing

Threshold

Representative bone-conduction ASSR threshold results for two infants and an adult with normal hearing are illustrated in Figure 11–1. Both infants have better thresholds at 500 and 1000 Hz compared to the adult, but poorer thresholds at 2000 and 4000 Hz compared with the adult. Also, both infants have thresholds

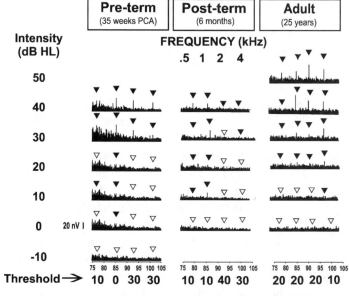

Figure 11–1. Representative bone conduction ASSR results for an individual pre-term infant (35 weeks postconceptional age), a post-term infant (6 months), and an adult (25 years). Shown are amplitude spectra resulting from FFT analyses (70 to 101 Hz) of the ASSRs. *Filled triangles* indicate responses that differ significantly from the background noise (*P* < .05). *Open triangles* indicate no response (*P* ≥ .05; EEG noise less than 11 nV). Threshold is defined as the lowest intensity that produced a significant response. (Reproduced with permission from Small & Stapells, 2006.)

at 500 and 1000 Hz that are 20 to 30 dB better than their thresholds at 2000 and 4000 Hz, in contrast with the adult subject, whose thresholds are the same at 500, 1000, and 2000 Hz and 10 dB better at 4000 Hz. A total of seven published studies to-date have reported bone conduction ASSR threshold data in individuals with normal hearing (Dimitrijevic et al., 2002; Jeng, Brown, Johnson, & Vander Werff, 2004; Lins et al., 1996; Small, Hatton, & Stapells, 2007; Small & Stapells, 2005, 2006, in press). Bone conduction ASSR thresholds from these studies are summarized in Table 11–1. Four of these studies investigated bone conduction ASSRs in adult subjects; the three remaining studies reported findings for pre-term and post-term infants.

One of the challenges of comparing bone conduction data from different studies is accounting for the variability due to differences in the following factors:

■ Placement of the bone oscillator (forehead versus mastoid)

■ Occluded versus unoccluded ears

■ Type of stimulus and calibration

■ Application of correction factors to allow comparisons across studies

For example, in adults, it is well established that bone conduction thresholds for forehead placement of the bone oscillator are higher compared with a mastoid placement, and that bone conduction thresholds are better in the low frequencies when ears are occluded compared with thresholds when ears unoccluded. Issues regarding bone conduction stimulus calibration and testing methods are discussed in more detail later in this chapter.

In order to allow comparisons across infant and adult studies, the adult bone conduction mean ASSR thresholds shown in Table 11–1 are presented in dB HL corrected to the mastoid (ANSI S3.6-1996) and for the occlusion effect. Comparison of bone conduction ASSR thresholds in adults across studies indicates values with considerable variability. In particular, the values reported by Jeng and associates (2004) are much higher than those reported in the other three studies of adults. However, if the Jeng et al. data are excluded, and the mean thresholds from these three studies (within 11 dB of each other) are averaged, bone conduction ASSR thresholds are 28, 24, 16, and 17 dB HL at 500, 1000, 2000, and 4000 Hz, respectively (Dimitrijevic et al., 2002; Lins et al., 1996; Small & Stapells, 2005).

The infant subjects were tested with a high temporal bone placement (equivalent to mastoid placement) with ears unoccluded. On average, bone conduction ASSR thresholds for post-term infants (0 to 11 months) are 15, 4, 25, and 15 dB HL at 500, 1000, 2000, and 4000 Hz, respectively. Note that ASSR thresholds at 4000 Hz obtained using mastoid electrodes were not significantly better compared with ASSR thresholds using a nape electrode (Small & Stapells, in press). Pre-term infants tested at the bedside in a neonatal intensive care unit (NICU) have, on average, bone conduction ASSR thresholds of 16, 17, 36, and 33 dB HL at 500, 1000, 2000, and 4000 Hz, respectively. Infant bone conduction ASSR thresholds in the studies by Small and colleagues were less variable, probably because they were estimated using the same stimuli and test conditions (Small & Stapells, 2006, in press; Small et al., 2007).

It is clear that ASSR thresholds to bone conduction stimuli differ in infants and adults. Overall, the bone conduction ASSR threshold data suggest that low-frequency bone conduction thresholds worsen and

Table 11–1. Across-study comparison of bone conduction ASSR thresholds in dB HL (corrected to the mastoid or temporal bone, unoccluded)

Study	Age Group (weeks)	Condition	Frequency (Hz)			
			500	1000	2000	4000
Small & Stapells (2006)	Pre-term infants; 32–43 PCA	High temporal bone; unoccluded[†*]	16	16	37	33
	Post-term infants; 0.5–27	High temporal bone; unoccluded[†]	14	2	26	22
Small, Hatton, & Stapells (2007)	Pre-term infants; 32–43 PCA	High temporal bone; unoccluded[†*]	16	17	35	33
	Post-term infants; 0.5–38	High temporal bone; unoccluded[†]	17	5	28	15
Small & Stapells (submitted)	Post-term infants; 8–44	High temporal bone; unoccluded[†m]	13	5	20	9
Lins et al. (1996)	Adults	Forehead; occluded[•]	31	29	20	19
Dimitrijevic et al. (2002)[1]	Adults	Forehead; occluded[†]	32	18	10	13
Jeng et al. (2004)	Adults	Forehead; occluded[•]	47	33	40	37
Small & Stapells (2005)	Adults	High temporal bone; unoccluded[•]	22	26	18	18

[•]Multiple AM tones.
[†]Multiple AM/FM tones.
[*]Tested in NICU.
[m]Inverting electrodes on ipsilateral mastoid; all other studies had inverting electrode at the nape.
PCA, post-conceptional age.
[1]Thresholds were calculated from ASSR (AM tones)–behavioral (AM tones) threshold differences (A. Dimitrijevic, personal communication).

high-frequency bone conduction thresholds improve with maturation. Bone conduction ASSR threshold differences between post-term infants and adults probably are due to skull and neurophysiological maturation. Differences between premature and older infants are likely explained both by skull and/or neurophysiological changes and the masking effect of high ambient noise levels in the NICU (and possibly to other issues related to prematurity), because both infant groups show the same frequency pattern.

It is noteworthy that the trend for infants' *bone conduction* ASSR thresholds to be better for low frequencies compared to high frequencies is the opposite of what is seen for *air conduction* ASSR thresholds. Mean air conduction ASSR thresholds in infants vary across studies (reviewed in Cone-Wesson, Dowell, Tomlin, Rance, & Ming., 2002; Picton, John, Dimitrijevic, & Purcell, 2003; Stapells, Herdman, Small, Dimitrijevic, & Hatton, 2005); however, air conduction ASSR thresholds at 500 Hz are consistently poorer than those at higher frequencies. Moreover, threshold and amplitudes changes with maturation are quite different for air versus bone conduction ASSRs, with air conduction showing improvement at all frequencies (lower threshold and larger ampitudes) with maturation, with larger changes for the higher frequencies (Savio, Cardenas, Perez-Abalo, Gonzalez, & Valdes, 2001).

Clinical Implications

Bone conduction ASSR findings indicate that different normal bone conduction ASSR levels are needed for infants of different ages. Based on our results for pre-term infants (Small & Stapells, 2006), and our more recent results for larger groups of post-term infants (0 to 11 months) and adults (Small & Stapells, submitted), we recommend the following preliminary "normal levels" for bone conduction ASSRs[1]:

- *Pre-term infants:* 30 dB HL at 500 and 1000 Hz, 50 dB HL or higher at 2000 Hz, and 50 dB HL at 4000 Hz

- *Post-term infants* (0 to 11 months): 30 dB HL at 500 Hz, 20 dB HL at 1000 Hz, 40 dB HL at 2000 Hz, and 30 dB HL at 4000 Hz

For comparison, adult normal levels are 50, 40, 30, and 30 dB HL for 500, 1000, 2000, and 4000 Hz, respectively. In addition, our recently submitted findings (Small & Stapells, submitted) suggest that normal levels for older infants (12 to 24 months) are not yet adult-like (40, 20, 40, and 30 dB HL at 500, 1000, 2000, and 4000 Hz, respectively).*

Bone Conduction Auditory Steady-State Response Amplitude and Phase versus Auditory Brainstem Response Amplitude and Latency Measurements

The pattern of amplitudes of bone conduction ASSRs in infants as a function of frequency (Small & Stapells, 2006) are similar to previously reported bone conduction auditory brainstem response (ABR) amplitudes in infants. Low-frequency bone conduction ABR amplitudes are larger than those at high frequencies (Cone-Wesson & Ramirez, 1997; Foxe & Stapells, 1993; Stapells & Ruben, 1989); low-frequency ASSR amplitudes also are larger than those responding to

---

[1]More than 90% of infants with normal hearing had responses present at these levels.

high-frequency stimuli (Small & Stapells, 2006). Adults have larger ASSRs than infants at 2000 and 4000 Hz, but little difference between infants and adults is seen at 500 and 1000 Hz (Small & Stapells, 2006); however, direct comparison of ABR and ASSR amplitude differences across age groups cannot be made because of the additional contribution of the 40-Hz response to the adult ABR (when using a 40/sec rate) that is not present in the infant ABR (Foxe & Stapells, 1993).

Comparison of infant- and adult-phase delay (in ms) in bone conduction ASSRs and wave V latencies in bone conduction ABRs is complicated because direct conversion of phase (circular data) to latency (linear data) can be problematic (John & Picton, 2000). Figure 11–2 shows bone conduction ASSR phase delay (in ms) for pre- and post-term infants and adults with normal hearing. Some ASSR phase delay values are similar to ABR latencies, but others are markedly different and difficult to explain (Small & Stapells, 2006). Figure 11–2 shows that bone conduction ASSR phase delays shorten with maturation at all frequencies, similar to what is expected for air conduction ASSRs; however, these results are different from bone conduction brief-tone ABR results.

To look at a specific example, mean ASSR phase delays for 2000 Hz are longer for infants than adults, similar to ABR results which show slightly longer wave V latencies for 2000-Hz brief tones in infants compared to adults (Foxe & Stapells, 1993), but mean ASSR phase delays (ms) for 500 Hz are much longer for infants than adults, in contrast to ABR results, which show much shorter wave V latencies for 500-Hz brief tones in infants compared to adults (where infant wave V latency is 1.02 ms shorter) (Foxe & Stapells, 1993; Nousak & Stapells,

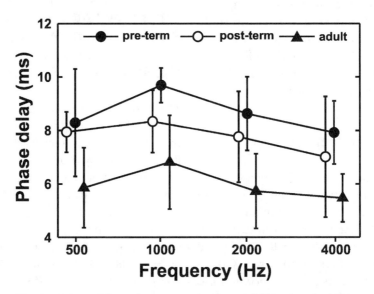

Figure 11–2. Mean bone conduction ASSR phase delays (±1 SD) across frequency for 29 pre-term infants (*filled circles*), 14 post-term infants (*open circles*) and 10 adults (*filled triangles*) with normal hearing. (Data from Small & Stapells, 2006.)

1992). In their study of adult air conduction ASSRs, John and Picton (2000) recommended adding an extra cycle in order to adjust for the number of cycles of the stimulus that may have occurred before the measured response; for example, adult phase delays reported by Small and Stapells (2006) would increase by 13, 12, 11, and 10 ms at 500, 1000, 2000, and 4000 Hz, respectively. The number of cycles to add for infants or with bone conduction ASSRs is not known; therefore comparisons of phase delay values between infants and adults are difficult.

Clinical Implications

Bone conduction ASSR amplitude is a straightforward measurement and can be interpreted in the same way as ABR amplitudes within and between age groups. Bone conduction ASSR phase measurements, however, must be interpreted with caution when comparing infant and adult results, because of the ambiguities associated with circular data.

Specific Issues with Bone Conduction Auditory Steady-State Responses

Artifact

It is well known that large-amplitude electromagnetic artifact is present in the electroencephalogram (EEG) when presenting bone conduction stimuli at moderate to high levels for ABR recording. Stimulus artifact in an ABRs is easily distinguished from an actual response because it is visible early in the time-domain waveform. Alternating the stimulus polarity is a common technique used to remove or reduce stimulus artifact when recording ABRs (e.g., see Hall, 1992, p. 319). When stimulus polarity is alternated, the polarity of the neural response is unchanged, but the stimulus artifact inverts in polarity; the inverted and noninverted artifact effectively cancels itself out when averaged together or at least is greatly reduced. A significant problem with bone conduction stimulus artifact in the EEG, when recording ASSRs, is that this energy can potentially alias to exactly the same frequency as the ASSR modulation rate and be interpreted as a response because the stimulus and response overlap in time, as shown in Figure 11–3. The top panel in the figure clearly shows that large stimulus artifact is present in the unfiltered EEG and is not removed by a 250-Hz low-pass filter when multiple bone conduction amplitude-modulated tones are presented.

Several studies have reported the presence of spurious responses during recording of high-intensity air or bone conduction ASSRs in persons with severe-to-profound hearing loss who were not able to hear the stimuli (Gorga et al., 2004; Jeng et al., 2004; Small & Stapells, 2004). Gorga and coworkers (2004) recorded air conduction ASSRs in 10 subjects with profound sensorineural hearing loss who could not hear the ASSR stimuli at the maximum limit of the equipment. Despite the severity of the hearing loss, they estimated ASSR thresholds at 100 dB HL, on average; these responses were obtained at levels at least 18–22 dB below the limits of the equipment. Gorga and associates concluded that these "responses" could not be auditory in nature. Jeng colleagues. (2004) recorded bone conduction ASSRs in five subjects with profound sensorineural hearing loss. They also found responses present

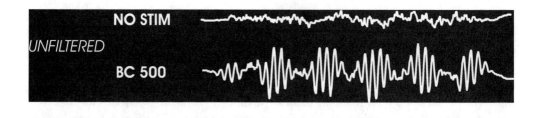

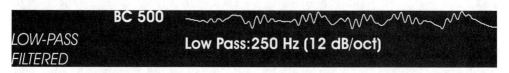

Figure 11–3. Stimulus artifact in the EEG. *Top panel:* The *first line* shows EEG signal when no stimulus is presented. The *second line* shows large stimulus artifact in the EEG when a 50 dB HL 500-Hz bone conduction stimulus is presented. *Lower panel:* The *first line* shows that stimulus artifact in the EEG is substantially reduced, but still preset, when a 12-dB/octave 250-Hz low-pass filter is used.

at levels considerably better than their behavioural thresholds for the same stimuli (53, 36, 54, and 53 dB HL at 500, 1000, 2000, and 4000 Hz, respectively) and concluded that the ASSRs were contaminated with stimulus artifact.

We also investigated the possibility of spurious ASSRs in individuals with severe-to-profound hearing loss who were not able to hear the stimuli (Small & Stapells, 2004). As mentioned previously, one potential source of spurious ASSRs is aliasing of stimulus artifact, which is of particular concern for ASSRs recorded using relatively slow analog-to-digital conversion (A/D) rates, such as 500 and 1000 Hz, which had commonly been used (Dimitrijevic et al., 2002; Herdman & Stapells, 2001, 2003). For these slow rates, aliasing of stimulus artifact is expected when the A/D rate is an integer multiple of the carrier frequency. For example, both 500- and 1000-Hz A/D rates are integer multiples of 500-, 1000-, 2000-, and 4000-Hz carrier frequencies. If these carrier frequencies are used, aliasing is

expected at the modulation rates for all of the carrier frequencies using a 500-Hz A/D rate, and at the modulation rates for 1000-, 2000-, and 4000-Hz carrier frequencies using a 1000-Hz A/D rate. If the A/D rate is not an integer multiple of these carrier frequencies (e.g., 1250 Hz), aliasing is not expected at any of the modulation rates for these frequencies (Small & Stapells, 2004). We recorded ASSRs in subjects with severe-to-profound hearing loss with both high-intensity air and bone conduction stimuli using different A/D rates (500, 1000, and 1250 Hz) and compared single versus alternated stimulus polarities. The purpose of the alternated stimulus polarity was to ascertain whether the spurious responses resulted from *stimulus* artifact aliasing to the modulation frequencies of the responses (i.e., cancellation or a significant decrease in response should occur) (Picton & John, 2004; Small & Stapells, 2004).

As predicted, the greatest number of spurious responses for both air and bone conduction ASSRs are found for 500-

and 1000-Hz A/D rates. Most of these responses were eliminated by either alternating the stimulus polarity or using the 1250-Hz A/D rate and a steep anti-aliasing filter (e.g., 300-Hz low-pass filter with a 115 dB/octave slope) (Small & Stapells, 2004). The results of this study proved that aliasing was a cause of this spurious response and led to an important modification of the Bio-Logic clinical ASSR system (which had used a 1000-Hz A/D rate) that was in the early stages of commercial implementation.

Not all ASSR equipment uses slow A/D conversion rates or rates that result in aliasing. For example, Hernández, Perez-Abalo, Rodriguez, and Rioja (2005) used the AUDIX system, which used a 932-Hz A/D rate to record multiple ASSRs to bone conduction stimuli in three children who had no residual hearing; these investigators found no spurious responses in this study. Other systems do not appear to use A/D rates that are likely to cause aliasing (i.e., Intelligent Hearing Systems SmartEP-ASSR; Viasys Audera); however, the possibility of spurious responses has not been investigated with these systems.

Spurious ASSRs are not always due to technical issues with stimulus artifact. We also observed many spurious responses to both, air and bone conduction 500-Hz stimuli that did not change in phase when the stimulus polarity was alternated (Small & Stapells, 2004) and were thus likely physiological in origin. In one case, the subject reported vestibular symptoms while we recorded ASSRs to high-intensity air conduction stimuli. Although these spurious ASSRs are most likely physiological, they are nonauditory in origin. One possibility is that these ASSRs are vestibular in origin. A number of studies have shown that high-level audi-

tory stimuli, particularly below 1000 Hz, can result in either vestibular-evoked myogenic responses (Bickford, Jacobson, & Cody, 1964; Geisler, Frishkopf, & Rosenblith, 1958; Townsend & Cody, 1971; von Békésy, 1935) or vestibular-evoked potentials (e.g., Rosengren & Colebatch, 2006; Sohmer, 2006; Todd, Rosengren & Colebatch, 2003). It is important to be aware that the possibility of eliciting a vestibular response to high-intensity air or bone conduction stimuli is not unique to ASSRs; nonauditory physiological responses also have been reported clinically using the ABR.

Clinical Implications

Stimulus artifact must be considered when ASSRs are recorded using bone conduction and high-intensity air conduction stimuli for threshold estimation. ASSRs to *single-polarity* bone conduction stimuli obtained using a 1250-Hz A/D rate can be recorded accurately for the following:

- 500-Hz stimuli up to 40 dB HL

- 1000-Hz stimuli up to 50 dB HL

- 2000-Hz stimuli up to at least 50 dB HL

- 4000 Hz stimuli up to 60 dB HL

ASSRs to single-polarity air conduction stimuli using a 1250-Hz rate can be recorded accurately for all frequencies, except perhaps at 1000 Hz, up to at least 114 to 120 dB HL. Other A/D conversion rates also can be used so long as they are selected to avoid aliasing.

The presence of spurious responses also affects the clinical use of ASSRs to assess residual hearing in persons with profound hearing loss. ASSRs can be elicited by stimuli at higher intensities than those used to elicit ABRs; for this reason, it was suggested that ASSRs may be a better method for detection of residual hearing (Rance, Dowell, Rickards, Beer, & Clark, 1998). It is common for persons with profound hearing loss to have residual hearing only in the low frequencies; consequently, if an ASSR is present to a low-frequency high-intensity stimulus, there is no way to know if it is auditory, physiological but nonauditory (e.g., vestibular), or due to aliasing of stimulus artifact in the EEG. Some of the ASSRs reported in the literature for individuals with profound loss *must be* due to aliasing or vestibular responses. Alternating stimulus polarity can help rule out stimulus artifact as a contributor, but not a nonauditory physiological response. Current clinical equipment designed to record multiple ASSRs, however, does not alternate stimulus polarity. It also must be emphasized that a safety issue must be considered in presenting high-level stimuli to the ear for as long as 5 minutes (a common length of time required to record threshold ASSRs). Exposure for this duration could cause a temporary threshold shift, tinnitus, and possibly permanent damage.

Dynamic Range for Bone Conduction Auditory Steady-State Responses

The testing range for a bone-conducted stimulus is limited by the output characteristics of the B-71 bone oscillator, particularly at low frequencies for behavioural, ABR, and ASSR testing. For a single bone conduction 500-Hz ASSR, the maximum allowable intensity is 60 dB HL.

For multiple bone conduction ASSRs (500- to 4000-Hz carrier frequencies), the maximum intensity without distortion is 50 dB HL (Small & Stapells, 2004). Beyond these maximum levels, the bone-conducted stimulus becomes nonlinear and distorted, and the oscillations can be asymmetrical. The dynamic range for ASSRs is more restricted than for pure-tone behavioural testing because more intense bone-conducted stimuli are needed to obtain ASSR thresholds. As mentioned earlier in this chapter, adult bone conduction ASSR thresholds are, on average, 28, 24, 16, and 17 dB HL at 500, 1000, 2000, and 4000 Hz, respectively. We also know that spurious nonauditory physiological responses can occur at intensities greater than 40, 50, 50, and 60 dB HL at 500, 1000, 2000, and 4000 Hz, respectively (Small & Stapells, 2004). This means that the dynamic ranges possible for adults at each carrier frequency are approximately 12, 26, 34, and 43 dB at 500, 1000 Hz, 2000 Hz, and 4000 Hz, respectively. For infants, the dynamic ranges are larger for the low frequencies but smaller for the high frequencies. For post-term infants (0–11 months) the dynamic ranges possible are approximately 24, 46, 23, and 41 dB at 500, 1000, 2000, and 4000 Hz, respectively. For pre-term infants (0.5-43 weeks post-conceptional age (PCA)) tested in the NICU, the maximum ranges possible are approximately 24, 33, 14, and 27 dB at 500, 1000 Hz, 2000 Hz, and 4000 Hz, respectively.

Clinical Implications

The dynamic ranges available at 500 Hz in adults and 2000 Hz in infants may limit clinical conclusions to statements that bone conduction thresholds are either "normal" or "elevated."

Bone Conduction Procedural Factors

It is a relatively straightforward procedure to deliver a calibrated air conduction stimulus to an infant or adult via earphones, although the sound pressure level at the tympanic membrane may vary (Rance & Tomlin, 2006; Sininger, Abdala, & Cone-Wesson, 1997; Voss & Hermann, 2005). For bone conduction testing, however, producing a predictable output of energy at the skull, and ultimately to the cochlea, is more complicated. Procedures are relatively standardized for estimating bone conduction behavioural thresholds in adults; in contrast, there are no standardized methods for bone conduction testing in infants, only recommended "best practices," many of which are based on assumptions rather than systematic investigation.

Bone Oscillator Coupling Method

Estimation of bone conduction hearing thresholds in young sleeping infants using auditory-evoked potentials poses unique challenges. Infants have smaller heads than adults, precluding the use of the standard adult or child steel headband. Also, infants must remain asleep during testing; disturbing the infant as little as possible while positioning the oscillator is critical, as is minimizing discomfort during a potentially longer testing time. One concern in bone conduction testing is that the amount of force applied to the oscillator is consistent. Yang, Stuart, Stenstrom, and Hollett (1991) measured wave V latencies and amplitudes for bone-conducted click-ABRs

using force levels of 225, 325, 425, and 525 g applied using an elastic band and concluded that 400 to 450 g was the most efficient amount of force to apply to the oscillator. They noted that coupling with a low force level (225 g) caused the oscillator to slip out of the elastic band, and that a high force level (525 g) caused the elastic band to slip off the oscillator.

For many years, coupling the oscillator to the infant's head using an elastic band has been a standard clinical method recommended by many researchers (Cone-Wesson, 1995; Stapells, 2000; Stapells & Oates, 1997; Yang & Stuart, 2000; Yang et al., 1991) because a known force can be applied to the elastic band and the amount of force verified using a spring scale (Yang & Stuart, 1990). It is important to keep in mind, however, that in many clinical settings the verification step is often omitted. The aim when testing sleeping infants is always to use sleep time efficiently and not to awaken the infant before the testing is complete.

Holding the oscillator in place by hand is also commonly done clinically because it is faster and is far less likely to awaken the infant than positioning an elastic band (which requires more manipulation of the infant's head). The hand-held method is also more comfortable for the infant because the oscillator can be removed and replaced easily between test conditions.

Despite the practical advantages of the hand-held method, its use has been discouraged (Yang & Stuart, 2000; Yang et al., 1991), based on the following assumptions:

- Potentially the applied force may vary during testing when using the hand-held method, resulting in inconsistent output from the transducer (Yang et al., 1991), poorer thresholds, and greater variability in thresholds.

■ Pressing down on the superior surface of the oscillator by hand (i.e., mass loading it) will dampen the response characteristics of the bone oscillator (Wilber, 1979).

Our recent study actually compared the force levels applied to the bone oscillator using the elastic-band and hand-held coupling methods, and estimated frequency-specific bone conduction *thresholds* in infants and adults using both of these coupling methods (Small et al., 2007). We found no significant difference in the mean force applied between coupling methods when using a trained assistant, although the variability in the amount of force applied by individual assistants was

slightly larger for the elastic-band compared to the hand-held method. The advantage of the elastic-band method is that the force applied can be measured; however, the disadvantage of verifying the force is that it takes extra time and may involve undoing the Velcro band several times, which often will awaken the baby.

As shown in Figure 11–4, bone conduction behavioural thresholds for adults are not significantly different for the two coupling methods (<3 dB difference across frequencies) (Small et al., 2007), suggesting that pressing down on the oscillator casing by hand, at least with approximately 425 g of force, does not significantly dampen the response characteristics of the oscillator (Yang et al., 1991). Bone conduction ASSR thresholds in young infants are also not significantly different using the two different coupling

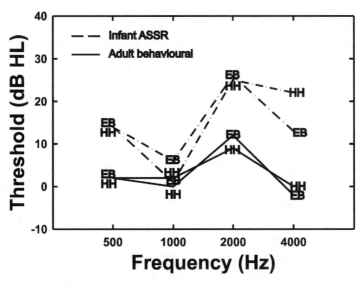

Figure 11–4. Bone oscillator coupling method. Comparison of bone conduction thresholds using the elastic-band (EB) and hand-held (HH) bone oscillator coupling methods in adults (*solid line* = pure-tone behavioral) and infants (*dotted line* = ASSR). (Data from Small & Stapells, 2007.)

methods (see Figure 11–4). However, we did find a small, albeit nonsignificant, elevation in threshold for the hand-held method for 4000 Hz, which may have some practical importance. Notably, threshold variability (i.e., standard deviations) is not greater for the hand-held method. Bone conduction ASSR amplitudes in young infants also are not significantly different (≤10nV difference) using the two different coupling methods (Small et al., 2007).

Of interest, the only other published study that compares bone conduction thresholds using different coupling methods was conducted in dogs by Munro, Paul, and Cox (1997). They compared bone conduction ABR thresholds to click stimuli in two species of dogs that had significantly different head sizes (Dalmations and Jack Russell terriers) holding the oscillator both by hand and using a 500-g weight. They also reported no difference in bone conduction thresholds using a hand-held coupling method compared with a method that applies a constant force (i.e., elastic band or 500-g weight).

Clinical Implications

Bone conduction thresholds can be obtained reliably in infants using either an elastic-band or hand-held coupling method, with the caveat that the clinician who is coupling the oscillator to the patient's head must have received appropriate training in whichever method is used.

There are clinical situations in which one method may be preferred. For example, the hand-held method may be a better choice if putting the elastic band on the infant's head is likely to awaken the infant. There are also clinical settings in

which holding the oscillator by hand is not practical—for example, when the evoked potential equipment is outside the sound booth and an assistant is not available to hold the oscillator.

Bone Oscillator Placement Location

A bone oscillator can be positioned in different locations on the skull, which can potentially affect the intensity of the signal reaching the cochlea (Stuart, Yang, & Stenstrom, 1990; Yang, Rupert, & Moushegian, 1987). It is well established that adult calibration values for bone conduction stimuli are different for mastoid and forehead bone oscillator placement location on the skull. On average, adult behavioural thresholds measured at the forehead are higher than at the mastoid by 14.0, 8.5, 11.5, and 8.0 dB at 500, 1000, 2000, and 4000 Hz, respectively (ANSI S3.6-1996).

Bone oscillator placement location also has been raised as an issue (Stuart et al., 1990; Yang & Stuart, 2000) when estimating bone conduction thresholds in sleeping infants because of the potential for thresholds to differ depending on where the oscillator is placed on the temporal (mastoid versus upper region) or frontal bone. When an elastic band is used to couple the oscillator to the skull, it typically is placed on the infant's temporal bone, posterior to the upper portion of the pinna so that the elastic band does not cover the infant's eyes or slide off the head; when the hand-held method is used, oscillator placement is not restricted to one area on the temporal bone. Earlier ABR studies that investigated bone oscillator placement in infants reported results that have been interpreted to suggest that bone oscillator location does affect the response in infants. Stuart and associates (1990) recorded ABRs to click stimuli at different intensities using different oscillator placements on the temporal bone and reported differences in ABR latencies for the different temporal placements. They found significant differences in wave V ABR latencies for different locations on the temporal bone and concluded that there are also significant differences in signal attenuation to the cochlea. They suggested that attenuation within the temporal bone occurs in infants because the temporal bone consists of several unfused components, thereby causing a reduction in signal transmission when areas of the temporal bone further away from the cochlea are used for oscillator placement.

The following issues affect the interpretation of these wave V ABR latency findings:

- Latency is not linearly related to signal attenuation (Mackersie & Stapells, 1994; Picton, Stapells, & Campbell, 1981); consequently, latency-intensity functions cannot be used to accurately estimate threshold changes (Mackersie & Stapells, 1994)

- Wave V amplitudes are better predictors of threshold than latency

- Threshold, the best measure for assessing attenuation, was not directly measured at the different placements on the temporal bone

- Attenuation may be frequency dependent, which cannot be assessed using click stimuli.

The assumption that attenuation would follow the same pattern as ABR latency differences appears to be incorrect based on our recent ASSR study (Small et al., 2007). We assessed the effects of placement on attenuation directly by comparing frequency-specific bone conduction ASSR thresholds in pre-term infants for three different bone oscillator placement locations—high temporal bone, mastoid, and forehead (Small et al., 2007). In agreement with the ABR studies, ASSR thresholds obtained with bone oscillator placement on the forehead are substantially elevated with respect to thresholds found with either the high temporal or mastoid oscillator placements. However, thresholds obtained at the high temporal and mastoid oscillator placements do not differ significantly. On average, thresholds for the forehead placement are significantly higher than both the high temporal and mastoid placements by at least 14, 11, 18, and 14 dB at 500, 1000, 2000, and 4000 Hz, respectively. These differences may be even greater because absent responses at the maximum intensity are seen more often with the forehead placement compared with the other two placements. The high temporal or mastoid placement should therefore be used to maximize the intensity range available to assess thresholds in infants.

We also found that the difference between bone conduction thresholds at the mastoid versus that at the forehead is the same at 500 Hz for adults and infants. However, at higher frequencies, the difference increases for infants compared with adults (infant forehead-mastoid differences are 3, 7, and 6 dB larger than adults at 1000, 2000, and 4000 Hz, respectively. Possible reasons for the larger attenuation differences at higher frequencies exhibited by infants compared with adults may result from the membranous sutures surrounding the temporal bone in the infant. Yang and coworkers (1987) suggested that the membranous sutures have the effect of attenuating the vibratory signal before it reaches the cochlea. When the forehead oscillator placement location is used, the vibratory energy must pass through two layers of membranous sutures before reaching the temporal bone to stimulate the cochlea and thereby initiate a physiological response (Yang et al., 1987). Consequently, the effective intensity that reaches the cochlea decreases as the distance between the bone oscillator and the cochlea increases (Stuart et al., 1990). Thresholds obtained at the forehead would, therefore, be worse (i.e., higher) than those obtained at either the temporal or mastoid locations, which is consistent with the findings of Small and associates. (2007). As noted by Yang and colleagues (1987), the membranous sutures in the infant skull may act like a low-pass filter, allowing low-frequency energy to pass the sutures with minimal attenuation, whereas the high-frequency energy is substantially attenuated. The idea that membranous sutures act like a low-pass filter in infants may explain why infants and adults have the same attenuation between placements at 500 IIz but demonstrate more attenuation than adults at 1000, 2000, and 4000 Hz.

Clinical Implications

Placement of the oscillator on either the high temporal bone or the mastoid does not significantly affect the bone conduction ASSR threshold; however, a forehead placement should be avoided in clinical testing.

Unoccluded versus Occluded Ears

Correcting for the occlusion effect when estimating bone conduction thresholds with occluded ears is well described in adults (Dirks & Swindeman, 1967; Elpern & Naunton, 1963; Hodgson & Tillman, 1966; Small & Stapells, 2003). For insert earphones, behavioural thresholds to brief tones improve by 3 to 5 dB at 500 to 1000 Hz (Small & Stapells, 2003), whereas pure-tone behavioral thresholds in the low frequencies (250-1000 Hz) improve by as much as 17 dB, depending on the insertion depth (Dean & Martin, 2000). As discussed earlier, any test protocols used to estimate thresholds in sleeping infants must be designed to minimize the possibility of waking the infant. Air conduction thresholds typically are assessed using insert earphones, followed by bone conduction testing (Stapells, 2000). A question that arises is whether insert earphones should be removed before assessing bone conduction thresholds. It is important to know whether occluding the ears increases, decreases, or has no effect on bone conduction thresholds in infants.

We investigated the occlusion effect in infants and found that bone conduction ASSR thresholds in infants younger than 6 months of age do not change when the ear canal is occluded (Small et al., 2007). Comparison of unoccluded and occluded bone conduction mean ASSR thresholds indicate no more than a 4-dB difference across frequency, in contrast with adults, whose bone conduction thresholds at 250 to 1000 Hz improve as much as 17 dB when the ear canal is occluded using insert earphones (Dean & Martin, 2000). Bone conduction mean

ASSR amplitudes and phase delays also are not significantly affected by occluding the ear canal in young infants.

In adults, the unoccluded ear acts as a high-pass filter—that is, low-frequency energy is lost through the open ear canal (Gelfand, 1981, p. 66; Tonndorf, 1966); in an occluded ear, the improvement in the bone conduction thresholds is due to the enhancement of the low frequencies. The underlying mechanism for the occlusion effect in adults is the osseotympanic pathway of bone-conducted sound (Tondorff, 1966). The mechanisms of bone conduction hearing in infants have not been investigated; the absence of an occlusion effect in infants suggests that there may be substantial differences between infants and adults in the way that bone-conducted sound reaches the cochlea.

Clinical Implications

The clinical implications of these occlusion findings are that it may be possible to do bone conduction testing, at least in infants younger than 6 months of age, with ears occluded without applying a correction factor. Further studies should be conducted in a larger group of infants to confirm these findings (Small et al., 2007). Also, it is important to investigate whether the occlusion effect is present in older infants and to determine at which age the occlusion effect should be compensated for in clinical testing.

Calibration of Bone-Conducted Stimuli

It is important to note that although "dB HL" is a convenient and easily un-derstood metric for calibrating bone-conducted ASSR stimuli, it does not actually represent "hearing level" in infants, particularly in the low frequencies. The ANSI S3.6 specifications (1996) recommended force levels based on adult data. In force levels (dB re: 1 μN), we know that adults are more sensitive to high- than to low-frequency stimuli transmitted by a bone oscillator, which is reflected in the Reference Equivalent Threshold Force Levels in dB re: 1 μN that correspond to 0 dB HL at the mastoid. For adults, in order to make the spectra of a bone oscillator equal cross frequency (i.e., converted to dB HL), force levels need to be 38.0, 22.5, 11.0, and 15.5 re: 1 μN at 500, 1000, 2000, and 4000 Hz, respectively (ANSI, 1996). Infant bone conduction ASSR threshold data support the observation that infants do not require the same boost in the low frequencies as adults to make bone-conducted ASSR stimuli detectable, but they require approximately the same force levels as adults to detect high frequencies. It must be further emphasized, that even if we correct dB HL for infants, physiological measures such as the ASSR still require a correction factor to be able to accurately predict behavioural thresholds for bone conduction stimuli (i.e., ASSR dB HL does not equal behavioral dB HL). This correction factor is not yet known for bone conduction stimuli.

Clinical Implications

It is appropriate to calibrate bone conduction ASSR stimuli in dB HL, keeping in mind that these dB HL values are adult-based and that threshold results are different for infants. Also, ASSR thresholds (in dB HL) must be corrected to accurately predict behavioural thresholds.

Interaural Attenuation to Bone-Conducted Stimuli in dB HL

Yang and associates (1987) reported the first estimate of interaural attenuation to a bone-conducted stimulus in infants. They estimated that signal attenuation from a temporal to frontal placement ranged from 30 to 35 dB in neonates and from 20 to 25 dB in 1-year-olds; attenuation from an occipital to temporal placement was 15 to 20 dB in both infant groups. By contrast, in adults the latency differences between responses to different placements were not significant, and the attenuation between oscillator placement was judged to be no more than 5 to 10 dB (Yang et al., 1987). This attenuation estimate in adults is smaller than the ANSI (1996) standards for mastoid and forehead placements discussed previously, and the estimated changes in signal attenuation as a function of location suggested by Yang and coworkers (1987) must be interpreted with caution for the same reasons outlined previously.

We recently estimated interaural attenuation to bone-conducted stimuli in infants using frequency-specific stimuli (Small & Stapells, in press). The differences between ipsilateral and contralateral ASSR thresholds (contralateral minus ipsilateral) for 500-, 1000-, 2000-. and 4000-Hz carrier frequencies provide a minimum estimate of interaural attenuation—that is, if a response were present in both EEG channels, both cochleae *may* have been stimulated (although it is also possible that only one cochlea was stimulated); however, if a response was present only in the ipsilateral EEG channel, we could assume that the signal stimulated only the ipsilateral cochlea, and a minimum estimate of interaural attenuation could thus be attained. We found that interaural attenuation for infants is 10 dB or greater in 79% of the ASSR recordings, 20 dB or greater in 44%, and 30 dB or greater in 6%. For adults, interaural attenuation is 10 dB or greater in only 19% of the ASSR recordings. These results are in the same range as those reported by Yang and colleagues (1987).

Clinical Implications

In infants with normal cochlear function, the "test" cochlea is likely to be the one closest to the bone oscillator when bone conduction stimuli are presented at levels near threshold.

Direct and Indirect Estimation of Bone Conduction Thresholds

Assessment of bone conduction hearing sensitivity using ASSRs can be achieved using direct and indirect methods. The direct method of estimating bone conduction thresholds, and the most common method, involves the presentation of a bone conduction stimulus to the skull at varying intensities; the lowest level at which there is a response to the stimulus is the bone conduction threshold. All of the bone conduction ASSR threshold data presented in this chapter up to this point were obtained using this direct method.

Cone-Wesson and colleagues (2002) estimated ASSR bone conduction thresholds indirectly using the "sensorineural acuity level" (SAL) test (Dirks, 1973;

Jerger & Tillman, 1960), which uses bone-conducted noise to mask an air conduction stimulus that is presented just above the subject's threshold. There are several steps in the SAL test. The first step is to determine, in a group of persons with normal hearing, the amount of bone-conducted masking noise that is needed to mask an air-conducted tone near threshold. If a conductive loss is present, the air-conducted threshold for the test stimulus will be elevated, but the amount of bone-conducted masking noise will be the same as for normal subjects. If the hearing loss is sensorineural in nature,

the amount of bone-conducted masking noise needed to mask the air-conducted stimulus will be elevated (the air conduction threshold also will be elevated). For mixed losses, the difference between the air conduction threshold and the bone-conducted masking level indicates the amount of conductive loss.

Figure 11–5 shows the results reported by Cone-Wesson and associates (2002) using ASSRs and the SAL method to identify infants with conductive and sensorineural hearing loss. Nine of these infants had elevated air conduction ABR and ASSR thresholds and absent distortion-

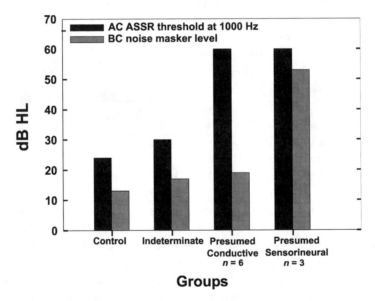

Figure 11–5. SAL technique: Comparison of ASSR thresholds for an air conduction 1000-Hz carrier frequency and bone conduction masker levels needed at ASSR + 10 dB. The infants in each group were separated on the basis of the following factors: (i) control: normal DPOAEs, ABRs, and tympanograms; (ii) indeterminate: absent DPOAEs, normal ABRs, and abnormal tympanograms; (iii) presumed conductive: absent DPOAEs, elevated ABR thresholds, and abnormal tympanogram (clinical history also suggested middle ear disorder); (iv) presumed sensorineural: absent DPOAEs, elevated ABR threshold, and normal tympanogram. (Adapted from Cone-Wesson et al., 2002.)

product otoacoustic emissions (DPOAEs). In three infants with elevated air conduction ABR and ASSR thresholds (greater than 40 dB HL) and normal tympanograms, the amount of bone conduction masking noise needed to mask the air-conducted signal was close to the air conduction ASSR threshold (consistent with a sensorineural hearing loss). In six infants with elevated ABR and ASSR thresholds, flat tympanograms, and absent DPOAEs, only 18 dB nHL of bone conduction masking noise was needed (infants with normal hearing needed 12 dB nHL of masking noise), which suggests a conductive hearing loss. This pattern of findings for ASSRs is similar to studies in which SAL techniques were assessed using the ABR (Webb & Greenberg, 1983; Ysunza & Cone-Wesson, 1987).

There are two suggested advantages of the SAL test in evoked potential testing:

1. The stimulus is delivered via air conduction and is therefore ear-specific; if there is any crossover of the bone-conducted noise masker, it would serve to mask the non-test ear.

2. Delivery of the test signal via air conduction minimizes the likelihood of stimulus artifact contaminating the ASSR; although artifact remains a concern for the bone-conducted masking noise, there is less chance that it will be mistaken as a response (Cone-Wesson et al., 2002).

The main disadvantage of the SAL test is that it is not a direct test of bone conduction hearing. It is an estimation of bone conduction hearing derived from two different threshold measures, which increases the likelihood of measurement error. At the time that the study by Cone-Wesson and colleagues was done, directly estimating bone conduction ASSR thresholds using modulated tones was not recommended by these researchers because there were unresolved technical issues with stimulus artifact and the ASSR. As discussed previously in this chapter, these issues have now been addressed and no longer appear to constitute a justification for not estimating infant bone conduction thresholds directly.

Clinical Implications

The majority of the bone conduction ASSR data has been and is currently being collected using direct threshold estimation. Preliminary ASSR results using SAL methods confirm that it is possible to differentiate between conductive, mixed, and sensorineural hearing losses in infants using this technique. Nevertheless, many more infants with hearing loss need to be tested using the SAL method (and using the direct method) before relative benefits can be determined; however, we believe that a direct estimation of threshold, because of its simplicity, will be the method of choice when using ASSRs to assess cochlear function.

Isolation of the Test Ear Using Bone-Conducted Stimuli

Because interaural attenuation in adults is much less for bone-conducted compared with air-conducted stimuli, it is difficult to determine how much each cochlea contributes to the resulting bone conduction response without using additional methods. Interaural attenuation to bone-conducted stimuli for adults is 10 dB on average at 250 to 4000 Hz (Nolan & Lyon, 1981); interaural attenuation for air-conducted stimuli is much higher—for example, for supra-aural earphones, attenuation is 40 to 50 dB on average at 250 to 4000 Hz (Goldstein & Newman, 1994, p. 117); for insert earphones with deep insertion, it is 69 to 94 dB on average at 500 to 4000 Hz (Sklare & Denenberg, 1987).

Presenting masking noise to the ear contralateral to the test ear often is used in adults to isolate the test ear; however, masking may not be practical when assessing infants because of the extra time required for testing, the difficulties of earphone placement, and the uncertainty about how much masking noise to use (Stapells & Ruben, 1989). The presence of wave I for a click-ABR also can be used to determine which cochlea is responding to the stimulus; however, wave I can be small and difficult to detect in infants with normal hearing and easily disappears if hearing loss is present (Jahrsdoerfer et al., 1985). Electrocochleography (N_1) using a transtympanic or tympanic electrode can also identify which cochlea is responding (Ferraro & Ferguson, 1989); the difficulty with this technique is that infants can only be tested using this method under general anesthesia.

Another method to determine which cochlea is responding to bone-conducted stimuli is to use the pattern of asymmetries in the ipsilateral and contralateral EEG channels of the bone conduction ABR or ASSR. Stapells and Ruben (1989) showed that contralateral ABRs to brief-tone bone conduction stimuli in infants have smaller wave V amplitudes and longer latencies for 500- and 2000-Hz stimuli compared with ipsilateral recordings. By contrast, adults have similar wave V amplitudes and latencies at 500 and 2000 Hz. Ipsilateral/contralateral asymmetries in the wave V region are robust at low levels; therefore, they can be used to assess the laterality of the response concurrently with threshold estimation in young infants. Stapells and Ruben (1989) found that these latency and amplitude asymmetries in infants are present at all intensity levels and persist beyond 1 year of age. These data support the observation that ipsilateral/contralateral asymmetries in the bone conduction ABR in infants can provide valuable ear-specific diagnostic information; based on the assumption that the cochlea closest to the channel that shows the largest and earliest wave V contributed to the recorded ABR.

Ipsilateral/Contralateral Asymmetries in Bone Conduction Auditory Steady-State Responses

Previous ABR studies have shown that two-channel recordings (i.e., EEG channels ipsilateral and contralateral to stimulus ear) of bone conduction ABRs show maturational differences (Foxe & Stapells, 1993; Stapells & Ruben, 1989; Stuart, Yang, & Botea, 1996). In our recent study, a similar pattern of ipsilateral/contralateral asymmetries was found for the bone-conducted ASSR (Small & Stapells, in press) and for air-conducted ASSRs (Small & Stapells, in press; van der Reijden, Mens, & Snik, 2005). Figure 11–6 shows individual results for a 6-month-old infant for two-channel ASSR recordings to a 2000-Hz bone conduction stimulus. The response is smaller and later in the contralateral EEG channel compared with the ipsilateral EEG channel when the

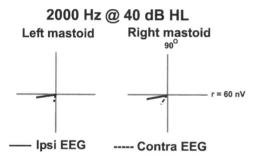

2000 Hz @ 40 dB HL

Left mastoid   Right mastoid

90°

r = 60 nV

—— Ipsi EEG   ----- Contra EEG

Figure 11–6. Ipsilateral/contralateral ASSR asymmetries. Representative polar plots for bone conduction (40 dB HL) ASSRs elicited by a 2000-Hz stimulus for an infant 6 months of age. The stimulus was presented to one mastoid while the ASSRs were simultaneously recorded in the ipsilateral (*solid line*) and contralateral (*dashed line*) EEG channels. ASSR amplitude is denoted by the length of the vector; ASSR phase delay is denoted by the angle of the vector (i.e., the larger the angle in a counterclockwise direction, the longer the phase delay). (Data from Small & Stapells, in press)

oscillator is placed on the left mastoid; the same pattern is seen for a stimulus presented at the right mastoid. Overall, many more infants than adults show these ipsilateral/contralateral asymmetries for both air and bone conduction stimuli (Small & Stapells, in press).

Clinical Implications

Infants have consistent ipsilateral/contralateral asymmetries in ASSRs to air and bone conduction stimuli that are not present to the same degree in adults. As with the ABR, these asymmetries in infants may be used clinically to determine which cochlea is responding to bone conduction stimuli by assuming that the EEG channel that contains the ASSR with the larger amplitude or shorter

phase delay is on the same side as the cochlea that is stimulated. This is very helpful in assessing infant hearing because clinical masking is time-consuming and may not be practical for recording auditory evoked potentials in a sleeping infant. Also, the appropriate amount of clinical masking that should be used for infants when using bone conduction stimuli is currently not known. The results of our study also indicate that the contralateral EEG channel should not be used to estimate air or bone conduction ASSR thresholds in infants.

Currently, normal levels for bone conduction ASSRs in infants of different ages are available and can be used clinically to screen for normal bone conduction hearing (Small & Stapells, submitted). On the basis of the findings of a recent study (Small & Stapells, in press), it is recommended that two-channel recordings always be used when eliciting bone conduction ASSRs, and that manufacturers incorporate this capability into all ASSR clinical equipment. However, it must be emphasized that there currently are no published bone conduction ASSR data for infants with hearing loss. Clinical use of bone conduction ASSR asymmetries will depend on future studies investigating these asymmetries in infants with conductive, mixed, and sensorineural hearing loss.

Results for Bone Conduction Auditory Steady-State Responses in Persons with Hearing Loss

There are no published bone conduction ASSR data for adults with sensorineural, conductive, or mixed hearing losses except for a study by Jeng and associates (2004) that simulated conductive hearing losses in adults and estimated the difference between their air and bone conduction ASSR thresholds. Also, there are no published bone conduction ASSR data for infants with hearing loss; however, researchers at the Cuban Neuroscience Center have been using multiple ASSRs to identify conductive losses in children 9 to 12 years of age (Hernández, Perez-Abalo, Rodriguez, & Rioja, personal communication). Their findings are very promising. Hernández and colleagues investigated the use of multiple ASSRs elicited by air and bone conduction stimuli to predict hearing threshold and the air-bone gap in children who had either normal hearing or conductive hearing loss. Figure 11–7a shows air and bone conduction ASSRs for a 7-year-old child with atresia of the right external auditory canal; the air conduction thresholds in dB HL are poorer than the bone conduction thresholds. Comparison of behavioural and audiometric results for this child, shown in Figure 11–7b, reveals a significant air-bone gap for both testing methods. These researchers' results indicated a significant correlation between air and bone conduction behavioural and ASSR thresholds and an even stronger correlation between their behavioural and ASSR air-bone gaps.

Clinical Implications

Air and bone conduction ASSRs can estimate air and bone conduction hearing thresholds and predict the audiometric air-bone gap in children 9 to 12 years of age with normal hearing or with conductive losses. These findings are very encouraging; this study needs to be repeated for infants with hearing loss to provide the necessary data to support the use of ASSRs to accurately identify and quantify conductive components in this population.

Recommendations for Bone Conduction Auditory Steady-State Responses and Bone Conduction Testing

This chapter has provided an overview of current bone conduction ASSR research and its clinical implications. At this time, the clinical use of bone conduction ASSRs for infants is limited to determining whether bone conduction hearing sensitivity is within normal limits or "elevated." "Normal levels" have been identified for infants up to 24 months of age that can be used clinically to identify normal cochlear function. At present, no data are available for infants with hearing loss; thus, it is not possible to interpret elevated bone conduction ASSR thresholds. The dynamic range for bone conduction ASSR also constrains interpretation of elevated thresholds, particularly at high frequencies.

Also presented in this chapter are data supporting the use of two-channel recordings in eliciting bone conduction ASSRs to determine which cochlea is responding to bone conduction stimuli; this line of evidence discounts the use of the contralateral EEG channel to estimate air or bone conduction ASSR thresholds in infants. It is recommended that manufacturers incorporate this capability into all ASSR clinical equipment.

This chapter also reviewed bone conduction testing issues and how recent

a.

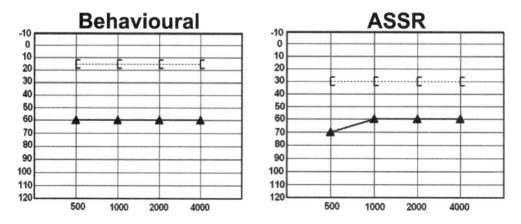

b.

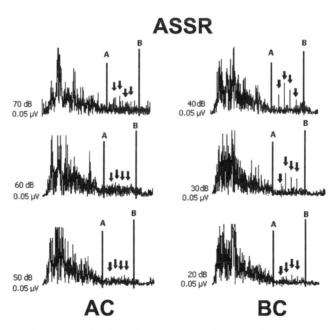

Figure 11–7. a., Bone conduction ASSRs for a 7-year-old child with atresia of the right external auditory canal. Shown are amplitude spectra resulting from FFT analyses (70 to 101 Hz) of the ASSRs. *Arrows* indicate responses that differ significantly from the background noise. The lowest levels (in dB HL) that produced significant responses are shown. **b.,** Behavioral and multiple ASSR audiograms for the right ear for the child described in part **a.** *Triangles* indicate air conduction thresholds; *square brackets* indicate bone conduction thresholds. (Results provided by Hernández et al. at the Cuban Neuroscience Center [personal communication].)

investigations have addressed procedural factors that are particularly important in assessing infants. The following recommendations are based on these recent findings:

■ Both the elastic band and the hand-held method are appropriate for coupling the bone oscillator to the head, with the important caveat that adequate training has taken place for the method used.

■ Either a temporal or mastoid placement location can be used (forehead placement should be avoided).

■ Ears may be unoccluded or occluded during bone conduction testing without significantly affecting threshold estimation.

■ Bone conduction stimuli should be calibrated in dB HL for ease of comprehension, with the awareness that this metric is adult-based.

■ Infants have greater interaural attenuation than adults to bone-conducted stimuli, which can help to isolate the test cochlea.

■ Direct estimation of bone conduction ASSR thresholds is the most straightforward method for assessing cochlear function.

Recommended Protocol

■ Ensure that stimuli (whether single or multiple) are correctly calibrated in dB HL at the mastoid.

■ Select a high-temporal-bone or mastoid placement location using either the elastic band or hand-held coupling method (ears may be occluded or unoccluded).

■ If response is absent at the normal screening level for air conduction ASSRs, record bone conduction ASSRs at normal levels. If the bone conduction response is present, there is a conductive component; if the bone conduction ASSR is absent at the normal level, there is a sensorineural component.

■ If ASSR thresholds are elevated, obtain air and bone conduction brief-tone ABR thresholds to complete diagnostic assessment of air and bone conduction hearing thresholds.

Future Research

To establish that bone conduction ASSR testing can differentially diagnose normal and elevated bone conduction thresholds, sufficient bone conduction ASSR threshold data for infant and adult subjects with conductive, mixed, and sensorineural hearing losses are needed. Estimation of air and bone conduction ASSR thresholds in infants with hearing loss (with both measures in the same subject) also is needed to determine how well ASSRs estimate air-bone gaps and to predict the audiogram.

The possibility of evoking vestibular responses when recording ASSRs (and ABRs) to bone conduction (and air conduction) stimuli is an area of research that needs to be explored. In particular, the development of a technique that allows clinicians to distinguish between auditory and vestibular responses would enhance the utility of using ASSRs (and other responses) to assess residual hearing in persons with profound hearing loss.

Some interesting theoretical questions emerge from infant-adult bone conduction hearing differences. For example, the apparent absence of an occlusion effect in young infants certainly suggests that the osseotympanic mode is not an important contributor to bone conduction hearing when ears are occluded, although it is for adults (Small & Stapells, submitted). The underlying mechanisms that contribute to bone conduction hearing in adults are not completely understood; however, much less is known about these mechanisms in infants. Clearly, further investigation is needed to describe and understand the mechanisms of infant bone conduction hearing.

Acknowledgments. This research was supported by a Canadian Institutes of Health Research (CIHR) Fellowship and a Michael Smith Foundation for Health Research Trainee Award to the first author, and grants from the CIHR and NSERC-Canada to the second author. We especially wish to thank M. Hernández, M. Perez-Abalo, E. Rodriguez, and L. Rioja for their generosity in providing an individual ASSR case study for a child with a conductive hearing loss.

References

ANSI. (1996). *American National Standard Specifications for Audiometers (ANSI S3.6-1996)*. New York: ANSI.

Bickford, R. G., Jacobson, J. L., & Cody, D. (1964). Averaged potentials to sound and other stimuli in man. *Annals of the New York Academy of Science, 112*, 201–223.

Cone-Wesson, B. (1995). Bone-conduction ABR tests. *American Journal of Audiology, 4*, 14–19.

Cone-Wesson, B., Dowell, R. C., Tomlin, D., Rance, G., & Ming, W. J. (2002). The auditory steady-state response: Comparisons with the auditory brainstem response. *Journal of the American Academy of Audiology, 13*(4), 173–187.

Cone-Wesson, B., & Ramirez, G. M. (1997). Hearing sensitivity in newborns estimated from ABRs to bone-conducted sounds. *Journal of the American Academy of Audiology, 8*, 299–307.

Dean, M. S., & Martin, F. N. (2000). Insert earphone and the occlusion effect. *American Journal of Audiology, 9*, 131–134.

Dimitrijevic, A., John, M. S., Van Roon, P., Purcell, D. W., Adamonis, J., Ostroff, J., et al. (2002). Estimating the audiogram using multiple auditory steady-state responses. *Journal of the American Academy of Audiology, 13*(4), 205–224.

Dirks, D. (1973). Bone-conduction measurements. In J. Jerger (Ed.), *Modern developments in audiology* (pp. 1–36). New York: Academic Press.

Dirks, D., & Swindeman, J. G. (1967). The variability of occluded and unoccluded bone-conduction thresholds. *Journal of Speech and Hearing Research, 10*(10), 232–249.

Elpern, B., & Naunton, R. F. (1963). The stability of the occlusion effect. *Archives of Otolaryngology, 77*, 376–384.

Ferraro, J. A., & Ferguson, R. (1989). Tympanic ECochG and conventional ABR: A combined approach for the identification of wave I and the 1-V interval. *Ear and Hearing, 3*, 161–166.

Foxe, J. J. & Stapells, D. R. (1993). Normal infant and adult auditory brainstem responses to bone-conducted tones. *Audiology, 32*, 95–109.

Geisler, C. D., Frishkopf, L. S., & Rosenblith, W. A. (1958). Extracranial responses to acoustic clicks in man. *Science, 128*, 1210–1211.

Gelfand, S. A. (1981). *Hearing: An introduction to psychological and physiological acoustics* (pp. 66). New York: Marcel Dekker.

Goldstein, B. A., & Newman, C. W. (1994). Clinical masking: A decision-making process. In J. Katz (Ed.), *Handbook of clinical audiology* (pp. 117). Baltimore: Williams & Wilkins.

Gorga, M. P., Neely, S. T., Hoover, B. M., Dierking, D. M., Beauchaine, K. L., & Manning, C. (2004). Determining the upper limits of stimulation for auditory steady-state response measurements. *Ear and Hearing, 25*, 302–307.

Hall, J. W. (1992). *Handbook of auditory evoked responses*. Needham Heights, MA: Allyn & Bacon.

Herdman, A. T, & Stapells, D. R. (2001). Thresholds of auditory steady-state responses in normal-hearing adults. *Scandinavian Audiology, 30*, 41–49.

Herdman, A. T, & Stapells, D. R. (2003). Auditory steady-state response thresholds of adults with sensorineural hearing impairment. *International Journal of Audiology, 42*, 237–248.

Hernández, M., Perez-Abalo M., Rodríguez, E., & Rioja, L. (2005). *Clinical usefulness of multiple auditory steady state responses elicited by bone- and air-conduction stimuli.* Paper presented at the XIXth Biennial Symposium of the International Evoked Response Audiometry Study Group, Havana, Cuba.

Hodgson, W. R. & Tillman, T. W. (1966). Reliability of bone conduction occlusion effects in normals. *Journal of Auditory Research, 6*, 141–151.

Jahrsdoerfer, R. A., Yeakley, J. W., Hall, J. W., Robbins, K. T., & Gray, L. C. (1985). High-resolution CT scanning and auditory brain stem response in congenital aural atresia: Patient selection and surgical correlation. *Otolaryngology—Head and Neck Surgery, 93*, 292–298.

Jeng, F.-C., Brown, C. J., Johnson, T. A., & Vander Werff, K. R. (2004). Estimating air-bone gaps using auditory steady-state responses. *Journal of the American Academy of Audiology, 15*, 67–78.

Jerger, J., & Tillman, T. (1960). A new method for the clinical determination of sensorineural acuity level (SAL). *Archives of Otolaryngology, 71*, 948–955.

John, M. S. & Picton, T. W. (2000). Human auditory steady-state responses to amplitude-modulated tones: Phase and latency measurements. *Hearing Research, 141*, 57–79.

Joint Committee on Infant Hearing (2000). Year 2000 position statement: Principles and guidelines for early hearing detection and intervention programs. *American Journal of Audiology, 9*, 9–29.

Lins, O. G., Picton, T. W., Boucher, B. L., Durieux-Smith, A., Champagne, S. C., Moran, L. M., et al. (1996). Frequency-specific audiometry using steady-state responses. *Ear and Hearing, 17*, 81–96.

Mackersie, C. L., & Stapells D. R. (1994). Auditory brainstem response wave I prediction of conductive component in infants and young children. *American Journal of Audiology 3*, 52–58.

Munro, K. J., Paul, B., & Cox, C. L. (1997). Normative auditory brainstem response data for bone conduction in the dog. *Journal of Small Animal Practice, 38*, 353–356.

Nolan, M. & Lyon, D. J. (1981). Transcranial attenuation in bone conduction audiometry. *Journal of Laryngology Otology, 95*, 597–608.

Nousak, J. K. & Stapells, D. R. (1992). Frequency specificity of the auditory brain stem response to bone-conducted tones in infants and adults. *Ear and Hearing, 13*, 87–95.

Picton, T. W. & John, M. S. (2004). Avoiding electromagnetic artifacts when recording auditory steady-state responses. *Journal of American Academy of Audiology 15*, 541–554.

Picton, T. W., John, M. S., Dimitrijevic, A., & Purcell, D. W. (2003). Auditory steady-state responses. *International Journal of Audiology, 42*, 177–219.

Picton, T. W., Stapells, D. R., & Campbell, K. B. (1981). Auditory evoked potentials from the human cochlea and brainstem. *Journal of Otolaryngology, 10*, 1–41.

Rance, G., Dowell, R. C., Rickards, F. W., Beer, D. E., & Clark, G. M. (1998). Steady-state evoked potential and behavioral hearing thresholds in a group of children with absent click-evoked auditory brain stem response. *Ear and Hearing, 19*(1), 48–61.

Rance, G., Tomlin, D. (2006). Maturation of auditory steady-state responses in normal babies. *Ear and Hearing, 27*(1), 20–29.

Rosengren, S. M., & Colebatch, J. G. (2006). Vestibular evoked potentials (VsEPs) in patients with severe to profound hearing loss. *Clinical Neurophysiology, 117,* 1145–1153.

Savio, G., Cardenas, J., Perez-Abalo, M., Gonzales, A., & Valdes, J. (2001). The low and high frequency auditory steady-state responses mature at different rates. *Audiology & Neuro-otology, 6,* 279–287.

Sininger, Y. S., Abdala, C., & Cone-Wesson, B. (1997). Auditory threshold sensitivity of the human neonate as measured by the auditory brainstem response. *Hearing Research, 104,* 27–38.

Sklare, D. A., & Denenberg, L. J. (1987). Interaural attenuation for tubephone insert earphones. *Ear and Hearing, 8,* 298–300.

Small, S. A., Hatton, J., & Stapells, D. R. (2007). Effects of bone oscillator coupling method, placement location, and occlusion on bone-conduction auditory steady-state responses in infants. *Ear and Hearing, 28*(1), 83–98.

Small, S. A., & Stapells, D. R. (2003). Normal brief-tone bone-conduction behavioural thresholds using a B-71 transducer: Three occlusion conditions. *Journal of the American Academy of Audiology, 14*(10), 556–562.

Small, S. A., & Stapells, D. R. (2004). Artifactual responses when recording auditory steady-state responses. *Ear and Hearing, 25*(6), 611–623.

Small, S. A., & Stapells D. R. (2005). Multiple auditory steady-state response thresholds to bone-conduction stimuli in adults with normal hearing. *Journal of the American Academy of Audiology, 16,* 172–183.

Small, S. A., & Stapells, D. R. (2006). Multiple auditory steady-state response thresholds to bone-conduction stimuli in young infants with normal hearing. *Ear and Hearing, 27*(3), 219–228.

Small, S. A., & Stapells, D. R. (in press). Normal ipsilateral/contralateral asymmetries in infant multiple auditory steady-state responses to air- and bone-conduction stimuli. *Ear and Hearing.*

Small, S. A., & Stapells, D. R. (submitted). Maturation of bone-conduction multiple steady-state responses. Manuscript submitted for publication.

Sohmer, H. (2006). Sound induced fluid pressures directly activate vestibular hair cells: Implications for activation of the cochlea. *Clinical Neurophysiology, 117,* 933–934.

Stapells, D. R. (2000). Frequency-specific evoked potential audiometry in infants. In R. C. Seewald (Ed.), *A sound foundation through early amplification* (pp. 13–31). Basel: Phonak AG.

Stapells, D. R., Herdman, A., Small, S. A., Dimitrijevic, A., & Hatton, J. (2005). Current status of the auditory steady-state responses for estimating an infant's audiogram. In R. C. Seewald & J. M. Bamford (Eds.), *A sound foundation through early amplification: Proceedings of an international conference* (pp. 43–59). Stafa, Switzerland: Phonak AG.

Stapells, D. R., & Oates, P. (1997). Estimation of the pure-tone audiogram by the auditory brainstem response: A review. *Audiology & Neuro-otology 2,* 257–280.

Stapells, D. R., & Ruben, R. J. (1989). Auditory brain stem responses to bone-conducted tones in infants. *Annals of Otology, Rhinology, and Laryngology, 98,* 941–949.

Stuart, A., Yang, E. Y., & Botea, M. (1996). Neonatal auditory brainstem responses recorded from four electrode montages. *Journal of Communication Disorders, 29,* 125–139.

Stuart, A., Yang E. Y., & Stenstrom, R. (1990). Effect of temporal area bone vibrator placement on auditory brain stem response in newborn infants. *Ear and Hearing 11,* 363–369.

Tonndorf, J. (1966). Bone conduction: Studies in experimental animals. *Acta Oto-laryngologica. Supplementum, 213,* 1–132.

Todd, N. P., Rosengren, S. M., & Colebatch, J. G. (2003). A short latency vestibular evoked potential potential (VsEP) produced by bone-conducted acoustic stimulation. *Journal of the Acoustical Society of America*, *114*, 3264–3272.

Townsend, G. L., & Cody, D. (1971). The averaged inion response evoked by acoustic stimulation: Its relation to the saccule. *Annals of Otology*, *80*, 121–132.

von Békésy, G. (1935). Uber Akustische Reizung des Vestibularapparates. *Archiv für die gemaste Physiologie des Menschen und der Tiere*, *236*, 59–76.

van der Reijden, C. S., Mens, L. H., & Snik, A. F. (2005). EEG derivations providing auditory steady-state responses with high signal-to-noise ratios in infants. *Ear and Hearing*, *26*(3), 299–309.

Voss, S. E., & Herrmann, B. S. (2005). How does the sound pressure generated by circumaural, supraural, and insert earphones differ for adult and infant ears? *Ear and Hearing*, *26*, 636–650.

Webb, K. C., & Greenberg, H. J. (1983). Bone-conduction masking for threshold assessment in auditory brainstem response testing. *Ear and Hearing*, *4*(5), 261–266.

Wilber, L. A. (1979). Pure-tone audiometry: Air and bone conduction. In W. F. Rintelmann (Ed.), *Hearing assessment* (pp. 27–42). Baltimore: University Park Press.

Yang, E. Y., & Stuart, A. (1990). A method of auditory brainstem response testing of infants using bone-conducted clicks. *Journal of Speech-Language Pathology and Audiology 14*, 69–76.

Yang, E. Y., & Stuart, A. (2000). The contribution of the auditory brainstem responses to bone-conducted stimuli in newborn hearing screening. *Journal of Speech Language Pathology and Audiology*, *24*, 84–91.

Yang, E. Y., Stuart, A., Stenstrom M. A., & Hollett, S. (1991). Effect of vibrator to head coupling force on the auditory brain stem response to bone-conducted clicks in newborn infants. *Ear and Hearing 12*, 55–60.

Yang, E. Y., Rupert, A. L., & Moushegian, G. (1987). A developmental study of bone conduction auditory brainstem responses in infants. *Ear and Hearing 8*, 244–251.

Ysunza, A., & Cone-Wesson, B. (1987). Bone conduction masking for brainstem auditory-evoked potentials (BAEP) in pediatric audiological evaluations. Validation of the test. *International Journal of Pediatric Otorhinolaryngology*, *12*, 291–302.

CHAPTER 12

Auditory Steady-State Responses and Suprathreshold Tests of Auditory Ability

ANDREW DIMITRIJEVIC
BARBARA CONE-WESSON

The vast majority of auditory steady-state response (ASSR)-related research studies in the past 30 plus years have examined pure-tone threshold estimation. Although this is an extremely valuable aspect of clinical application of ASSRs, more recent work over the past several years has revealed that we need not limit ourselves to pure-tone thresholds. A separate area of ASSR research has begun to emerge in which *suprathreshold* measures of hearing function, such as speech audiometry, and temporal processing are being investigated. This chapter provides a brief review of these novel applications of ASSRs.

Speech Audiometry

"Audiologic tests using speech stimuli are essential . . . because speech represents a class of sounds most important to effective daily communication. Results from routine pure tone tests often do not reflect either the potential or the limitations in receptive auditory communication of adults and children with hearing loss" (Olsen & Matkin, 1991).

There are two main categories of speech audiometry: (1) the determination of sensitivity for speech and

(2) suprathreshold measures of speech recognition. The former usually are referred to as speech (or word) recognition thresholds (SRTs), and the latter as word (or phoneme) recognition tests. SRTs can be estimated from the pure-tone threshold, using the average thresholds at 500, 1000, and 2000 Hz. Given that ASSRs can be used to estimate threshold at these frequencies, it is logical to assume that the SRT also could be estimated from ASSRs. Although this has been empirically demonstrated for click-evoked auditory brainstem responses (ABRs) (Sininger & Cone-Wesson, 2001), it has not yet been shown for ASSRs.

Word recognition tests are given to estimate the amount of speech information (word or phoneme) that a subject can understand. In clinical procedures, a list of words is read to the patient, and the score is determined as the percentage of correct words (or phonemes) repeated. A *performance-intensity* (P-I) function also can be determined in which the percentage score is plotted as a function of presentation level. The slope and asymptote of the P-I function provide information regarding the possible etiology of the hearing loss (conductive, sensorineural, or neural) and information that may be helpful for fitting amplification.

Is it possible to gain an estimate of word recognition ability or the performance intensity function from ASSRs? A number of potential ASSR-based approaches exist for this type of speech audiometry. One approach may be simply to multiply an ongoing speech waveform with an AM envelope (at 80 or 40 Hz). Using this approach, it is conceivable that speech ASSRs could be recorded at the AM envelope rate. It is difficult, however, to tell how much the response is specifically related to speech processing, rather than

just acoustic "envelope following," a concept described later in the chapter (T. W. Picton, personal communication, 2007). Another approach has been to record ASSRs to the natural "steady-state" portions of vowel stimuli. Speech acoustic elements also can be modeled as tonal modulations in the 40- and 80-Hz range. Both of these approaches are discussed next.

Auditory Steady-State Responses for Steady-State Vowels

Dajani, Purcell, Wong, Kunov, and Picton (2005) demonstrated a method for obtaining steady-state responses to slight variations in the fundamental frequency (F0) of the vowel sound /a/. The stimulus token was a 2-s recording of /a/, spoken by a male voice, with an F0 of 165 Hz. A second stimulus, in which the F0 was suppressed (using a high-pass filter), leaving only formants remaining, also was used to test seven normally hearing subjects.

Several signal processing methods, including development of a fine-structure spectrogram, were used to extract the "pitch contour"—characterized by small frequency fluctuations in the acoustic waveform (usually less than 5 Hz)—from the averaged evoked response. The averaged response showed a strong signal at the F0, along with those at the first formant. There also was a significant response to the pitch contour.

These results showed that some slight pitch (frequency) variations are evident in the neural response to vowels. This response was present even when the F0 was filtered out—that is, there was a response to the "missing fundamental." The investigators suggested that these neural responses to the pitch contour of a vowel may be useful in evaluating peripheral (cochlear and brainstem) mechanisms of vowel pitch perception. Because the response to the F0 probably was due to phase-locking responses of brainstem neurons, it also was suggested that the response might be used to evaluate brainstem temporal processing deficits that may occur in elderly persons, affecting speech perception. Neural phase-locking, the ability of auditory nerve and brainstem neurons to respond at a characteristic "phase" of a stimulus, provides a mechanism for pitch perception in the low and middle frequencies. Thus, it is implicated in measures of low- to mid-frequency sensitivity and the perception of pitch, and also of the F0, and possibly even F1, and F2. Because vowels are identified on the basis of their formant structure, accurate phase-locking would enhance vowel perception. Steady-state responses that follow the acoustic amplitude envelope of the vowel also have been obtained (Aiken & Picton, 2006). The vowel tokens /i/, /a/, and /u/ were used to evoke the response, and these had little variation in F0. In a second experiment, the vowel /^/ was used, with intentional pitch variation, to evoke this envelope following response (EFR). In a third experiment, three contiguous vowels, /^/, /u/, and /i/, were presented. Finally, the effects of vowel bandwidth on EFR responses were evaluated.

As in Dajani and coworkers' (2005) study, considerable signal processing was used to extract the EFR to the vowel tokens. Strong responses were obtained to the F0 of each vowel. Responses to the vowel formants (that is, integral multiples of the F0), F1, F2, and F3 also were present. The spectral analysis used also was able to detect the responses to the changing F0, a characteristic of natural speech, of the vowel /^/ used in the second experiment. When three contiguous vowels were used, responses were present at the F0, also, the responses varied in amplitude according to the type of vowel. The investigators suggested that the formant structure (i.e., placement of formants relative to one another) and the phase of the formants would have an effect on the amplitude of the EFR, thereby contributing to vowel identity at the neural level.

These two studies provided signal processing methodologies (frequency domain analyses) for for extracting information about the (brainstem) neural response to vowel components (i.e., F0 and formants) and vowel type. The investigators used natural (as opposed to synthesized) speech tokens as stimuli, encompassing the natural variation in vowel pitch. The techniques developed and demonstrated in these papers hurdled some substantial technical barriers. There is a growing and body of work on the clinical relevance of brainstem evoked responses to speech (Cunningham, Nicol, Zecker, & Kraus, 2000; Cunningham, Nicol, Zecker, Bradlow, & Kraus, 2001) and also their implications for speech reception (Galbraith et al., 2004; Krishnan, Xu, Gandour, & Carriani, 2004). Aiken and Picton (2006) discuss the implications of their work in terms of developing an objective method for assessing the benefits of amplification for speech perception. It is possible that these EFRs for hearing aid–amplified vowels could be used to demonstrate how amplification improved the neural representation of the vowel pitch contour, thereby resulting in improved vowel perception.

Modeled Speech: Independent Amplitude and Frequency Modulation

Natural speech is a complex acoustic waveform that contains inherent AM and FM properties. As described in Chapter 3, ASSRs can be recorded to AM and FM modulations of a pure tone. Therefore, the basic idea is that AM- and FM-elicited ASSRs may relate to a subject's ability to perceive speech. An important point, however, is that assessment of these ASSRs will not measure speech perception per se but rather examine the initial stages of acoustic processing that are required for speech perception. Perception of speech is a very complex process involving coordinated efforts between multiple brain regions (Hickok & Poeppel, 2004). As noted in Chapter 4, the neural generators of 80 and 40 Hz ASSRs are the brainstem and auditory cortex, respectively. Therefore, recordings of responses that are primarily generated in relatively early stages in the auditory pathway cannot encompass the complex cortico-cortical interactions necessary for speech perception. Tonal AM and FM stimuli do not "sound" like speech and do not activate the same complex auditory pathway involved in speech perception. Nonetheless, if there are problems in this early stage of processing, we most likely will observe deficits more "upstream" from brainstem and auditory cortex.

The first study examining speech audiometry and ASSRs was performed by Dimitrijevic, John, Van Roon, and Picton (2001). In that study, multiple *independent amplitude and frequency modulation (IAFM)* stimuli were used (see Chapter 3). The nature of the IAFM stim-ulus is such that there are two modulation rates per carrier frequency. One modulation rate is for AM, and the other modulation rate is for FM. Therefore, although the same carrier is used, two ASSR responses are elicited, one for AM and one for FM. With the multiple IAFM stimuli used in Dimitrijevic and coworkers' 2001 study, four carriers with the IAFM were examined, and therefore eight potential responses could be elicited (four AM and four FM). The depths of the AM and FM were set at 50% and 20%, respectively, and this was a reasonable estimation of AM and FM in speech. Carrier frequencies spanning speech frequencies of 500 to 4000 Hz were presented at equal intensity. The relationship between monosyllabic word recognition as a function of level (i.e., performance intensity function) and ASSRs was examined by presenting IAFM stimuli at intensities ranging from 20 to 70 dB SPL, as well as determining word recognition scores at the same intensities. Correlations between ASSRs and word recognition were carried out in multiple ways. The amplitudes of the AM and FM components (both alone and summed together) showed a statistically significant relationship with word recognition (ranging from 0.38 to 0.71, $P < .05$). The relationship with FM amplitudes and word recognition was better than for AM. When all of the amplitudes for all the carrier frequencies (AM and FM separate) were combined, correlations improved compared with when compared to single frequencies. This inherently makes sense because speech is made up of multiple stimuli, and combing responses across all carrier frequencies relates to more "real" speech.

One potential drawback of using ASSR amplitude data in this type of analysis is that such data are variable. An electrically recorded response (as opposed to magnetic responses) will vary with volume conduction. In other words, different people with different head sizes and skull thicknesses will show different ASSR amplitudes that are not at all related to auditory processing but rather differences due to current flow through the brain and skull. There are two potential solutions to this problem. One is to measure a reference ASSR (for example, an ASSR in response to 1000 Hz modulated at 80 Hz) and use this ASSR amplitude as a baseline for normalization of all other IAFM responses. Using this approach, it may be possible to "cancel" intersubject volume conduction differences. Another approach is to measure the presence or absence of a response. This type of measure will not vary across subjects (assuming that the signal-to-noise ratios are comparable). Using this response present–response absent method, Dimitrijevic and coworkers (2001) found correlations with word recognition scores were the highest (0.74; $P < .05$). One important caveat with this first study is that audibility plays an important role in both word recognition and ASSRs. Therefore, it is possible that some relationships between word recognition and ASSRs may have been due to level (because both were measured at increasing levels). Even controlling for the effects of level by way of partial correlations, however, significant relationships still existed.

The second study examining IAFM and word recognition (Dimitrijevic, John, & Picton, 2004) used stimuli constructed to more closely resemble the acoustics of normal speech. This was done in a number of ways. First, the depths of FM and AM were based on an extensive speech acoustics literature survey. The depth of FM was based on frequency changes for consonant-vowel and vowel-vowel transitions taken from the literature. Figure 12–1a illustrates an example used in the derivation. Similarly for AM, relative changes in amplitude were used derive AM estimates. This process is shown in Figure 12–1b. Another aspect of IAFM that was modeled after speech was the long-term speech spectra (LTSS). The LTSS shows that lower frequencies (associated with vowels) often are 30 to 40 dB louder than high frequencies (associated with fricatives). The IAFM stimuli therefore reflected relative amplitudes (across speech frequencies) for high and low frequencies (Figure 12–2). The IAFM stimuli were modulated at 40 and 80 Hz. It would have been ideal to go even lower (below 20 Hz) because most of the most speech envelope is in this range. ASSRs at this modulation rate, however, are particularly prone to noise compared with those at the higher modulation rates. Nonetheless, consonant-vowel transitions can have durations of 5 to 50 ms, resulting in effective modulation rates of 20 to 200 Hz (Blumstein & Stevens, 1980; Ohde & Abou-Khalil, 2001). Using 40- and 80-Hz modulation rates will encompass the modulation rate of most of these consonant-vowel transitions and also evoke neural responses from the brainstem and cortex (Chapter 4). The carrier frequencies also were based on mean formant frequencies and fricatives and accordingly the carrier frequencies were 500, 1500, 2500, and 4000 Hz. The experimental paradigm also was varied. In the original IAFM study, word recognition and IAFM were presented at levels varying from 20 to 70 dB SPL, whereas in the follow-up study, audibility was decreased by the use of speech

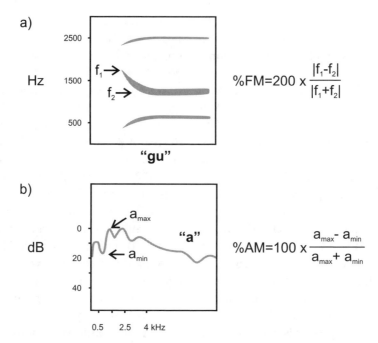

Figure 12–1. Sample derivations of the IAFM stimulus parameters using real speech. **a.,** Depth of FM using the consonant-vowel "gu." A spectrogram of "gu" shows the change in frequency over time. The change in frequency is shown in the *gray lines* for each formant. The initial frequency f_1 and final frequency f_2 illustrate the range of frequencies used for the second formant. The equation on the *right* illustrates how these changes in frequency can be used to derive the depth of FM. **b.,** Depth of AM using the vowel "a." The plot shows the amplitude as a function of frequency. Peaks (a_{max}) and valleys (a_{min}) are used to calculate the depth of AM.

noise maskers. Additionally, whereas the original study used only young, normal-hearing subjects, the follow-up study used young, normally hearing, elderly normal-hearing, and elderly hearing-impaired subjects. The correlations between word recognition and IAFM were improved compared with those in the original study (Figure 12–3). ASSR amplitude correlations were at 0.39 to 0.77, and the response presence–response correlations ranged from 0.65 to 0.85. The use of the novel stimuli improved

the relationship between ASSRs and word recognition scores; however, the correlations obtained, although statistically significant, do not yet appear to be robust enough to guide hearing aid fitting protocols for individual listeners. Nevertheless, the approach has great theoretical and practical implications. Cone-Wesson and Garinis (2005) and Alaerts, Luts, Van Dun, and Wouters (2007) also report on the use of suprathreshold ASSR to predict speech perception abilities. Cone-Wesson and coworkers used IAFM

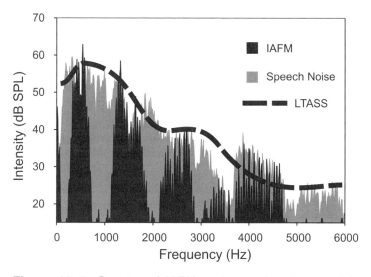

Figure 12–2. Spectra of IAFM and speech noise used in the study by Dimitrijevic and colleagues (2004). The *black-shaded area* shows the spectra of IAFM stimulus. Note the four prominent bands, each representing the formants using the modeled carriers. The *gray shading* shows the spectra of speech noise. The *black dotted line* shows the long-term average speech spectra (LTASS).

stimuli similar to those used by Dimitrijevic and colleagues (2004) to obtain ASSRs from infants aged 5 to 13 months. They plotted the "percent of responses present" as a function of stimulus level (20 to 70 dB SPL). They also obtained behavioural measures of speech feature discrimination, by measuring the infants' ability to detect a change in a consonant-vowel token /ba/ versus /da/ (place-of-articulation) and /ba/ versus /sa/ (manner). They found that the average response present function for the 1500 Hz carrier had a correspondence with the average speech-feature discrimination function. They interpreted this finding as indicative of the importance of frequency information in the region of the second formant transition, which is near 1500 Hz, for the discrimination of place and manner cues.

Alaerts and colleagues (2007) compared ASSRs for speech-modulated noise presented in stationary noise to the ability of normal hearing adults and those with hearing loss to perceive speech in noise. The ASSRs were obtained using modulation rates of 4, 10, 20, and 38 Hz at signal-to-noise ratios of −10, −5, 0, and +5 dB. Speech perception tests used sentence materials, presented in stationary and fluctuating noise, and and word recognition tests, presented in stationary noise. Correlations between the 20- and 38-Hz ASSR signal-to-noise ratio and speech perception scores ranged from 0.64 to 0.80, with *P* values ranging from less than 0.01 to 0.05. These findings suggest that the brainstem and cortical neural substrates reflected in the ASSRs also may be used in speech-in-noise perception abilities.

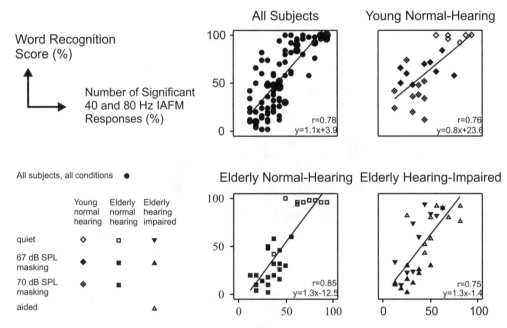

Figure 12–3. Correlations between IAFM and word discrimination found in the study by Dimitrijevic and colleagues (2004). The number of significant responses (percentage of 16) are plotted on the x-axis, and the y-axis shows the word discrimination score. The *top left plot* shows the relationship pooled across all subjects (the size of the circle is related to the number of overlapping data points). The *top right plot* shows the IAMF-word discrimination relationship in the young normal hearing population. The *bottom left* and *right plots* show the relationship in elderly normal-hearing and hearing-impaired populations, respectively.

Temporal Processing

The ability to process temporal cues in speech or music is an important part of everyday listening. Shannon, Zeng, Klamath, Wygonski, and Ekelid (1995) demonstrated that speech understanding is possible while listening to only the temporal envelope of speech without any spectral cues. Processes that disrupt temporal processing and temporal acuity such as sensorineural hearing loss, aging or auditory neuropathy (Zeng, Kong, Michalewski, & Starr, 2005) will disrupt speech perception abilities. These deficits can be measured psychoacoustically using techniques such as gap detection, or temporal modulation transfer functions (TMTFs) (Viemeister & Plack, 1993). Gap detection often is measured as the smallest duration needed to detect a pause in white noise or a pure tone. Temporal modulation transfer functions measure the ability to detect modulation both as a function of depth and rate (Viemeister & Plack). TMTFs indicate the just detectable modulation depth (expressed as 20 log m, where m varies from 0 to 1.0) as a function of modulation frequency (in Hz). The TMTF expresses the highest modulation frequency at which the auditory pathway can no longer accurately encode amplitude changes in the signal.

The auditory system is more sensitive to amplitude change (modulation) for lower modulation frequencies (up to 80 Hz or so) and then this sensitivity is reduced dramatically. In listeners with temporal processing difficulties (e.g., auditory neuropathy) the TMTF is abnormal. Although these psychoacoustic measures provide good correspondence with speech understanding, they do require active cooperation of the subject and therefore are problematic in attempts to test infants or cognitively impaired persons. The following discussion explains how auditory steady state responses can potentially overcome these issues.

In developing the TMTF, the modulation rate is varied and the listener is asked to make a detection of the modulated stimulus. To estimate the TMTF electrophysiologically, ASSRs to many different modulations must be recorded. This would be a very laborious task indeed. Fortunately, borrowing techniques from visual steady-state research (Regan, 1989), an investigator can gradually sweep through various parameters such level or modulation rate (Linden, Campbell, Hamel, & Picton, 1985). Sweeping (or ramping) basically means that a stimulus parameter can be slowly changed and the evoked response examined as a function of that parameter. Technically, these responses are not ASSRs because the latter's "steady-state" aspect implies that the stimulus is not changing; rather, these responses to ramped or swept stimuli have been called *envelope following responses* (EFRs) (Purcell, John, Schneider, & Picton, 2004).

Purcell and coworkers (2004) used a white noise stimulus that swept in modulation rate from 20 to 600 Hz at a depth of 25%. The sweep (one cycle) occurred over a period of 30 seconds; during the first 15 seconds, the modulation rate slowly and linearly increased to a maximum, and then the second 15-second interval decreased in modulation rate to the starting modulation rate. This enabled averages of the first and second halves of the stimulus. The EFR was recorded for 50 to 100 of these ramped stimuli in each subject. The carrier was white noise modulated at 25%. The stimulus was presented at suprathreshold levels at 60 dB SPL. In addition to recording these EFRs, the investigators also carried out psychophysical measures of gap detection and modulation detection using white noise carriers. Two subject populations were used: young and elderly normal-hearing listeners. The EFRs showed local peaks near 40 and 80 Hz (see Chapter 4) and continued to decrease thereafter. The highest modulation rate eliciting a statically significant response (i.e., response-to-noise ratio meeting a predefined criterion) was used for the correlation with psychophysical data. Significant correlations with gap detection ($r = -0.43$) and with modulation detection ($r = 0.72$) were noted. Very little overlap was observed between the two populations with respect to the the highest modulation rate that evoked a significant EFR. This evidence confirms previous work by Snell (1997) in which elderly listeners demonstrated poorer temporal acuity.

Cone-Wesson, Garinis, Varrichio, and Wong (2007) attempted to correlate suprathreshold ASSRs for amplitude-modulated tones that varied in modulation depth, with detection of modulation. Infant subjects were tested using modulation depths of 100%, 50%, 20%, and 10% at rates of near 80 Hz. A control group of adults was tested with these stimuli, and also with stimuli modulated at the same depth, but using rates near 40 Hz. Infants and adults also performed a modulation detection task in which they were taught to discriminate between modulated and unmodulated tones. ASSR thresholds increased and amplitudes decreased with decreasing modulation depths, whereas behavioural modulation detection was constant for detection of 100%, 50%, and 20% modulations. There appeared to be little correspondence between ASSR amplitude or threshold and modulation detection abilities.

Summary

ASSRs (or EFRs) can be evoked by speech-modeled IAFM tones and natural vowel segments, and as a function of modulation rate and depth. Tests using these stimuli presented at a suprathreshold level are still the domain of the research laboratory. The findings from the laboratory suggest that the ASSRs contain information about neural representations of vowel pitch and formants (Aiken & Picton, 2006; Dalmani et al., 2005), and about neural correlates of sensitivity for AM and FM used in phoneme perception (Cone-Wesson et al., 2005; Dimitrijevic et al., 2001, 2004) and for perception of speech in noise (Alaerts et al., 2007). Temporal processing abilities are fundamental to speech understanding and can be disrupted by neural-type hearing loss, such as found in elderly persons, or those with auditory neuropathy. ASSRs may be used to assay an aspect of temporal processing, the TMTF, by using "ramped" modulated noise (Purcell et al., 2004).

Audiologic assessment is more than pure-tone audiometry. Audiologic assessment involves assessment of speech perception in quiet and in noise, and increasingly, of "central auditory processing" abilities that may inform clinicians regarding rehabilitation, including the provision of hearing aids. Auditory evoked potentials from the brainstem and cortex, including those evoked by modulated tones, noise, or vowels, should eventually provide clinicians with information about the underlying neural integrity for speech understanding and temporal processing.

References

Alaerts, J., Luts, H., Van Dun, B., & Wouters, J. (2007). *Evaluating speech understanding by means of suprathreshold ASSR.* International Evoked Response Audiometry Study Group, XX Biennial Symposium, June 10–14, Bled, Slovenia.

Aiken, S. J., & Picton, T. W. (2006). Envelope following responses to natural vowels. *Audiology and Neurotology, 11,* 213–232.

Blumstein, S. E., & Stevens, K. N. (1980). Perceptual invariance and onset spectra for stop consonants in different vowel environments. *Journal of the Acoustical Society of America, 67*(2), 648–662.

Cone-Wesson, B., & Garinis A. (2005). *Infant ASSRs and speech feature discrimination.* International Evoked Response Audiometry Study Group, XIX Biennial Symposium, June 12–16, Havana, Cuba.

Cone-Wesson, B., Garinis, A., Varrichio, S., & Wong, A. (2007). *Infant ASSR and the detection of amplitude modulation.* International Evoked Response Audiometry Study Group, XX Biennial Symposium, June 10–14, Bled, Slovenia.

Cunningham, J., Nicol, T., Zecker, S., Bradlow, A., & Kraus, N. (2001). Neurobiologic responses to speech in noise in children with learning problems: deficits and strategies for improvement. *Clinical Neurophysiology, 112,* 758–767.

Cunningham, J., Nicol, T., Zecker, S., & Kraus, N. (2000). Speech-evoked neurophysiologic responses in children with learning problems: Development and behavioral correlates of perception. *Hearing Research, 21*, 554–568.

Dajani, H. R., Purcell, D., Wong, W., Kunov, H., & Picton, T. W. (2005). Recording human evoked potentials that follow the pitch contour of a natural vowel. *IEEE Transactions on Biomedical Engineering, 52*(9), 1614–1618.

Dimitrijevic, A., John, M. S., van Roon, P., & Picton, T. W. (2001). Human auditory steady-state responses to tones independently modulated in both frequency and amplitude. *Ear and Hearing, 22*(2), 100–111.

Dimitrijevic, A., John, M. S., & Picton, T. W. (2004). Auditory steady-state responses and word recognition scores in normal-hearing and hearing-impaired adults. *Ear and Hearing, 25*(1), 68–84.

Galbraith, G. C., Amaya, E. M., de Rivera, J. M., Donan, N. M., Duong, M. T., Hsu, J. N., et al. (2004). Brain stem evoked response to forward and reversed speech in humans. *Neuroreport, 15*, 2057–2060.

Hickok, G., & Poeppel, D. (2004). Dorsal and ventral streams: A framework for understanding aspects of the functional anatomy of language. *Cognition, 92*(1–2), 67–99.

Krishnan, A., Xu, Y., Gandour, J. T., & Cariani, P. A. (2004). Human frequency-following responses: representation of pitch contours in Chinese tones. *Hearing Research, 189*, 1–12.

Linden, R. D., Campbell, K. B., Hamel, G., & Picton, T. W. (1985). Human auditory steady state evoked potentials during sleep. *Ear and Hearing, 6*(3), 167–174.

Moore, B. C. J. (2003). *An introduction to the psychology of hearing* (5th ed.). New York: Elsevier.

Olsen, W. O., & Matkin, N. D. (1991). Speech audiometry. In W. F. Rintelmann (Ed.), *Hearing assessment* (2nd ed., pp. 39–140). Austin, TX: Pro-Ed.

Ohde, R. N., & Abou-Khalil, R. (2001). Age differences for stop-consonant and vowel perceptions in adults. *Journal of the Acoustical Society of America, 110*(4), 2156–2166.

Purcell, D. W., John, S. M., Schneider, B. A., & Picton, T. W. (2004). Human temporal auditory acuity as assessed by envelope following responses. *Journal of the Acoustical Society of America, 116*(6), 3581–3593.

Regan, D. (1989). *Human brain electrophysiology: Evoked potentials and evoked magnetic fields in science and medicine.* New York: Elsevier.

Shannon, R. V., Zeng, F. G., Kamath, V., Wygonski, J., & Ekelid, M. (1995). Speech recognition with primarily temporal cues. *Science, 270*(5234), 303–304.

Sininger, Y. S., & Cone-Wesson, B. (2002). Threshold prediction using auditory brainstem response and steady-state evoked potentials with infants and young children. In J. Katz, R. F. Burkard, & L. Medwetsky (Eds.), *Handbook of clinical audiology* (pp. 298–322). Philadelphia: Lippincott Williams & Wilkins.

Snell, K. B. (1997). Age-related changes in temporal gap detection. *Journal of the Acoustical Society of America, 101*(4), 2214–2220.

Viemeister, N. F., & Plack, C. J. (1993). Time analysis. In W. A. Yost, N. Popper, & R. R. Fay (Eds.), *Human psychophysics*. New York: Springer-Verlag.

Zeng, F. G., Kong, Y. Y., Michalewski, H. J., & Starr, A. (2005). Perceptual consequences of disrupted auditory nerve activity. *Journal of Neurophysiology, 93*(6), 3050–3063.

CHAPTER 13

Auditory Steady-State Responses and Hearing Device Fitting

Part A
The Role of Auditory Steady-State Responses in Fitting Hearing Aids

FRANZ ZENKER-CASTRO
JOSÉ JUAN BARAJAS DE PRAT

The advent of universal hearing screening programs has ensured early detection of hearing impairment at birth. This involves the fitting of hearing aids at the earliest stage possible. Hearing aid fittings constitute the most frequent method of hearing impairment habilitation in newborns and very young infants. Early hearing aid fitting in infants contributes to acquisition and development of oral language. For this reason, it is important to have hearing aid fitting protocols specifically designed for very young infants.

These protocols will be dependent on electrophysiological methods, because behavioural audiometry is not viable until the age of 5 to 6 months and, in some infants or young children with developmental delay, not possible at all.

In infants and in the adult population, hearing aid fitting consists of three stages: the assessment of hearing sensitivity, the selection of adjustment parameters to restore the hearing perception, and the verification of the prescribed gain for each patient (Scolie & Seewald, 2001).

241

Assessing hearing implies the establishment of hearing thresholds and maximum comfort and discomfort levels at different frequencies for each ear independently. The prescription of adjustment parameters requires the establishment of the gain in such a way that the speech spectrum (Cornelisee, Gagné, & Seewald, 1991; Zenker, Delgado, & Barajas, 2003) is amplified within the dynamic hearing range of the patient (Cornelisse, Seewald, & Jamieson, 1995; Zenker & Barajas, 1999). Finally, the verification of amplification allows the clinician to check that the objectives set in the prescription of adjustment parameters have been achieved (Stelmanchiwiccz, Kopun, Mace, Lewis, & Nittrouer, 1995).

For certain difficult-to-test populations, hearing thresholds can be obtained only through electrophysiological measures that do not require any voluntary response from the individual (Goldstein & Aldrich, 1999). Moreover, electrophysiological tests can assist those involved in the adaptation of hearing aids, because these tests can measure auditory function objectively (Picton et al., 2002). Assessment of auditory steady-state responses (ASSRs) provides a quick and objective way to establish electrophysiological hearing thresholds at different frequencies. The ASSRs have several advantages in their application in hearing aid fitting: First, they provide assessment of hearing thresholds at different frequencies. Second, from these measurements it is possible to infer the adjustment parameters of hearing aid devices. Third, the acoustic characteristics of the ASSR's stimuli allow verification that the hearing aid is functioning and that the subject perceives and discriminates sounds at a brain level (Picton et al., 2002).

Recent studies (Cone-Wesson, Parker, Swiderski, & Rickards, 2002; Picton et al., 1998; Zenker, Fernández, & Barajas, 2006) have proposed that assessment of auditory evoked potentials, and specifically ASSRs, could serve as an useful tool in the fitting and verification of the function of hearing aids. The application of electrophysiological techniques in hearing aid fitting requires measures of (1) the stimuli, (2) the acoustic characteristics of external auditory canal, and (3) the frequency-specific hearing threshold assessment. These aspects are reviewed in the following sections.

Estimating Pure-Tone Audiometric Threshold Through Auditory Evoked Potentials

Hearing aid amplification is based on the individual characteristics of each patient. In this regard, individual amplification is established by gain prescription methods. Cornelisse and colleagues (1995) defined this prescription process as "a function that prescribes hearing devices' gain at different frequencies related to the patient's audiometric values." The first gain prescription methods were established by Watson and Knudsen (1940) and later by Lybarger (1944). At present, prescription methods can be provided either by hearing aid manufacturers or through independent procedures such as the "Desired Sensation Level" (Seewald, Ross, & Spiro, 1985) or the National Acoustic Laboratory approach (Byrne & Tonnisson, 1976).

The manufacturer modules for fitting hearing aids require knowledge of the patient's hearing sensitivity. Once this information is obtained from electrophysiological procedures, an estimation of behavioural thresholds must be carried out. In the case of ASSRs, the estimation of hearing thresholds can be inflenced by certain measurement conditions such as the stimulus frequency, the degree of hearing loss, the age of the subject, and the duration of the electrophysiological test. Some studies indicate that the physiological thresholds may be more accurate in hearing-impaired individuals than in normal-hearing subjects (Dimitrijevic et al., 2002; Rance & Briggs, 2002). Two main procedures are used to estimate audiogram thresholds: The first consists of obtaining the average difference between ASSRs and behavioural thresholds; the second procedure consists of determining the regression function between the physiological and the psychoacoustic thresholds for different values of hearing loss (Rance & Briggs, 2002; Rance et al., 1995). The ways in which behavioural hearing thresholds can be predicted from ASSR findings are discussed in detail in Chapter 7.

Frequency Specificity

The adjustment of hearing aids requires frequency specific information at hearing threshold level. The thresholds obtained from the ASSR are at least as accurate and have the same frequency-specificity as that for tone-burst evoked auditory brainstem responses (ABRs) (Herdman, Picton, & Stapells, 2002). Moreover, they offer the advantage that thresholds for several carrier frequencies can can be measured simultaneously (Lins & Picton,

1995). Up to eight thresholds can be obtained in a significantly shorter time than is typical with use of techniques based on sequential testing using one stimulus at a time (John et al., 2002).

Stimulus Calibration

The prescription of amplification from behavioural testing must take into account the calibration of the stimuli employed. In this regard, electrophysiological and behavioural responses can significantly differ for the same patient. These dissimilarities can be ascribed to differences in the type of stimulus and physiological generators involved in the detection of tone.

Modulated tones used during ASSR testing are similar to warble tones used in behavioural testing (Rance et al., 1998). This implies that calibration corrections associated with tone burst and clicks (used for ABR) are not required, and the stimuli can therefore be presented at levels that extend to 120 dB HL. Calibration of ASSR stimuli can be carried out with the same standards used for pure tones employed in audiometers. This procedure makes it possible to obtain the thresholds in dB HL and thereby to directly introduce these values into hcaring aid fitting modules. It should be noted that the values used in hearing aid fitting algorithms are based on behavioural thresholds. An additional step, therefore, is needed to convert the ASSR thresholds (in dB HL) to estimated behavioural thresholds (also in dB HL). This can be done by using regression formulas or correction factors. These methods and their benefits and limitations are reviewed in Chapter 7.

Ear Canal Acoustics

Sininger and coworkers (1997) have demonstrated that part of the differences found between the physiological and behavioural thresholds in infants and adults may be due to the large ear canal resonances associated with small infant ear canals. The effect of the ear canal resonance on the gain prescription of the hearing aid can be minimized by the measurement of the real ear to couple difference (RECD). Bagatto and associates (2005) proposed the following equation to obtain the finally estimated dB SPL thresholds at the ear canal level.

dB SPL threshold (ear canal level) = dB HL threshold + insert earphone RETSPL + RECD

Table 13-1 provides an example of how hearing threshold, in dB SPL, is calculated from ASSR threshold. In this case, the estimated behavioural thresholds at the eardrum in dB HL can be converted into dB SPL by using the *real-ear coupler-difference* (RECD) plus the *reference equivalent threshold sound pressure levels*

(RETSPLS) according to ANSI S3.6-1996. In the example case, values reflect the RECD for a newborn 6 months of age.

Applications of Auditory Evoked Potentials in Hearing Device Fittings

Several studies have proposed the application of electrophysiological techniques at the different stages of hearing aid fittings. An essential contribution of the electrophysiological technique consists of the verification of the prescribed gain and the calculations of the adjustment parameters of the hearing aid derived from the amplitude or latency of the AEPs.

The Amplitude Projection Procedure

Kiessling (1982, 1983) published several articles describing the clinical applications of the ABRs in hearing aid fitting. He established an objective method based on the amplitude of the ABR especially indicated for noncooperative subjects

Table 13–1. Example worksheet to calculate the hearing threshold, in dB SPL, at the ear canal from the ASSR thresholds in dB HL

	500 Hz	1000 Hz	2000 Hz	4000 Hz
Thresholds (dB HL) (estimated from ASSR)	40.0	45.0	45.0	50.0
RECD	6.0	13.0	14.0	18.0
RETSPL correction	5.5	0.0	3.0	5.5
dB SPL threshold (ear canal)	51.5	58.0	62.0	73.5

and infants with multiple disabilities. The *amplitude projection procedure* (APP) is an attempt to establish the adjustment parameters of hearing aids such as the dynamic range, gain, or compression factor. These parameters are derived from the wave V amplitude intensity function of the ABRs. The methodology is based on the assumption proposed, and never demonstrated, by Kiessling, that wave V amplitude of the ABR correlates with the sensation of loudness. The steepness of the amplitude intensity function of the ABR described the amount of compression needed for a listener with hearing loss. For example, a patient with a severe-to-profound hearing loss will have elevated ABR (or ASSR) thresholds, but the amplitude growth of the response above threshold will be minimal. This would correspond to the limited dynamic range of hearing, that is, the difference between threshold and uncomfortably loud sounds, associated with severe-to-profound hearing loss. In such cases, greater compression would be indicated, compared with that for the patient who has a mild-to-moderate loss, with a considerably greater dynamic range, and who demonstrates some growth of ABR (or ASSR amplitude) over a 30- to 40-dB stimulus range. In a subsequent study, Davidson, Wall, and Goodman (1990) studied the relationship between loudness and the ABR wave V amplitude. In this study, great individual variation in the amplitude was found. As expected, variability was reduced as soon as the number of sessions increased. This is because variability in background EEG noise causes great variability in the ABR amplitude. If background noise levels are held constant (and low), such as by measuring the estimated noise from a statistic like Fsp (Don

et al., 1996), then ABR amplitude data become less variable and more reliable. Davidson and colleagues reported no significant differences in the prescription of the hearing aid gain and compression settings for two out of three hearing-impaired subjects when the APP fitting procedure was compared with conventional prescription methods. Given that hearing aid compression technologies today are much different than those existing in 1990, it may be difficult to replicate this result. Yet the underlying physiological principles are sound: The evoked potential threshold can be used to estimate the amount of gain needed, and the amplitude growth function provides information relevant to the listener's dynamic range of hearing, for which compression can be used as compensation.

Electrophysiological Gain Verification

Functional gain is one of the most used procedures in the verification of the prescribed parameters of hearing aids. Measurement of the amount of functional gain is calculated as the difference between aided and unaided thresholds at each specific frequency obtained through free field testing (Mueller, Hawkins, & Northen, 1992) and is defined as the relative decibel difference between the aided and unaided thresholds. Because this technique is based on voluntary behavioural procedures, the inherent degree of variability to which behavioural thresholds measurements are subjected will also influence functional gain measurements (Mueller et al., 1992). Interaction between the test stimuli, the transducer employed, the hearing aid and the test room acoustics are well known limitations that interfere with the accurate determination of hearing thresholds. Moreover, verifying the hearing aid in the free field does not provide ear specific information. Several attempts have been made in order to reproduce the functional gain test through electrophysiological procedures. Electrophysiology testing has been seen as a procedure that may provide an objective method to verify the adjustment of a hearing aid.

Mokotoff and Krebs (1976) published a pioneer study in which ABR measurements were obtained from adult hearing aid users. Results indicated that aided ABR measurement compared favorably with aided audiological data. Several authors have used the ABR with click or tone burst in order to obtain an objective measurement of the hearing aid response. As described by Mahoney (1985), however, obtaining ABR in the sound field with amplification is a complex issue. In general, the brief nature of the stimulus employed during ABR testing shows high susceptibility to distortion in both: the sound field speaker and the hearing aid amplifier (Hall & Ruth, 1985).

Picton and colleagues (1998) demonstrated that ASSRs can be recorded when multiple stimuli are presented simultaneously through a sound field speaker and amplified with a hearing aid. Therefore, this procedure seems more useful than procedures using transient stimuli. Its application is limited, however, because ASSR cannot provide information regarding how well the nonlinear processing of the hearing aid is benefiting the listener (Picton et al., 2002). Even though ASSR can be used to assess suprathreshold hearing, it does not provide information regarding to how the aided sound is perceived, following processing in the brain (Picton et al., 2002).

Fitting Hearing Aids from the Auditory Steady-State Response Testing

Loudness and Auditory Steady-State Responses

Loudness measurement serves two important clinical functions in audiological practice: to determine the adjustment of hearing aids (Fabry & Schum, 1994) and to distinguish the site-of-lesion in sensorineural hearing loss (Hall, 1991). Subjective judgements of loudness are often obtained to define the *most comfortable level* (MCL) or the *loudness discomfort level* (LDL). Another method often employed is to obtain loudness judgement over a range of stimulus levels providing information on how listeners perceive the growth of loudness. Finally, a loudness growth function can be derived from the intensity values of the stimulus by the loudness magnitude.

Nonlinear circuits found in digital or wide dynamic range compression (WDRC) hearing aids have incorporated new fitting strategies that provide information about the loudness growth function over the range of intensities amplified (Serpanos, O'Malley, & Gravel, 1997). The adjustment of non linear hearing aids involves the concept of loudness growth normalization, where hearing aid features would be adjusted for a particular hearing loss in order to normalize the perception of loudness (Byrne et al., 2001). From this kind of loudness judgment it is possible to derive electroacoustic characteristics of hearing aids such as average gain, maximum output, compression ratio and onset level (Kiessking, 1982). Much effort has been made in order to develop adequate methods to measure loudness, and a series of different loudness scaling procedures have been especially proposed for hearing aid fitting, rather than for diagnostic purposes.

Objective methods for estimating loudness growth have been proposed using electrophysiological measures. Several studies have revealed that loudness growth could be estimated using click-evoked ABR (Davidson et al., 1990; Galambos & Hecox, 1977; Picton et al., 1977; Thornton, 1987). In these studies, the wave V latency (Rosenhamer et al., 1981), the slope of the latency-intensity function (Galambos & Hecox, 1977; Picton et al., 1977; Thorton, 1987), interaural latency differences (Rosenhamer et al., 1981), and thresholds of the ABR (Conjin, Brocaar, & van Zanten, 1990) have been used as indicators of loudness. ABR amplitude has not been used as latency since it has greater intersubject variability (Schwartz, Morris, & Jacobson, 1994). The major disadvantage of the procedure based on ABR measurements is the lack in frequency specificity of these responses.

Assessment of ASSRs partly overcomes the limitations of ABR testing. Because the amplitude of the ASSR decreases as the intensity of the stimulus decreases, ASSRs can be used as an indicator of loudness. The major limitation of this procedure is the variability of the amplitude of the ASSRs, because recordings at a given intensity vary from subject to subject. The recorded amplitude of the ASSRs depends on several parameters. Among those the most important are the amount of synchronized current in the generators, the orientation of these generators in relation to the recording electrodes, and the impedance of the volume conductor.

An electrophysiological measure of loudness growth could assist audiologists in estimating discomfort levels and determining hearing aid features. Objective measurement of loudness could be included in the prescription of gain in order to fit hearing aids within the first few month of age.

In a recent contribution of our group (Zenker, Barajas, & Fernández, 2005), an attempt was made to prove whether it is possible to establish a relationship between subjective loudness growth derived from the contour test and the physiological responses obtained from the ASSR. The *contour test* is a clinical method to quantify loudness perception (Cox, Alexander, Taylor, & Gray, 1997). This test was designed to develop a function that describes the growth of loudness perception as input levels increase from near threshold to uncomfortably loud levels. In the contour test, tonal stimuli were 5% warble tones presented at .5, 1, 2, and 4 kHz. Verbal judgement from the subject of the perceived loudness was required by rating the loudness in seven categories ranging from very soft to uncomfortably loud.

The amplitude of the ASSR for each level as a function of frequency is illustrated in Figure 13–1.

There are differences in the slope of the amplitude growth function as a function of frequency. The slopes of the functions vary from 0.002 µV/dB (right ear, 4000 Hz) to 0.0005 µV/dB (left ear, 1000 Hz). (Right-versus-left ear ASSR amplitude differences are observed among normal hearing listeners [John, personal communication, 2007], but the application of this knowledge to clinical diagnosis is yet unclear.) Not only do the slopes vary with frequency, but overall amplitude does as well. The largest amplitude responses are found for 500 and 4000 Hz (at 80 dB HL). The variability between

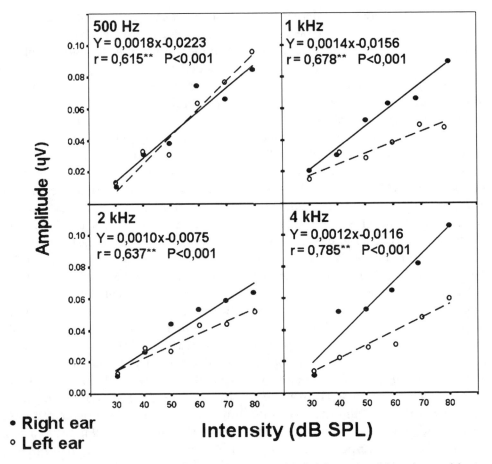

Right ear
Left ear

Figure 13–1. ASSR amplitude as a function of level in normal-hearing subjects. Amplitude growth functions are derived by means of linear regression. As expected, the amplitude of the responses increases with increasing level above threshold.

subjects was fairly similar for a given stimulus level across carrier test frequencies. The variability increased as the intensity level increased. Table 13–2 provides the mean amplitude (and standard deviation) of ASSR amplitude as a function of frequency, ear, and level.

Figure 13–2a shows the amplitude spectra of ASSRs and the loudness growth functions (Figure 13–2b) (from the contour test) obtained in a 29-year-old subject with normal hearing. The amplitude growth functions as a function of frequency and the loudness growth functions are correlated.

A multiple regression analysis was performed using the data from the contour test (sensation of loudness), level of the stimulus and amplitudes of the ASSR. The multiple regression analysis resulted in a prediction of loudness estimated from the ASSR amplitude and amplitude growth functions (Figure 13–3a). This relationship can be defined by the equation

$$Y_{(f)} = B_0 + B_1 * \text{level} + B_2 * \text{AMPLITUDE}$$

where B_0 = y-intercept
B_1 = level (dB HL) coefficient
B_2 = ASSR amplitude coefficient

Table 13–2. Mean amplitude and standard deviations of ASSRs for each carrier frequency and each ear (R and L). The corresponding modulation rate for each carrier frequency also is indicated. Response amplitude increases as the stimulus intensity increases for all carrier frequencies.

Intensity (dB HL)	500		1000		2000		4000	
	R (81 Hz)	L (77 Hz)	R (89 Hz)	L (85 Hz)	R (97 Hz)	L (93 Hz)	R (105 Hz)	L (101 Hz)
80	0.120 (0.089)	0.759 (0.065)	0.074 (0.040)	0.056 (0.034)	0.055 (0.031)	0.077 (0.049)	0.124 (0.066)	0.122 (0.066)
70	0.110 (0.081)	0.842 (0.068)	0.064 (0.028)	0.056 (0.030)	0.053 (0.024)	0.050 (0.035)	0.084 (0.045)	0.063 (0.036)
60	0.093 (0.090)	0.065 (0.070)	0.056 (0.023)	0.050 (0.027)	0.047 (0.025)	0.054 (0.031)	0.067 (0.037)	0.059 (0.037)
50	0.070 (0.067)	0.052 (0.064)	0.047 (0.025)	0.039 (0.025)	0.053 (0.022)	0.043 (0.018)	0.041 (0.020)	0.043 (0.025)
40	0.044 (0.039)	0.029 (0.030)	0.035 (0.020)	0.026 (0.019)	0.037 (0.017)	0.038 (0.017)	0.030 (0.018)	0.031 (0.019)
30	0.036 (0.030)	0.020 (0.015)	0.026 (0.019)	0.024 (0.015)	0.033 (0.019)	0.028 (0.018)	0.047 (0.086)	0.025 (0.014)
20	0.013 (0.011)	0.016 (0.010)	0.025 (0.013)	0.018 (0.011)	0.022 (0.015)	0.021 (0.012)	0.020 (0.009)	0.024 (0.013)
10	0.020 (0.012)	0.017 (0.014)	0.0218 (0.014)	0.020 (0.009)	0.015 (0.009)	0.014 (0.009)	0.022 (0.012)	0.014 (0.009)

ASSR Modulated Tones (Hz)

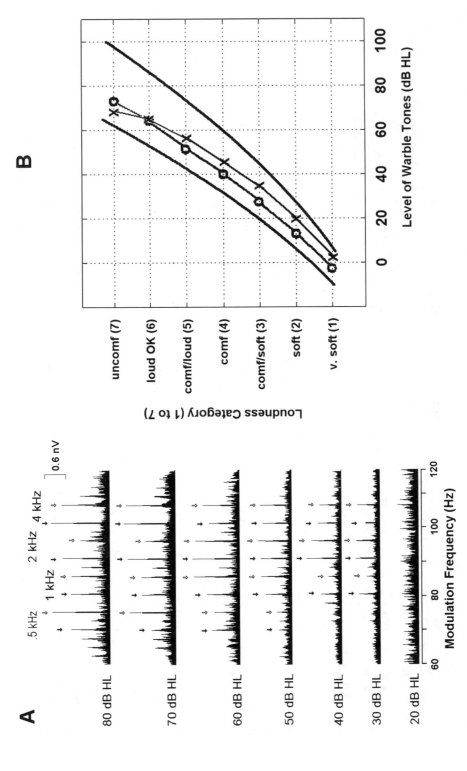

Figure 13–2. A, ASSR amplitude spectra recorded at levels ranging from 80 to 20 dB HL for the four carrier frequencies presented to each ear. *Arrows* indicate a significant response. As level increases, so does the amplitude of the ASSR. **B,** Loudness Contour Test results are for the same subject.

A

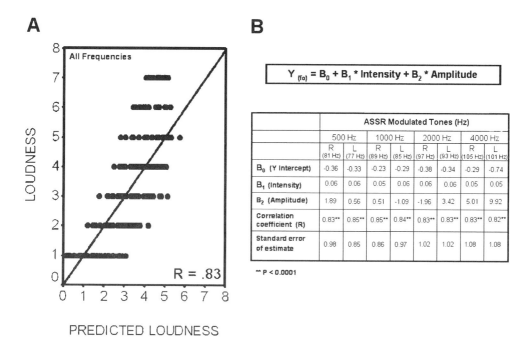

B

$$Y_{(fo)} = B_0 + B_1 * Intensity + B_2 * Amplitude$$

	ASSR Modulated Tones (Hz)							
	500 Hz		1000 Hz		2000 Hz		4000 Hz	
	R (81 Hz)	L (77 Hz)	R (89 Hz)	L (85 Hz)	R (97 Hz)	L (93 Hz)	R (105 Hz)	L (101 Hz)
B_0 (Y Intercept)	-0.36	-0.33	-0.23	-0.29	-0.38	-0.34	-0.29	-0.74
B_1 (Intensity)	0.06	0.06	0.05	0.06	0.06	0.06	0.05	0.05
B_2 (Amplitude)	1.89	0.56	0.51	-1.09	-1.96	3.42	5.01	9.92
Correlation coefficient (R)	0.83**	0.85**	0.85**	0.84**	0.83**	0.83**	0.83**	0.82**
Standard error of estimate	0.98	0.85	0.86	0.97	1.02	1.02	1.08	1.08

** $P < 0.0001$

Figure 13–3. A, Loudness judgements plotted as a function of predicted loudness from the equation derived from the multiple regression analysis of ASSR amplitude with loudness contour. (The regression equation accounts for 70% of total variance.) **B**, The table shows the result of the multiple regression analysis predicting loudness, with a high correlation index regardless of carrier frequency and ear.

B0, B1, and B2 are coefficient values obtained from the multiple regression analyses (Figure 13–3b). The sensation of loudness showed a significant correlation with ASSR amplitude growth of between 0.82 and 0.85 regardless of the carrier frequency. The regression line for all frequencies has a slope of −0.43 loudness/amplitude * level.

In summary, these data suggest that loudness growth can be reasonably well predicted from ASSR amplitude (at least in subjects with normal hearing).

Hearing Aid Selection

Regardless of the fitting formula employed to adjust a hearing aid, all procedures must give information about some critical parameters. First, hearing dynamic range must be established from the pure tone hearing loss and loudness discomfort level; second, the hearing aid is supposed to amplify the whole range of speech into the dynamic range of a particular hearing loss; third, the difference between the hearing loss and the lower limit of the speech dynamic range provide the amount of gain required by the hearing aid; fourth, the compression factor will be determined by the degree of hearing loss to relative to the *long-term average speech spectrum* (LTASS) and finally, the *maximum power output* (MPO), the hearing aid power may be established from the amplitude growth function of the electrophysiological response.

In a recent study, Zenker and colleagues (2006) proposed an ASSR prescription method based on the APP presented earlier in this chapter. Dynamic range, gain, compression, and MPO of the hearing aid were established from the level amplitude function of the ASSRs. ASSRs were obtained in a 27-month-old infant diagnosed with bilateral moderate sensorineural hearing impairment. ASSR thresholds were 50 dB SPL for 0.5Hz and 1.0 kHz; 60 dB SPL for 2 kHz; and 70 dB SPL for 4 kHz. (Converted to dB HL, the thresholds were 55, 50, 63, and 75 dB for 0.5, 1.0, 2.0, and 4.0 kHz, respectively.)

Dynamic Range

Figure 13-4 shows the APP from which the dynamic range is obtained. In this figure, the previously established amplitude level function from a group of normal-hearing subjects (continuous line) is presented with the amplitude level function obtained from a group of hearing-impaired children (dashed line). In the same figure, the dynamic range of speech (40 to 80 dB) for the 500 Hz is projected upward from the abscissa to the normal amplitude intensity function. Then, horizontally, it is projected to the function obtained from the hearing-impaired individual and, finally, projected vertically upward to yield the output dynamic range. Hence, the equivalent dynamic range for this child with a moderate hearing loss is 27 dB (84 − 57 dB) for a 40-dB input range.

Gain and Compression Factor

The difference between the initial point of the output dynamic range (in this case, 57 dB) and the initial point of the input dynamic range (40 dB) define the gain (57 − 40 = 17 dB) of the hearing aid. The width of the output dynamic range is determined from the output range (in this case, 57 to 84 dB, or 27 dB). The need for compression is determined by the ratio of the output dynamic range (27 dB) to the input dynamic range (40 dB); that is, 27/40 = 0.67.

Maximum Power Output

From the ASSRs obtained for this patient, the MPO can be derived from the loudness sensation levels estimated from the amplitude level function. The MPO of the hearing aid is determined from the formula

$$MPO = [L_{oud} − B0 − (B2 * amplitude)]/B1$$

The values of the regression coefficients (determined from the multiple regression analysis described previously) are shown in Figure 13-3b. The MPO must be fitted to the category of uncomfortably loud, that is, contour test category 7. The amplitude data (Table 13-3) used in the formula are those obtained at the highest test level (80 dB SPL) for this patient. The MPO settings for this patient are 103, 110, 123, and 121 dB SPL for 0.5, 1.0, 2.0, and 4.0 kHz, respectively (see Table 13-3).

Finally, curves describing hearing aid output as a function of input are shown for each carrier frequency in Figure 13-5. These curves are shown with respect to threshold (estimated from ASSR threshold) and the maximum output (estimated from ASSR amplitude). As shown in the figure, using these fitting procedures, speech is amplified within the dynamic range of this patient's hearing.

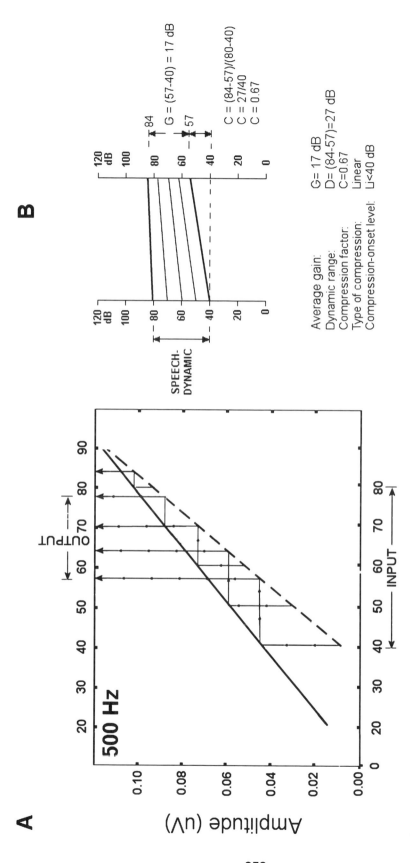

Figure 13–4. A, The amplitude projection procedure (APP). *Solid line* indicates the amplitude level function for normal-hearing subjects; *dashed line* indicates the amplitude level function for infants and children with sensory hearing loss. The input speech dynamic range of 40 to 80 dB is projected upward on the normal curve. Then the projection from the curve for ears with hearing loss yields the output dynamic range for this patient. **B,** The gain requirement is estimated as the difference between hearing loss (57 dB) and the lower limit of the LTASS (40 dB), or 57 − 40 = 17 dB. The compression factor (C) is given by the ratio of the dynamic range of the patient to the normal speech dynamic range (80 − 40 = 40 dB), so C = 0.67.

Table 13–3. MPO values prescribed from the ASSR for a 27-month-old infant diagnosed with bilateral moderate sensorineural hearing impairment (see text)

Feature	ASSR Modulated Tones (Hz)			
	500 (81 Hz)	1000 (89 Hz)	2000 (97 Hz)	4000 (105 Hz)
Amplitude (µV)	0.07	0.066	0.061	0.058
Loudness category	7	7	7	7
B0	−0.36	−0.26	−0.38	−0.29
B1	4.8	4	6.18	5
B2	1.89	0.51	−1.96	5.01
B2 × amplitude	0.13	−0.03	−0.12	0.29
MPO	103	110	123	121

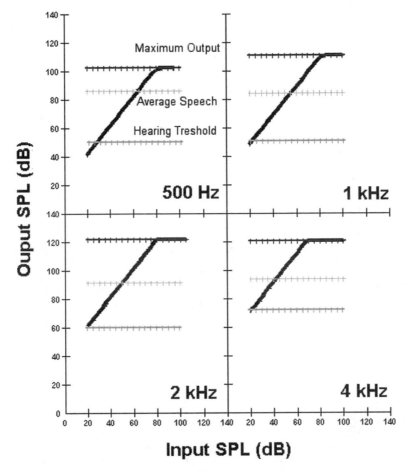

Figure 13–5. Input-output curves prescribed for each carrier frequency studied. The patient's hearing threshold, average speech for each carrier frequency, MPO, and final insertion gain calculated are shown.

Summary

The treatment of those with hearing loss involves the selection and fitting of amplification devices. In difficult-to-test individuals, such as young infants, subjective and objective measures such as functional gain and real-ear probe measurements, are not always possible. For those subjects who do not provide reliable responses to behavioural audiometry, the appropriate selection and fitting of hearing aids requires the establishment of accurate hearing thresholds by other means. ASSR can be used in the characterization of hearing loss to estimate the auditory threshold. In addition, the ASSR can provide information at threshold and also at suprathreshold levels. ASSRs can be used to verify and select the adjustment of hearing aids.

The role of ASSR in hearing aid fittings outlined in this chapter are: the estimation of hearing thresholds that can be introduced in the fitting software and the prescription of hearing aid features such as MPO, gain and the compression ratio. The procedures described in this chapter need further empirical demonstration of their effectiveness and accuracy. As well, the the estimation error of hearing threshold from the ASSR can be unacceptably large when applied to hearing aid fittings, but in cases where no other information is available, the ASSR thresholds provide a valuable starting point.

The APP method described provides estimates of loudness sensation derived from the amplitude level function of the ASSR. This procedure provides frequency specific information about features of hearing aids, such as average gain, compression factor, onset level, and output limitation. This procedure, based directly on the ASSR amplitudes, could deliver an initial adjustment of the hearing aid until other behavioural responses can be obtained.

References

Aoyagi, M., Kiren, T., Furuse, H., Fuse, T., Suzuki, Y., Yokota, M., et al. (1994). Pure-tone threshold prediction by 80-Hz amplitude-modulation following response. *Acta Otolaryngologica Suppl, 511*, 7-14.

Bagatto, M., Moodie, S., Scollie, S., Seewald, R., Moodie, S., Pumford, J., et al. (2005). Clinical protocols for hearing instrument fitting in the Desired Sensation Level method. *Trends in Amplification, 9*(4), 199-226.

Burkard, R. F., & Secor, C. (2002). Overview of auditory evoked potentials. In J. Katz (Ed.), *Handbook of clinical audiology* (pp. 233-248). New York: Lippincott Williams & Wilkins.

Byrne, D., Dillon, H., Ching, T., Katsch, R., & Keidser, G. (2001). NAL-NL1 procedure for fitting nonlinear hearing-aids: Characteristics and comparisons with other procedures. *Journal of the American Academy of Audiology, 12*(1), 37-51.

Cone-Wesson, B., Parker, J., Swiderski, N., & Rickards, F. (2002). Full-term and premature neonates. *Journal of the American Academy of Audiology, 13*, 260-269.

Conjin, E. A. J. G., Brocaar, M. P., & van Zanten, G. A. (1990). Frequency specificity of the auditory brainstem response elicited by 1000 Hz filter clicks. *Audiology, 29*, 181-195.

Cornelisse, L. E., Seewald, R. C., & Jamieson, D. G. (1995). The input output formula: A theoretical approach to the fitting of personal amplification devices. *Journal of the Acoustical Society of America, 97*, 1854-1864.

Cornelisse, L. E., Gagné, J. P., & Seewald, R. C. (1991). Ear level recordings of the long-term average spectrum of speech. *Ear and Hearing, 12,* 47–54.

Cornelisse, L. E., Seewald, R. C., & Jamieson, D. G. (1995). The input/output formula: A theoretical approach to the fitting of personal amplification devices. *Journal of the Acoustical Society of America, 97,* 1854–1864.

Cox, R. M., Alexander, G. C., Taylor, I. M., & Gray, G. A. (1997). The contour test of loudness perception. *Ear and Hearing, 18*(5), 388–400.

Davidson, S. A., Wall, L. G., & Goodman, C. M. (1990). Preliminary studies on the use of an ABR projection procedure for hearing-aid selection. *Ear and Hearing, 11,* 332–339.

Dimitrijevic, A., John, M. S., van Roon, P., Purcell, D. W., Adamonis, J., Ostroff, J., et al. (2002). Estimating the audiogram using multiple auditory steady-state responses. *Journal of the American Academy of Audiology, 13*(4), 205–224.

Don, M. & Elberling, C. (1996). Use of quantitative measures of auditory brainstem response peak amplitude and residual background noise in the decision to stop averaging. *Journal of the Acoustical Society of America, 99*(1), 491-499.

Fabry, D. A., & Schum, D. J. (1994). The role of subjective measurement techniques in hearing-aid fittings. In M. Valente (Ed.), *Strategies for selecting and verifying hearing-aid fittings* (pp. 136–155). New York: Thieme.

Galambos, R., & Hecox, K. (1977). Clinical applications of the brain stem auditory evoked potentials. In J. E. Desmedt (Ed.), *Auditory evoked potentials in man. Psychopharmacology correlates of EPs. Progress in Clinical Neurophysiology, 2,* 1–19. Basel, Switzerland: S. Karger.

Goldstein, R., & Aldrich, W. M. (1999). *Evoked potential audiometry: Fundamentals and applications.* Boston: Allyn & Bacon.

Hall, J. W., & Ruth, R. A. (1985). Acoustic reflexs and auditory evoked responses in hearing-aid selection. *Seminars in Hearing, 6,* 251–277.

Hayes, D., & Jerger, J. (1982). Auditory brainstem response (ABR) to tone-pips: Results in normal and hearingimpaired subjects. *Scandinavian Audiology, 11,* 133–142.

Herdman, A. T., Picton, T. W., & Stapells, D. R. (2002). Place specificity of multiple auditory steady-state responses. *Journal of the Acoustical Society of America, 112,* 1569–1582.

John, M. S., Purcell, D. W., Dimitrijevic, A., & Picton, T. W. (2002). Advantages and caveats when recording steady-state responses to multiple simultaneous stimuli. *Journal of the American Academy of Audiology, 13*(5), 246–259.

Kiessling, J. (1982). Hearing-aid selection by brainstem audiometry. *Scandinavian Audiology, 11*(4), 269–275.

Kiessling, J. (1983). Clinical experience in hearing-aid adjustment by means of BER amplitudes. *Archives of Otorhinolaryngology, 238*(3), 233–240.

Lins, O. G., Picton, T. W., Boucher, B. L., Durieux-Smith, A., Champagne, S. C., Moran, L. M., et al. (1996). Frequency-specific audiometry using steady-state responses. *Ear and Hearing, 17,* 81–96.

Lybarger, S. (1944). *Method of fitting hearing-aids.* U.S. Patent Applications S.N. 543, 278, July 3, 1944.

Mahoney, T. M. (1985). Auditory brainstem response hearing-aid applications. In J. T. Jacobson (Ed.), *The auditory brainstem response* (pp. 349–370). San Diego, CA: College-Hill Press.

Mokotoff, B., & Krebs, D. F. (1976). Brainstem auditory-evoked responses with amplification [Abstract]. *Journal of the Acoustical Society of America, 60,* S16.

Muller, H. G., Hawkins, D. B., & Northern, J. L. (1992). *Probe microphone measurements: Hearing-aid selection and assessment.* San Diego, CA: Singular.

Picton, T. W., Dimitrijevic, A., van Roon, P., John, M. S., Reed, M., & Finkelstein, H. (2002). Possible roles for the auditory steady state responses in fitting hearing-aids. In R. C. Seewald & J. S. Gravel (Eds.), *A sound foundation through early amplification*

2001. Proceedings of the 2nd International Conference (pp. 63–73). Basel: Phonak.

Picton, T. W., Durieux-Smith, A., Champagne, S., Whittingham, J., Moran, L., Giguére, C., et al. (1998). Objective evaluation of aided thresholds using auditory steady state responses. *Journal of the American Academy of Audiology*, *9*, 315–331.

Picton, T. W., Ouellette, J., & Hamel, G. (1979). Brainstem evoked potentials to tone pips in notched noise. *Journal of Otolaryngology*, *8*, 289–314.

Picton, T. W., Woods, D. L., Barbeau-Braun, J., & Healey, T. M. G. (1977). Evoked potential audiometry. *Journal of Otolaryngology*, *6*, 90–119.

Purdy, S. C., & Abbas, P. J. (1989). Auditory brainstem response audiometry using linearly and Blackman gated tonebursts. *American Speech-Language-Hearing Association*, *31*, 115–116.

Rance, G., & Briggs, R. J. (2002). Assessment of hearing in infants with moderate to profound impairment: The Melbourne experience with auditory steady-state evoked potential testing. *Annals of Otology, Rhinology, and Laryngology Supplement*, *189*, 22–28.

Rance, G., Rickards, F. W., Cohen, L. T., De Vidi, S., & Clark, G. M. (1995). The automated prediction of hearing thresholds in sleeping subjects using auditory steady-state evoked potentials. *Ear and Hearing*, *16*, 499–507.

Rance, G., Rickards, F. W., Beer, D. E., & Clark, G. M. (1998). Steady state evoked potential and behavioural hearing thresholds in a group of children with absent click evoked auditory brainstem response. *Ear and Hearing*, *19*, 48–61.

Rosenhamer, H. J., Lindstrom, B., & Lundborg, T. (1981). On the use of click-evoked electric brainstem responses in audiological diagnosis. IV: Interaural latency differences (wave V) in cochlear hearing loss. *Scandinavian Audiology*, *10*, 67–73.

Savio, G., Cardenas, J., Perez-Abalo, M., Gonzalez, A., & Valdes, J. (2001). The low and high frequency auditory steady state responses mature at different rates. *Audiology and Neuro-Otology*, *6*, 279–287.

Schwartz, D. M., Morris, M. D., & Jacobson, J. T. (1994). The normal auditory brainstem response and its variants. In J. T. Jacobson (Ed.), *Principles and applications in auditory evoked potentials* (pp. 123–154). Needham Heights, MA: Allyn & Bacon.

Seewald, R. C., Ross, M., & Spiro, M. K. (1985). Selecting amplifications characteristics for young hearing-impaired children. *Ear and Hearing*, *6*, 48–51.

Serpanos, Y. C., O'Malley, H., & Gravel, J. S. (1997). The relationship between loudness intensity functions and the Clic-ABR wave V latency. *Ear and Hearing*, *18*(5), 409–419.

Sininger, Y. A., Abdala, C., & Cone-Wesson, B. (1997). Auditory threshold sensitivity of the human neonate as measured by the auditory brainstem response. *Hearing Research*, *104*, 27–38.

Stapells, D. R. (2000). Threshold estimation of the tone evoked auditory brainstem response. A literature meta-analysis. *Journal of Speech-Language Pathology and Audiology*, *24*(2), 74–82.

Stapells, D. R., Gravel, J. S., & Martin, B. E. (1995). Thresholds for auditory brain stem responses to tones in notched noise from infants and young children with normal hearing or sensorineural hearing loss. *Ear and Hearing*, *16*, 361–371.

Stapells, D. R., Picton, T. W., & Durieux-Smith, A. (1994). Electrophysiological measures of frequency-specific auditory function. In J. T. Jacobson (Ed.), *Principles and applications in auditory evoked potentials* (pp. 251–282). Needham Heights, MA: Allyn & Bacon.

Stelmachowicz, P. G., Kopun, J., Mace, A., Lewis, D. E., & Nittrouer, S. (1995). The perception of amplified speech by listeners with hearing loss: Acoustic correlates. *Journal of the Acoustical Society of America*, *98*, 1388–1399.

Thorton, A. R. D. (1987). Electrophysiological measures of hearing disorders. *British Medical Bulletin*, *43*, 926–939.

Vander Werff, K. R., & Brown, C. J. (2005). Effect of audiometric configuration on threshold and suprathreshold auditory steady-state responses. *Ear and Hearing, 26*(3), 310–326.

Watson, N., & Knudsen, V. (1940). Selective amplification in hearing-aids. *Journal of the Acoustical Society of America, 18,* 401–408.

Zenker, F., Barajas, J. J., Meco, G., & Espinosa, S. (1996). *Auditory brainstem response to 1000 Hz filtered tone burst in normal hearing subjects*. Presented at the XXIII International Congress of Audiology, Bari, Italy.

Zenker, F., Fernández, R., & Barajas, J. J. (2005). *The contour test electrified*. Presented at the VII European Federation of Audiology Societies (EFAS) Congress, Goteborg, Sweden.

Zenker, F., Delgado, J., & Barajas, J. J. (2003). Acoustic characteristics and audiological applications of the Long-Term Speech Spectrum. *Revista de Logopedia, Foniatría y Audiología, 23*(2), 13–20.

Zenker, F., Fernández, R., & Barajas, J. J. (2006). Fitting hearing-aids in early childhood based on auditory evoked potentials in steady states. *Acta Otorrinolaringológica Española, 57*(9), 388–393.

Part B
Fitting Cochlear Implants Using Electrically Evoked Auditory Steady-State Responses

BARBARA CONE-WESSON

Infants with severe to profound congenital hearing loss are now undergoing cochlear implant surgery at the age of 12 months or younger. This sophisticated hearing technology requires a fair amount of "input data" about the user's hearing sensitivity, comfortable and uncomfortable listening levels, and, ideally, speech perception abilities. The limitations of behavioural techniques in the infant population have spurred research aimed at determining auditory abilities from electrophysiological responses including transiently evoked (click and tone-burst) and steady-state evoked brainstem and cortical auditory evoked potentials (CAEPs). A large part of this research has used acoustic stimuli, although there is now an evidence base for using electrical stimulation (through the implant electrode) to evoke these responses for use in estimating hearing abilities in persons with cochlear implants.

Vander Werff and associates (Chapter 7) discuss the strengths and weaknesses of using ASSRs to determine hearing sensitivity, the starting point for any hearing aid or cochlear implant prescriptive procedure. Dimitrijevic and Cone-Wesson (Chapter 12) describe ways in which ASSR may be used to infer suprathreshold hearing abilities, some of which may be relevant to determining the benefits of amplification or cochlear implantation. In the first segment of this chapter ("The Role of Auditory Steady-State Responses in Fitting Hearing Aids"), Zenker and Barajas propose a procedure for using (acoustically evoked) ASSR testing for fitting hearing aids. This method uses ASSR threshold, amplitude, and amplitude growth data to estimate the hearing aid

259

gain, maximum power output (MPO), and compression as a function of frequency.

Would there be any benefit to using electrically evoked ASSRs for the purpose of fitting ("mapping") a cochlear implant? Have there been any attempts to do so? The answer to the first question is best considered in light of the experience with other electrically evoked auditory potentials, such as eighth nerve action potentials (Abbas, Brown, Hughes, & Gantz, 1999; Brown, 2003; Hughes, Brown, Abbas, Wolaver, & Gervais, 2000a), ABR (Hughes, Brown, Abbas, Wolaver, & Gervais, 2000b; Kileny & Zwolan, 2004), middle latency and cortical evoked potentials (Kileny, 1991; Kileny, Zwolan, Boerst, & Telian, 1997; Sharma, Dorman, & Spahr, 2002). The answer to the second question is a qualified yes, and the one published attempt is described subsequently.

The need for electrophysiological methods for the purposes of verification of implant function and to determine electrical stimulation levels (i.e., threshold, comfortable and uncomfortable loudness settings) has been addressed by cochlear implant manufacturers. The manufacturers have developed the hardware and software for recording eighth nerve action potentials through the implant itself in conjunction with a computer interface used for the implant device programming. That is, the surgically implanted cochlear implant electrode to provide an electrical stimulus to the auditory nerve (spiral ganglion cells) and also as the recording electrode for the compound nerve action potential resulting from the electrical stimulus. The computer interface provides a method for display of the potentials and some rudimentary analyses. It is possible to determine the (electrical stimulus) threshold of the auditory nerve action potential for a given electrode location. Such electrically-evoked auditory nerve-action potential (E-AP) thresholds can be used to guide initial stimulation settings. It is the case that the E-AP threshold does not approximate perceptual (electrical stimulation) threshold, but the presence of the E-AP indicates that the eighth nerve is stimulable at that electrode site. Furthermore, the E-AP threshold and the perceptual threshold have a fairly constant relationship across the electrode array, so determination of the amount of "offset" of the electrical from the perceptual threshold at one electrode site can be used to estimate the perceptual threshold across the array (i.e., set the "T" level). This is the major clinical application of the E-AP: to estimate perceptual threshold for the purpose of mapping. In research, the E-AP also can be used to investigate refractoriness/adaptation for electrical stimulation, and to estimate the spread of current in the cochlea which has implications for designing more (spectrally) precise stimulation schemes.

Given the fact that E-AP technologies are well developed, is there a need for electrically evoked ASSR (E-ASSR)? The ASSR for modulation rates of 70 Hz and above is primarily a brainstem response. But is there any advantage for E-ABR over E-AP? The experience with E-ABR (Brown, 2002; Hughes et al., 2000b) is similar to that with E-AP: The threshold of the E-ABR falls within the dynamic range of the listener but may well be closer to the comfortable listening levels than it is to perceptual threshold. Yet the presence of an E-ABR indicates that the stimulus provided by the implant is stimulating brainstem auditory nuclei and pathways. So the presence of an E-ASSR (for high modulation rates), in conjunction with an E-AP, would give additional information with regard to brainstem auditory function but probably would not provide any additional information that could be used for device programming. Furthermore, unlike acoustically evoked ABRs or action potentials, in comparison with the ASSR, the issue of frequency specificity is not relevant, because the cochlear place of stimulation is determined by the choice of implant electrode stimulated.

Firzst and associates have completed seminal work on electrically evoked ABR (E-ABR), middle latency response (E-MLR), and E-CAEP in deaf adults who use implants to hear (Firszt, Chambers, & Kraus, 2002; Firszt, Chambers, Kraus, & Reeder, 2002). The work of these investigators shows that the latency and amplitude of the E-MLR had the highest correlations (among the E-AEPs) with speech perception abilities. This finding suggests that the E-ASSR for carriers modulated at 40 Hz, for which the generators are thought to be the same as those for MLR, may provide some information relevant to speech perception abilities. This is speculative at best.

The overriding technical issue in recording an evoked potential using electrical stimulation is that of electrical artifact created by the implant. Single or several cycles of biphasic electrical pulses are used to evoke transient potentials such as the E-AP or E-ABR. Even then, the stimulus artifact often swamps the electrophysiological response. To overcome artifact issues, the E-AP is derived from a forward masking paradigm in which the electrical artifacts of both the masker and the probe are subtracted from the average containing a response to the probe stimulus. In the case of E-ABR, the stimulus artifact obscures early components of the response, and wave V may be the only component visualized. E-ABRs and later responses such as E-MLR and E-CAEP also require the use of radiofrequency filters and electrophysiological preamplifiers that are not overloaded by the electrical artifact created by the implant. For E-ASSR, the biphasic pulses must be presented in a steady-state (continuous) manner. This means that the stimulus artifact is present during the entire recording epoch and is orders of magnitude greater than the response.

Menard and colleagues (2004) tackled the technical problem of recording ASSRs for electrical stimulation provided by an implant. The Lyon group recorded ASSRs to amplitude-modulated steady-state biphasic pulses electrical pulses provided by an MXM Digisonic cochlear implant. The modulation rates were between 70 and 85 Hz. These investigators varied both pulse width (duration) and intensity to derive thresholds and response amplitude input-output functions. They reasoned that stimulus artifact would show a linear growth with intensity and duration, whereas physiological responses would show nonlinear growth functions. In this way, they estimated the portion of the response that was physiological versus the artifactual portion. This method took advantage of the charge density basis of neural excitability. Of note, this method of estimating the portion of response due to stimulus artifact and that portion due to neural excitation was used only for higher-intensity and longer-duration stimuli. The investigators made an assumption that the responses obtained for short pulse width durations were free of artifact. They compared the

E-ASSR thresholds (in this case, the minimum pulse width duration that resulted in an ASSR) with perceptual thresholds obtained as a function of pulse width duration. A linear relationship was observed between perceptual threshold and ASSR threshold, and the differences between the two measures were on the same order of magnitude as those seen for E-ABR. This is not surprising: With the modulation rates used, the E-ASSR was generated primarily at the brainstem. The investigators further suggest that the E-ASSR input-output functions show saturation, and this saturation point may prove useful in the estimation of comfortable listening levels but is yet untested. (This concept is similar to that underlying the Zenker and Barajas method [see Chapter 13] of using ASSR amplitude to estimate MPO for hearing aids.)

The question remains: Is there an advantage to using E-ASSR over other evoked potential methods? One advantage may be that several electrode sites could be tested simultaneously by using different modulation rates for each. Given that programming cochlear implants requires the setting of threshold and comfortable listening levels for up to 22 electrodes, this could be advantageous in comparison with the single electrode test techniques (such as E-AP or E-ABR). This advantage may be outweighed by the technical demands of separating the steady-state stimulus artifact from the steady-state response.

References

Abbas, P. J., Brown, C. J., Hughes, M. L., & Gantz B. J. (2000). Electrically evoked compound action potentials (EAP) recorded from subjects who use the Nucleus C124M device. *Annals of Otology, Rhinology, and Laryngology, 185*, 6-9.

Brown, C. J. (2003). Clinical uses of electrically evoked auditory nerve and brainstem responses. *Current Opinion in Otolaryngology and Head & Neck Surgery, 11*(5), 383-387.

Firszt, J. B., Chambers, R. D., & Kraus, N. (2002). Neurophysiology of cochlear implant users. II: Comparison among speech perception, dynamic range and physiological measures. *Ear and Hearing, 23*, 516-531.

Firszt, J. B., Chambers, R. D., Kraus, N., & Reeder, R. M. (2002). Neurophysiology of cochlear implant users. I: Effect of stimulus current level and electrode site on the electrical ABR, MLR and N1-P2 response. *Ear and Hearing, 23*, 502-515.

Hughes, M. L., Brown, C. J., Abbas, P. J., Wolaver, A. A., & Gervais, J. P. (2000a). Comparison of EAP thresholds with MAP levels in the Nucleus 24 cochlear impant: Data from children. *Ear and Hearing, 21*, 164-174.

Hughes, M. L., Brown, C. J., Abbas, P. J., Wolaver, A. A., & Gervais, J. P. (2000b). The relationship between EAP and EABR thresholds and levels used to program the Nucleus 24 speech processor: Data from adults. *Ear and Hearing, 21*, 151-163.

Kileny, P. R. (1991). Use of electrophysiologic measures in the management of children with cochlear implants: Brainstem, middle latency and cognitive (P300) responses. *American Journal of Otology, 12*, 37-41.

Kileny, P. R., & Zwolan, T. A. (2004) Preoperative transtympanic electrically evoked auditory brainstem response in children. *International Journal of Audiology, 43*(Suppl. 1), S16-S21.

Kileny, P. R., Zwolan, T. A., Boerst, A., & Telian, S. A. (1997) Electrically evoked auditory potentials: Current clinical applications in children with cochlear implants. *American Journal of Otology, 18*, S90-S92.

Menard, M., Gallego, S., Truy, E., Berger-Vashon, C., Durrant, J. D., & Collet, L. (2004). Auditory steady-state thresholds in cochlear implant patients. *International Journal of Audiology*, *43*(Suppl. 1), S39–S43.

Sharma, A., Dorman, M. F., & Spahr, A. J. (2002). A sensitive period for the development of the central auditory system in children with cochlear implants: Implications for age of implantation. *Ear and Hearing*, *23*, 532–539.

CHAPTER 14

Case Studies in Application of Auditory Steady-State Response Testing

Case Study 1
Auditory Evoked Potential Assessment of a Child with Multiple Disabilities

Author: Gary Rance
Affiliation: University of Melbourne

Subject History

Subject A was born at 27 weeks postconceptual age. Her weight at delivery was 930 g. She spent 6 weeks in neonatal intensive care (requiring oxygen support for 5 weeks) and then remained in hospital for an additional 6 weeks in a special care environment. Subject A was subsequently diagnosed with athetoid cerebral palsy, thought to be a consequence of her prematurity and rocky neonatal course.

Results

Hearing assessment was undertaken at the University of Melbourne School of Audiology Clinic when Subject A was 19 weeks of age (6 weeks corrected). Initial testing was carried out with the child awake but resting quietly on her mother's lap. Behavioural observation assessment revealed no obvious response to a range of speech and noisemaker stimuli presented in the free field at maximum levels of approximately 70 to 80 dBA. A repeatable "eye widening" response was observed to a drum beat at 95 dBA and above, but no aural palpebral reflex could be elicited at 105 dBA. These findings are difficult to interpret in a 2-month-old child (particularly one with cerebral palsy) but are broadly consistent with conductive or mixed loss of mild degree or greater, or significant sensorineural deficit of at least moderate degree. Impedance audiometry (1000-Hz probe tone) showed type A tympanograms, suggesting normal middle ear function bilaterally.

Evoked potential testing was carried out using systems custom built at the University of Melbourne Department of Otolaryngology, as detailed by Rance and colleagues (Rance, Dowell, Beer, Rickards, & Clark, 1998).[1] The assessments took place in a sound-treated room with the child in natural sleep, using the procedures outlined by the investigators in (Rance et al., 1998). For auditory brainstem response (ABR) testing, alternating-polarity, 100 s clicks were presented at a rate of 11 Hz. Auditory steady-state responses (ASSRs) were elicited by amplitude- and frequency-modulated (AM/FM) tones at octave frequencies from 500 Hz to 4 kHz. The modulation rate for each carrier tone was 90 Hz. Response threshold (for both ABR and ASSR testing) was established by increasing stimulus presentation level in 10-dB steps from 60 dB HL until a response could be detected, and then decreasing the level in 5-dB steps until the auditory evoked potential (AEP) was no longer recordable.

Click-ABR assessment in this case showed response waveforms to air conducted stimuli at left levels 75 dB nHL and above for the left ear and 80 dB nHL and above for the right ear. These results are consistent with mid- to high-frequency hearing loss of moderate-to-severe degree bilaterally (Stapells et al., 1994). No response was observed to unmasked, bone-conducted clicks at the maximum presentation level (50 dB nHL), indicat-

ing that the loss in each ear was primarily of sensorineural origin.

ASSR testing showed thresholds at levels around 70 to 80 dBHL for test frequencies across the audiometric range (Figure 14–1.1). As such, the findings were consistent with the click-ABR (and behavioural) results and suggested flat-configuration hearing loss at moderate-to-severe levels bilaterally.

Based on these results, Subject A was referred for hearing aid fitting and early intervention support. Behind-the-ear devices were fit bilaterally at the (corrected) age of 3 months, with amplification levels set conservatively, assuming hearing levels 10 to 15 dB better than the ASSR thresholds. (Data generated in the 15 years since this child was assessed would suggest that her hearing levels were most likely to be only about 5 dB better than ASSR threshold [see Chapter 7], but at the time, there was only limited data correlating ASSR and behavioural threshold in hearing-impaired babies.) Subject A tolerated her hearing aids well and by 6 months of age was reported by the family and teacher of the deaf to be showing consistent responses to speech at normal voice levels.

By 17 months of age however, Subject A's responses had become sporadic, and her family and clinicians began to doubt that she was receiving optimal input from the hearing aids. Attempts to carry out conditioned audiometric testing had been unsuccessful because of her severe physical difficulties. She was at this point unable to sit without support, had very limited head control, and showed mixed muscle tone (a combination of hyper-

---

[1]Assessment of this child (in the early 1990s) predated the development of commercial ASSR systems.

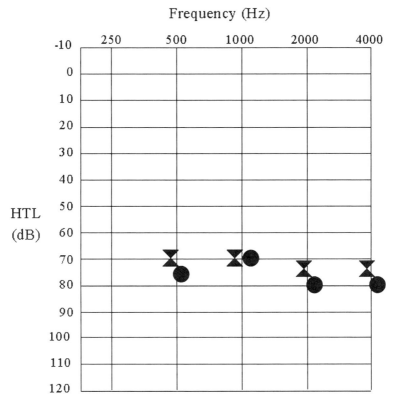

Figure 14–1.1. ASSR threshold levels obtained at the age of 6 weeks for the left (*filled crosses*) and right (*filled circles*) ears.

and hypotonia) with involuntary movements. As such, objective hearing assessment was organized.

ASSR testing was repeated at the age of 18 months. Subject A was not inclined to fall asleep in the clinical setting, so the assessment was carried out with the child under sedation (with chloral hydrate in a dose of 50 mg/kg of body weight).[2] ASSR thresholds for each ear were consistent with those obtained previously, suggesting stable hearing levels bilaterally (Figure 14–1.2).

At 12 years of age, Subject A was a consistent hearing-aid wearer who was reportedly more comfortable when aided than when not. Her physical limitations had continued to make conditioned audiometric assessment difficult, and only approximate behavioural hearing levels could be determined. A further AEP assessment was therefore undertaken.

---

[2]The effect of sedation (and general anesthetic) on the high rate ASSR is yet to be fully explored. If there is a response threshold difference between sedated and natural sleep, it appears to be minimal (Rance et al., 1995). Response sensation levels in sedated subjects may, if anything, be slightly reduced, because EEG noise levels are comparatively low.

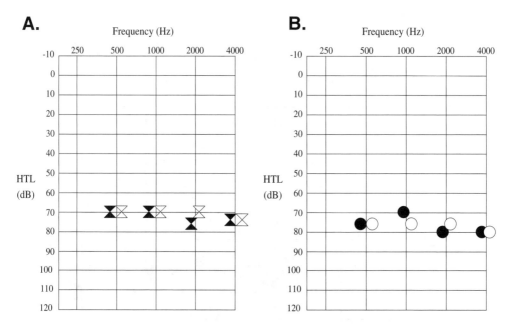

Figure 14–1.2. A, ASSR threshold levels obtained for the left ear at 6 weeks (*filled crosses*) and at 18 months (*unfilled crosses*). **B,** ASSR threshold levels obtained for the right ear at 6 weeks (*filled circles*) and at 18 months (*open circles*).

On this occasion she was tested awake using ASSR and cortical auditory evoked potentials (CAEP).

These assessments were carried out using the GSI Audera system. The stimuli for ASSR testing were AM/FM tones modulated at a rate of 40 Hz. CAEPs were elicited by Blackman-gated tone bursts (5:40:5 cycles) presented at a rate of 0.7 Hz. Stimulus step size (around threshold) for both tests was 5 dB.

Movement- and muscle-related artifact did hamper response recording at times. However, repeatable 40 Hz ASSR response thresholds were obtained at levels around 70 to 75 dB HL (Figure 14–1.3). CAEP thresholds were obtained at similar levels. Figure 14–1.4 shows the averaged electroencephalogram (EEG) tracings for 500-Hz tone bursts presented to each ear. The lowest presentation level at which

the P1/N1 waveform complex could be identified in each case was 70 dB nHL. Thus, the 40-Hz ASSR and CAEP findings were consistent with each other and match the evoked potential findings for this child across the first decade of life.

Outcomes

Subsequent behavioural hearing tests (performed when she was 15 years of age) have confirmed the AEP findings for Subject A, indicating a flat configuration, sensorineural hearing loss of moderate degree (see Figure 14–1.3). She remains a consistent hearing aid user, is responsive to familiar voices and has shown evidence of receptive understanding. Expressive (spoken) language development has, however, been limited.

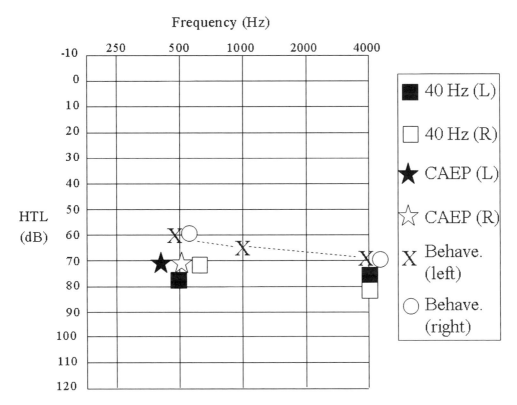

Figure 14–1.3. 40-Hz ASSR and CAEP thresholds (recorded at the age of 12 years) and conditioned behavioural hearing thresholds (recorded at the age of approximately 14 to 15 years).

Comments

This study provides an example of the way in which a battery of tests can be used to estimate hearing level in a child unable to provide an accurate audiogram. Converging evidence from multiple sources (both behavioural and electrophysiological) in this case provided a solid basis for intervention at a young age.

One of the features of this study was the consistency of the ASSR findings across an extended (12-year) assessment period. Almost identical response thresholds were obtained when the child was tested at 6 weeks of age and then again at 18 months. This result is consistent with the (limited) clinical evidence, suggesting that ASSRs can be recorded at consistently low sensation levels in neonates and young babies with sensorineural hearing loss (Luts, Desloovere, & Wouters, 2006; Rance, Rickards, Cohen, De Vidi, & Clark, 2005).[3] Infants with normal hearing, by contrast, show significant maturational changes and would

---

[3] The observation that ASSR sensation levels have not changed across assessments assumes that Subject A's hearing has been stable.

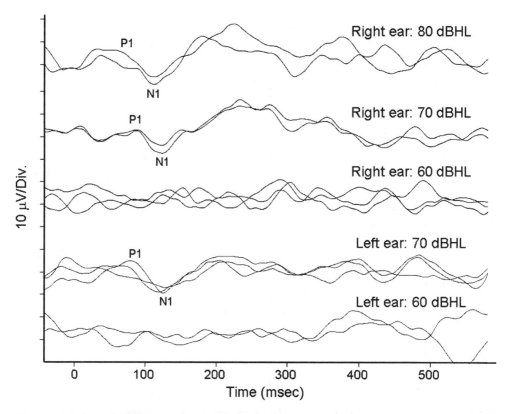

Figure 14–1.4. CAEPs to 500-Hz tone bursts presented to the left and right ears.

for, example, be expected to show a threshold decrease between assessments at 6 weeks and 18 months of up to 10 dB (particularly for low-frequency stimuli). See Chapter 9 for details.

When the child was tested at 12 years of age, 40-Hz ASSR and CAEP thresholds were obtained at similar levels. This result is consistent with recent studies comparing these tests in hearing-impaired adult subjects who have shown equivalent response thresholds (particularly to low-frequency [500-Hz] stimuli) (Tomlin, Rance, Graydon, & Tsialios, 2006; Van Maanen & Stapells, 2006). Maturation studies involving the CAEP and 40-Hz ASSR have in both cases suggested that the developmental course of the poten-

tial is not complete until adolescence (Pethe, Muhler, Siewert, & von Specht, 2004; Ponton, Egermont, Kwong, & Don, 2000). This child's auditory pathway, however, appeared (at the age of 12 years) mature enough to produce responses at levels close to hearing threshold.

The AEP findings for the multiply disabled child described in this study were "normal" or at least consistent with the degree of her hearing loss. That is, there was no suggestion that central factors had influenced the results. Because cerebral palsy is a motor disease, sensory responses such as the AEPs are expected to be unaffected. The impact of other forms of neurological compromise (which can affect the central auditory pathways) on the ASSR is yet to be fully explored and may need to be considered by clinicians in some circumstances.

References

Luts, H., Desloovere, C., & Wouters, J. (2006). Clinical application of dichotic multiple-stimulus auditory steady-state responses in high-risk newborns and young children. *Audiology and Neurotology, 11*, 24–37.

Pethe, J., Muhler, R., Siewert, K., & von Specht, H. (2004). Near-threshold recordings of amplitude modulation following responses (AMFR) in children of all ages. *International Journal of Audiology, 43*, 339–345.

Ponton, C. W., Egermont, J. J., Kwong, B. & Don, M. (2000). Maturation of human central auditory system activity: Evidence from multi-channel evoked potentials. *Clinical Neurophysiology, 111*(2), 220–236.

Rance, G., Dowell, R. C., Beer, D. E., Rickards, F. W., & Clark, G. M. (1998). Steady-state evoked potential and behavioural hearing thresholds in a group of children with absent click-evoked auditory brain stem response. *Ear and Hearing, 19*, 48–61.

Rance, G., Rickards, F. W., Cohen, L. T., De Vidi, S., & Clark, G. M. (1995). The automated prediction of hearing thresholds in sleeping subjects using auditory steady-state evoked potentials. *Ear and Hearing, 16*, 499–507.

Rance, G., Roper, R., Symonds, L., Moody, L. J., Poulis, C., Dourlay, M., et al. (2005). Hearing threshold estimation in infants using auditory steady state responses. *Journal of the American Academy of Audiology, 16*, 293–302.

Stapells, D. R., Picton, T. W., & Durieux-Smith, A. (1994). Electrophysiologic measures of frequency-specific auditory function. In J. T. Jacobsen (Ed), *Principles and applications in auditory evoked potentials* (pp. 251–283). Boston: Allyn & Bacon.

Tomlin, D., Rance, G., Graydon, K., & Tsialios, I. (2006). A comparison of 40 Hz ASSR and CAEP thresholds in awake adult subjects. *International Journal Audiology, 45*, 580–588.

Van Maanen, A., & Stapells, D. R. (2005). Comparison of auditory steady-state responses (80 versus 40 Hz) and slow cortical potentials for threshold estimation in hearing impaired adults. *International Journal of Audiology, 44*, 613–624.

Case Study 2
An Infant with Sensorineural Hearing Loss Following Meningitis

Author: Gary Rance
Affiliation: University of Melbourne

Subject History

Subject M was born at 40 weeks post-conceptual age after an uneventful pregnancy. The neonatal course was normal, and the child's health was good until he suffered a bout of bacterial meningitis at 5 weeks of age. Subject M was born before the advent of newborn hearing screening in Australia, so no formal assessment of hearing acuity was made before his illness. His parents did, however, report rudimentary behavioural responses (e.g., stilling, aural palpebral reflex) to sound at levels consistent with normal hearing.

Results

Initial hearing testing took place at the University of Melbourne School of Audiology Clinic after discharge from hospital. At the time of testing, 18 days after his illness, the child was 8 weeks of age. Auditory evoked potential (AEP) assessment was carried out using a GSI Audera system in a sound-treated room with the child in natural sleep. Differential recordings were made between electrodes placed on the high forehead (Fz) and the ipsilateral mastoid. A third electrode on the contralateral mastoid served as a ground.

Auditory brainstem response (ABR) assessment showed no recordable response to alternating click stimuli at maximum presentation levels (100 dB nHL) in each ear. The tracings are shown in Figure 14–2.1. Testing was also carried out using unipolar clicks at 80 dB nHL to investigate the possibility of auditory pathway disorder (Rance et al., 1999). Cochlear microphonic responses were absent bilaterally suggesting significant peripheral (cochlear) insult. Together, these results suggested the presence of mid- to high-frequency hearing loss of at least severe degree (Rance, Dowell, Beer, Rickards, & Clark, 1998). ABR testing to

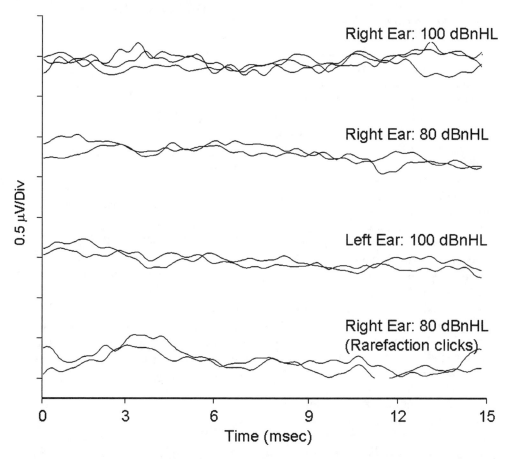

Figure 14–2.1. Averaged EEG findings for Subject M at 8 weeks of age. The *top* and *middle* tracings show no ABR to alternating-click stimuli for the left and right ears. The *bottom* tracing shows absence of ABR and cochlear microphonic responses to rarefaction clicks presented to the right ear at 80 dB nHL.

bone-conducted clicks at maximum levels (50 dB nHL) also showed no repeatable response, which indicated that the loss was at least in part cochlear (rather than middle ear) in origin.[4]

Auditory steady-state response (ASSR) assessment was undertaken using the clinical protocols outlined by Rance and colleagues (2005). The stimuli were single amplitude- and frequency-modulated (AM/FM) tones with centre frequencies at 500 Hz, 1 kHz, 2 kHz, and 4 kHz. Modulation rates varied with carrier tone and were between 70 and 100 Hz. These signals were presented monaurally via mu-metal-shielded TDH-39 headphones that allowed a maximum presentation level of 120 dB HL. To obtain ASSR thresholds, the level of the stimulus was decreased in 10-dB steps until the response could no longer be identified. It was then increased in 5-dB increments until the potential was again detected. ASSR thresholds obtained for Subject M in this way were at levels consistent with profound bilateral hearing loss. See Figure 14–2.2 for details.

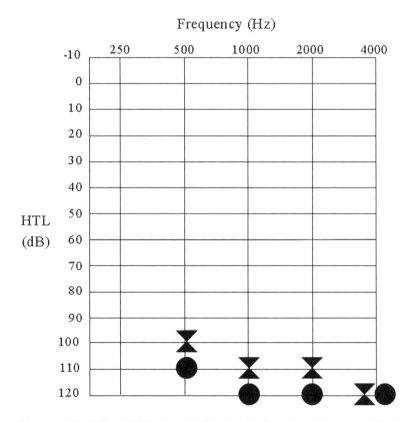

Figure 14–2.2. ASSR threshold levels for the left ear (*filled crosses*) and right ear (*filled circles*) at the age of 8 weeks.

---

[4]Multiple-probe tone impedance audiometry showed type A tympanograms consistent with normal middle ear function on this occasion. Middle ear assessments on each of the subsequent test occasions described in this study also showed no evidence of abnormality.

In summary, the findings from the evoked potential test battery at this initial assessment point were consistent with each other and indicated the presence of significant sensorineural hearing loss. As such, Subject M was referred for hearing aid fitting and early intervention support. High-powered behind-the-ear devices were administered bilaterally, with amplification levels set assuming hearing levels 10 dB better than the ASSR thresholds for each test frequency. These 10-dB corrections broadly correspond to the typical ASSR-behavioural difference (5 dB in the severe to profound range) plus another 5 dB to account for the variability in the difference across subjects (Rance & Briggs, 2002). No tolerance problems or resistance to hearing aid use were observed, and Subject M began (over the course of 1 or 2 months) to show

consistent responses to auditory stimuli. He was also subsequently referred to the Melbourne Cochlear Implant Clinic, where radiological investigation of his cochleae showed no evidence of post-meningitic structural changes such as scar tissue or calcification.

The estimates of Subject M's hearing levels made on the basis of ASSR findings at the age of 8 weeks were subsequently shown to be accurate. Conditioned audiometric testing (visual response audiometry) at the age of 7 months showed profound hearing loss bilaterally (see Figure 14–2.3A and B).

Repeat audiological assessment carried out as part of Subject M's pre-cochlear implant workup were unremarkable until, at 9 months of age, he appeared to show some hearing recovery in the right ear. A change in his general responsive-

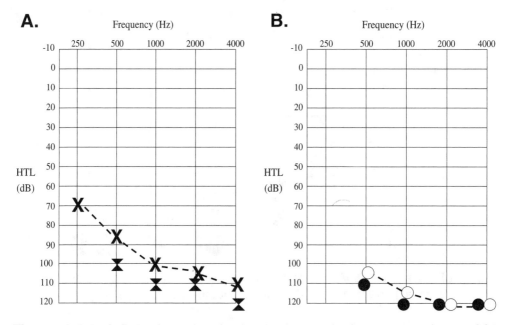

Figure 14–2.3. A, Behavioural hearing levels at 7 months (*open crosses*) and ASSR thresholds at 8 weeks (*filled crosses*) for the left ear. **B**, Behavioural hearing levels at 7 months (*open circles*) and ASSR thresholds at 8 weeks (*filled circles*) for the right ear.

ness to sound (when wearing his hearing aids) also was reported by his parents and teacher of the deaf at this time. Reports of improvement in children with little residual hearing are not uncommon at around this age and often can reflect general developmental changes that allow demonstration of sound awareness at levels closer to their "true" hearing levels. Therefore, a repeat electrophysiological assessment was arranged, and Subject M again underwent ASSR testing in natural sleep. Response thresholds in the right ear were consistent with his improved behavioural detection levels and were 20 to 25 dB better at some frequencies than those obtained in the

period immediately after his illness (see Figure 14-2.4 for details). The ASSR threshold at 1 kHz for the left ear remained stable at 120 dB HL.

Further hearing level improvements were subsequently observed for the right ear until around 11 months of age (10 months after the meningitis), when Subject M's audiogram stabilized in the severe-loss range (Figure 14-2.5). A final ASSR evaluation was carried out with the child under general anesthesia when, at 26 months of age, he was hospitalized for a minor surgical procedure. As can be seen in Figure 14-2.5, the findings again closely mirrored the behavioural audiogram.

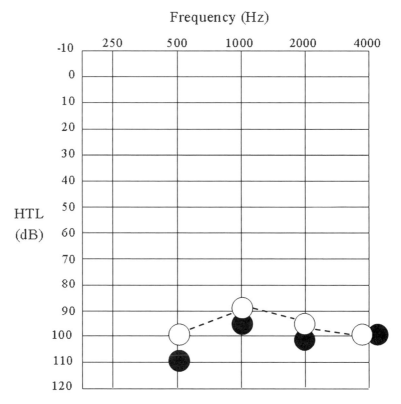

Figure 14–2.4. Behavioural hearing levels (*open circles*) and ASSR thresholds (*filled circles*) at 9 months of age for the right ear.

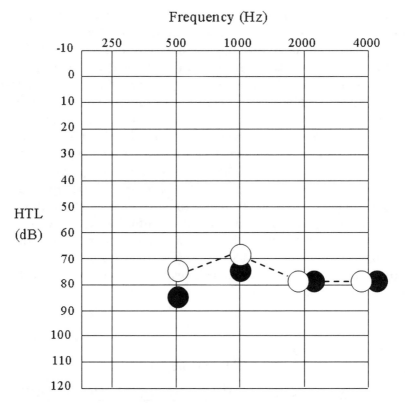

Figure 14–2.5. Behavioural hearing levels (*open circles*) and ASSR thresholds (*filled circles*) at 26 months of age for the right ear.

Outcomes

As a result of his acuity changes, Subject M was not considered a suitable cochlear implant candidate in his infant years. The improved hearing in his right ear eventually afforded him near-complete access to the 70 dB SPL speech spectrum with amplification, and his speech and language progress to 3 years of age were only mildly delayed. Recent improvements in pediatric cochlear implant performance have, however, brought Subject M within the realm of candidacy for this procedure, and his parents are considering this option.

Comments

This case demonstrates the utility of the ASSR technique for quantification of significant hearing loss. The continuous modulated tones used to elicit the response could be presented at levels as high as 120 dB HL at each test frequency allowing assessment of residual hearing in the profound range. ABR testing in contrast was restricted by a maximum presentation level of 100 dB nHL. This limitation is due to the brevity of the acoustic click stimulus. Because the duration of the click is only 100 ms, the threshold advantage for pure tones arising from the temporal integration mechanism is not obtained. As a result, behavioural thresholds for clicks (at the presentation rates used for clinical evoked potential testing) are typically around 30 to 35 dB SPL (peak) (Klein & Teas, 1978; Stapells, Picton, & Smith, 1982). Because the maximum output level for most transducers is approximately 135 dB SPL (peak), click-ABR testing is restricted to corrected presentation levels of 100 dB nHL or less, so the possibility of residual hearing at profound levels cannot be thoroughly explored.[5]

This study also provides an example of the degree to which insights generated by AEP assessment in infancy can inform the intervention process in young hearing-impaired children. ABR and ASSR testing in concert at the age of 8 weeks established the likely form of hearing loss and offered a detailed enough picture of the degree and configuration of Subject M's hearing loss to provide a basis for his amplification strategy.

Finally, this case study clearly demonstrates the phenomenon of post-meningitic hearing recovery. Although meningitis-related sensorineural hearing loss detected at hospital discharge typically remains stable over time, a number of cases showing hearing deterioration, fluctuation and improvement in the months or even years following the illness have appeared in the literature (Brookhauser & Auslander, 1989; Ozdamar, Kraus, & Stein, 1983; Rosenhaal & Kankkunen, 1981). Some of these reports of hearing recovery may, however, have been spurious, particularly when audiometric findings have been the sole measure of change. Comparing behavioural hearing levels from the immediate post-illness phase with subsequent findings may, for example, simply be measuring improvements in the child's ability to produce an accurate audiogram. This is always an issue when testing young children, but is particularly relevant in meningitis cases, because the coexisting neurobehavioral sequelae of the disease (Taylor, Michaels, & Mazur, 1984) can significantly impair a child's ability to perform conditioned audiometric tasks in the initial post-illness period. For Subject M, by contrast, changes in the behavioral audiogram have been objectively tracked from profound to moderate-severe levels using the ASSR technique.

References

Brookhauser, P. E., & Auslander, M. C. (1989). Aided auditory thresholds in children with postmeningitic deafness. *Laryngoscope, 99,* 800–808.

Klein, A. J., & Teas, D. C. (1978). Acoustically dependent latency shifts of BSER (wave V) in man. *Journal of the Acousicalt Society of America, 63,* 1887–1895.

Ozdamar, O., Kraus, N., & Stein, L. (1983). Auditory brainstem responses in infants recovering from bacterial meningitis. Audiological evaluation. *Archives of Otolaryngology, 109*(1), 8–13.

Rance, G., Beer, D. E., Cone-Wesson, B., Shepherd, R. K., King, A., Rickards, F. W., & Clark, G. M. (1999). Clinical findings for a group of infants and young children with auditory neuropathy. *Ear and Hearing, 20*(3), 238–252.

Rance, G., & Briggs, R. J. S. (2002). Assessment of hearing level in infants with significant hearing loss: The Melbourne experience

---

[5]Tone-burst stimuli also are limited in their presentation range. Maximum levels vary with frequency and are around 100 to 110 dB nHL (Stapells et al. 1990).

with steady-state evoked potential threshold testing. *Annals of Otology, Rhinology, and Laryngology, 111*(5), 22–28.

Rance, G., Dowell, R. C., Beer, D. E., Rickards, F. W., & Clark, G. M. (1998). Steady-state evoked potential and behavioural hearing thresholds in a group of children with absent click-evoked auditory brain stem response. *Ear and Hearing, 19,* 48–61.

Rance, G., Roper, R., Symonds, L., Moody, L. J., Poulis, C., Doural, M. & Kelly, T. (2005). Hearing Threshold Estimation in Infants Using Auditory Steady-State Responses. *Journal American Academy Audioliology, 16,* 293–302.

Rosenhall, U., & Kankkunen, A. (1981). Hearing alterations following meningitis. 1. Hearing improvement. *Ear and Hearing, 1*(4), 185–190.

Stapells, D. R., Picton, T. W., & Smith, A. D. (1982). Normal hearing thresholds for clicks. *Journal of the Acoustical Society of America, 72,* 74–79.

Taylor, H. G., Michaels, R. H., & Mazur, P. M. (1984). Intellectual, neuropsychological, and achievement outcomes in children six to eight years after recovery from *Haemophilus influenzae* meningitis. *Pediatrics, 74*(2), 198–205.

Case Study 3
Infant with Steeply Sloping High-Frequency Hearing Loss

Author: Gary Rance
Affiliation: University of Melbourne

Subject History

Subject S was referred to the University of Melbourne School of Audiology Clinic after bilateral "fail" results on her newborn hearing screening assessment. She showed no identifiable waveform on automated auditory brainstem response (ABR) to acoustic clicks at 35 dB nHL when tested 2 days after birth. She had no neonatal risk factors for hearing loss but did have a family history of congenital sensorineural deficit (an older sister has mild-to-moderate loss and wears hearing aids bilaterally).

Results

Initial diagnostic hearing testing was carried out when Subject S was 3 weeks of age. Otoacoustic emission and auditory evoked potential (AEP) assessments were undertaken using a GSI Audera system in a sound-treated room with the child in natural sleep. Differential recordings (for the electrophysiological assessment) were made between electrodes placed on the high forehead (Fz) and the ipsilateral mastoid. A third electrode on the contralateral mastoid served as a ground. Otoscopic examination and multiple-probe tone impedance showed no evidence of middle ear abnormality in either ear.[6]

Click-ABR assessment revealed repeatable but poor morphology waveforms for each ear (Figure 14–3.1A and B). Response thresholds were 40 dB nHL, consistent with mild mid- to high-frequency hearing loss bilaterally (Stapells, Gravel, & Martin, 1994). An incomplete bone conduction ABR assessment showed no repeatable waveform to clicks at 35 dB nHL, suggesting that the loss was of primarily sensorineural origin.

---

[6]Tympanometric testing subsequently showed type A response patterns consistent with normal middle ear function on each of the test occasions reported in this study.

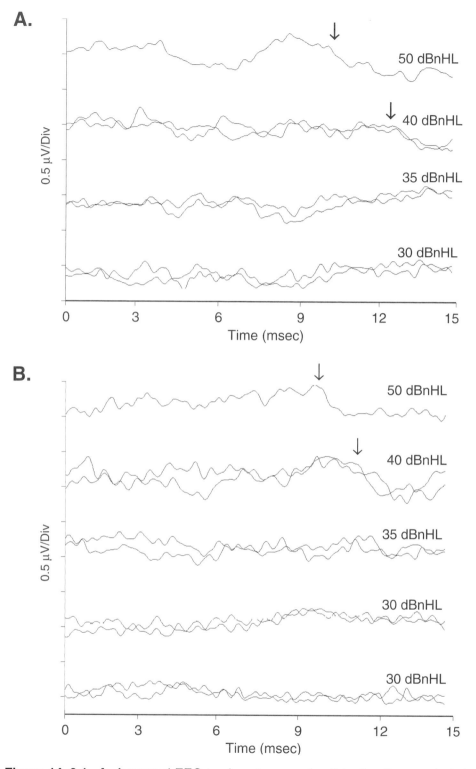

Figure 14–3.1. A, Averaged EEG tracings to acoustic click stimuli presented via air conduction to the left ear. *Arrows* represent ABR wave V. **B**, Averaged EEG tracings to acoustic click stimuli presented via air conduction to the right ear. *Arrows* represent ABR wave V.

Distortion-product otoacoustic emission testing of the left ear was then undertaken. (Subject S became unsettled before testing of the right ear could be performed.) Interestingly, responses were obtained to mid-frequency tone pairs, suggesting normal or near-normal (outer hair cell) function in this region (Figure 14–3.2). Emissions were absent to high-frequency stimuli.

In summary, results obtained on this first test occasion were consistent with high-frequency sensorineural hearing loss of mild degree in both ears. Therefore, a review appointment for frequency specific evoked potential assessment was organized. Subject S was reassessed at 4 weeks of age, when she underwent auditory steady-state response and tone-burst ABR testing.

Auditory steady-state response assessment was carried out using the protocols described by Rance and colleagues (2005). The stimuli were amplitude- and frequency-modulated tones at octave frequencies between 500 Hz and 4 kHz. Modulation rate varied with carrier frequency and was in the range of 70 to 100 Hz. Amplitude modulation depth was 100%, and the breadth of frequency

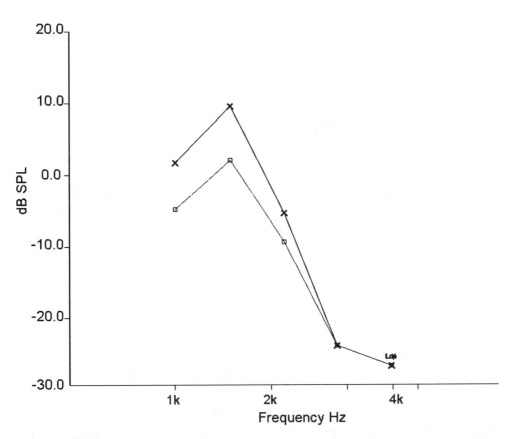

Figure 14–3.2. Distortion product otoacoustic emission responses obtained for Subject S (left ear).

modulation was ±10% of the carrier tone. ASSR response threshold was determined for each test frequency using a stimulus step size of 5 dB.

Tone-burst ABR assessment used positive polarity Blackman-gated stimuli (2:1:2 cycles) presented at a rate of 39.09 Hz. The test frequencies in this case were 500 Hz, 2 kHz, and 4 kHz. Two runs, each consisting of averaged responses from 2000 samples, were obtained at presentation levels between 20 and 90 dB nHL. As with the ASSR testing, stimulus step sizes were 5 dB around threshold.

The ASSR and tone-burst ABR threshold levels obtained for each ear are shown in Figure 14–3.3A and B. These results suggested the presence of steeply sloping hearing loss bilaterally. As such, they were broadly consistent with the earlier click-ABR findings although losses of moderate-to-severe degree in the high-frequency range now seemed most likely.

Subject S awoke from the evoked potential assessment in a relaxed and quiet mood, so an unconditioned behavioural hearing evaluation was also attempted. Repeatable responses (typically eye widening and stilling) were observed to low-frequency stimuli such as the 500-Hz chime bar and reduplicated phoneme pattern /mʌ mʌ mʌ/ at levels consistent with normal hearing (40 to 50 dBA). No reactions were observed to high-frequency signals including the Manchester rattle (greater than 4 kHz energy range) and the phoneme pattern /sss/ (4 kHz and higher). As such, the results matched the pattern described by the evoked potential measures.

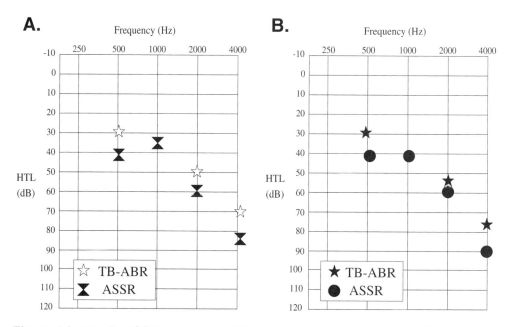

Figure 14–3.3. A, ASSR thresholds (*filled crosses*) and tone-burst ABR thresholds (*open stars*) obtained for the left ear at the age of 4 weeks. **B**, ASSR thresholds (*filled circles*) and tone-burst ABR thresholds (*filled stars*) obtained for the right ear at the age of 4 weeks.

As a result of these findings, Subject S was referred for hearing aid evaluation. She was subsequently fit bilaterally with behind-the-ear devices at 3 months of age. The amplification characteristics of the aids were set assuming hearing levels 10 dB below the ASSR thresholds at 2 and 4 kHz. Negligible gain was provided in the low-mid frequency range as ASSR and ABR thresholds were at levels consistent with normal hearing (in 4-week-old babies [Rance, Tomlin, & Rickards, 2006]) and because OAE responses (for the left ear) were present, indicating normal function (or at least normal cochlear outer hair cell function) in this region. Subject S was also referred to an early intervention center, where the family pursued an auditory-verbal–based habilitation program.

Subject S could be reliably conditioned for audiometric testing from 8 months of age. Figures 14–3.4A and B show her hearing levels established using the visual reinforcement technique. As can be seen in these figures, ASSR threshold levels (obtained 7 moths earlier) accurately mirrored the audiometric pattern in each ear.

Outcomes

This child became a consistent hearing aid user at a young age. She was subsequently fitted for an FM device at 4 years of age to optimize the signal-to-noise ratio of her teacher's voice in her mainstream kindergarten and primary schools.

At 5 years of age, Subject S has normal spoken language skills. Her vocabulary development as measured by the Pea-

body Picture Vocabulary Test (PPVT) has shown performance levels similar to those of her normally hearing peers on repeated measures from 2½ to 4½ years of age (Figure 14–3.5). Furthermore, despite her precipitous loss, her speech production is relatively normal. At 5 years of age she demonstrated a functional consonant repertoire of 21 (out of a possible 24) phonemes and correctly produced 92% of phonemes on the Diagnostic Evaluation of Articulation and Phonology (DEAP) speech production measure.[7]

Comments

Overall, the battery of tests used to assess this child in the early infant period built up an accurate picture of her hearing status. The sloping configuration of her audiogram did, however, reveal some of the weaknesses of the individual measures. Click-ABR assessment, for example, underestimated the degree of high-frequency deficit. Acoustic clicks are broadband stimuli containing energy at frequencies across the audiometric range. Physiological factors relating to the mechanics of cochlear transduction mean that the ABR elicited by the click is dominated by activity in the basal turn, but response thresholds can still reflect hearing in the range of 1 kHz and above (Stapells et al., 1994). In the case of Subject S, the response is likely to have been generated at the lower end of this range, as the signal would in fact have been inaudible at 2 kHz and 4 kHz when presented at the ABR threshold level (40 dB nHL).

---

[7]Mean score on this test for normally hearing children of her age is 97%.

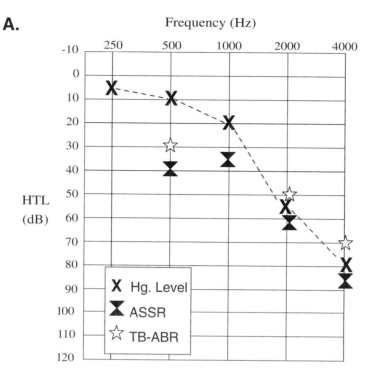

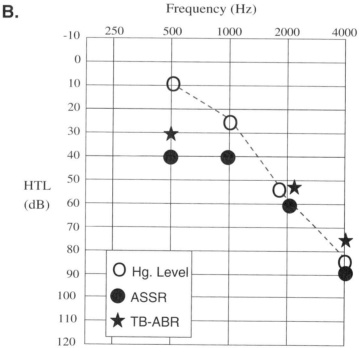

Figure 14–3.4. A, Left ear behavioural hearing levels (*open crosses*) for Subject S at 8 months of age. Also shown are ASSR thresholds (*filled crosses*) and tone-burst ABR thresholds (*open stars*) obtained at the age of 4 weeks. **B**, Right ear behavioural hearing levels (*open circles*) for Subject S at 8 months of age. Also shown are ASSR thresholds (*filled circles*) and tone-burst ABR thresholds (*filled stars*) obtained at the age of 4 weeks.

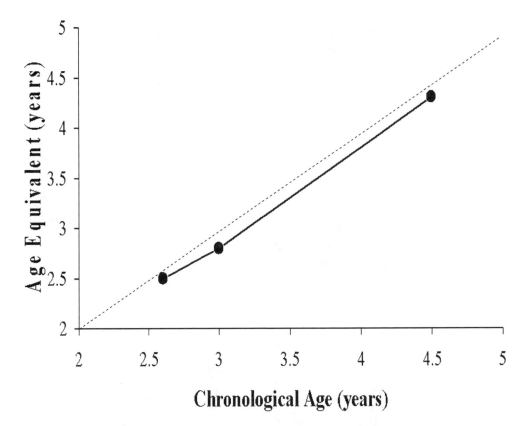

Figure 14–3.5. Receptive vocabulary development for Subject S from 2.5 to 4.5 years of age. Data points represent equivalent language age (relative to normally hearing children) as measured by the Peabody Picture Vocabulary Test (PPVT).

This case also illustrates the degree to which evoked potential threshold sensation levels vary with audiometric threshold. The fact that ASSRs can be recorded at levels closer to behavioural hearing level in subjects with significant hearing loss than in those with normal acuity is well established (and is discussed in detail elsewhere in this book). In Subject S, this relationship is demonstrated within an individual ear with relatively high sensation levels (approximately 30 dB) obtained for the low frequencies where the hearing was normal and comparatively low sensation levels (approxi-

mately 5 dB) for the high frequencies where the sensorineural hearing loss was pronounced, and where recruitment-like processes are likely to have come into play. Similar findings have been reported in other subjects with steeply sloping audiograms (Johnson & Brown, 2005).

Unlike the ASSR findings, tone-burst ABR thresholds underestimated the degree of high-frequency hearing loss in Subject S. Again, this result is consistent with previous TB-ABR findings for subjects with steeply sloping loss (Johnson & Brown, 2005; Purdy & Abbas, 2002) that have shown underestimations of

25 dB (or more) in some cases with precipitous slopes. As with the findings reported by Johnson and Brown, the results for Subject S suggest that in some instances, ASSRs thresholds to AM/FM tones are able to offer a more accurate representation of audiometric configuration than ABR thresholds evoked by Blackman-gated tone bursts. This is presumably because the energy spectra of the modulated tones are narrower than those of the tone bursts. Johnson and Brown measured the frequency responses of AM/FM tones and Blackman-gated tone bursts and concluded that the main energy lobe was broader for the tone bursts, and that as a result, these stimuli were more likely to elicit responses from regions of better hearing beyond that of the nominal test frequency.[8] The use of a masking paradigm such as the "notched-noise" technique proposed by Stapells and associates (Stapells, Gravel, & Martin, 1990; Stapells, Picton, Durieux-Smith, Edwards, & Moran, 1995) to minimize responses from frequencies distant to the test region may have improved the specificity of the tone burst-elicited responses obtained for Subject S. Johnson and Brown, however, found no improvement in predictive accuracy in their adult subjects with similar hearing configurations when they measured ABRs to tone bursts in notched noise masking.

In summary, the relatively frequency-specific AM/FM tones used to elicit the ASSRs in this case allowed accurate prediction of the behavioural audiogram and successful intervention at an early age for this child with steeply sloping hearing loss.

References

Johnson, T. A., & Brown, C. J. (2005). Threshold prediction using the auditory steady-state response and the tone burst auditory brain stem response; a within subject comparison. *Ear and Hearing, 26,* 559–576.

Purdy, S. C., & Abbas, P. J. (2002). ABR thresholds to tone bursts gated with Blackman and linear windows in adults with high frequency sensorineural hearing loss. *Ear and Hearing, 23,* 358–368.

Rance, G., Roper, R., Symonds, L., Moody, L. J., Poulis, C., Dourlay, M., et al. (2005). Hearing threshold estimation in infants using auditory steady state responses. *Journal of the American Academy of Audiology, 16,* 293–302.

Rance, G., Tomlin, D., Rickards, & F. W. (2006). Comparison of auditory steady-state response and tone burst auditory brainstem response thresholds in normal babies. *Ear and Hearing, 27*(6), 751–762.

Stapells, D. R, Gravel, J. S., & Martin, B. A. (1995). Thresholds for auditory brain stem responses to tones in notched noise from infants and young children with normal hearing or sensorineural hearing loss. *Ear and Hearing, 16,* 361–371.

Stapells, D. R., Picton, T. W., & Durieux-Smith, A. (1994). Electrophysiologic measures of frequency-specific auditory function. In J. T. Jacobsen (Ed), *Principles and applications in auditory evoked potentials* (pp. 251–283). Boston: Allyn & Bacon.

Stapells, D. R., Picton, T. W., Durieux-Smith, A., Edwards, C. G., & Moran, L. M. (1990). Thresholds for short-latency auditory evoked potentials to tones in notched noise in normal-hearing and hearing-impaired subjects. *Audiology, 29,* 262–274.

---

[8]The stimuli investigated by Johnson and Brown (2005) were similar but not identical to those used in this case study.

Case Study 4
Hearing Screening Follow-up in an Infant with Mild Hearing Loss

Author: Heleen Luts*
Affiliation: ExpORL, Department of Neurosciences, University of Leuven, Leuven, Belgium

Subject History

A baby girl (born at 38 weeks postconceptional age) was referred at 25 days of age for audiological assessment after a failed hearing screening at the left ear; the right ear passed. The screening was done by means of automated auditory brainstem responses (A-ABR) at 35 dB nHL. The mother has hearing loss, diagnosed at the age of 11 years. The infant had no other risk factors for hearing impairment.

Findings

An appointment was scheduled at the Ear-Nose-Throat (ENT) Department of the University of Leuven 3 days after the hearing screening (at 4 weeks of age). Otoscopy showed a normal appearance of the left ear but an opaque tympanic membrane in the right ear. Transiently evoked otoacoustic emissions (OAEs) were absent in both ears. The "pass" of the right ear with A-ABR was thus not confirmed by the OAEs.

Auditory steady-state response (ASSR) thresholds were assessed with a binaural multiple-stimulus technique using the MASTER software (John & Picton, 2000). Carrier frequencies were 500, 1000, 2000,

and 4000 Hz, and modulation rates were between 82 and 110 Hz. Thresholds were determined at 10-dB accuracy. Stimuli were presented through ER-3A insert phones. The eight signals were calibrated in dB SPL. For ease of comparison, threshold values are reported in dB HL. Recording electrodes were placed at the forehead (+), the inion (−), and the clavicle (ground). For each stimulus intensity, 32 sweeps (16.4 seconds each) for a total of 8.8 minutes were recorded. The significance of the responses was evaluated using F-ratio statistics ($P < .05$).

Recordings were started at 60 dB SPL. All responses reached significance after only four sweeps for the left ear and ten sweeps for the right ear. The second recording at 40 dBSPL resulted in no significant responses. At 50 dB SPL, three out of eight responses reached significance. The frequency spectra of the ASSR recordings are shown in Figure 14–4.1. This combination of highly significant responses to all stimuli at the first evaluated intensity and no significant responses at an intensity 20 dB lower is rather unusual. To double-check the results, the recording at 60 dBSPL was repeated. Again, the responses rapidly reached significance.

For threshold assessment, the level of significance of the responses is determined only at the end of the recording. The *change* of the significance level during the recording, however, can be informative (as shown in Figure 14–4.2). If the *P* value is decreasing but does not reach .05 by the 32nd sweep, it may be wise to prolong the recordings. In this example, however, the significance level remained high, and the response would not be expected to reach significance by extending the recording.

For the left ear, ASSR thresholds were 45, 50, 57, and 55 dB HL for 500, 1000,

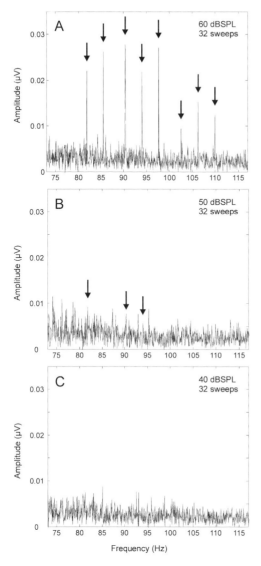

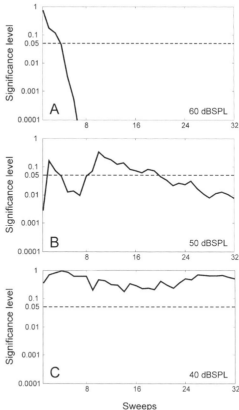

Figure 14–4.2. Significance level as a function of number of sweeps for the response to the 1000-Hz stimulus in the left ear. The *dashed line* represents a significance level of $P = .05$. At 60 dB SPL (**A**), the significance level is lower than 0.0001 from sweep 7 on. At 50 dB SPL (**B**), the P value decreases gradually, whereas at 40 dB SPL (**C**), the P value remains high for the complete recording. The threshold for this stimulus is 50 dB SPL.

Figure 14–4.1. Frequency spectra of ASSR recordings of 32 sweeps at 60 dB SPL (**A**), 50 dBSPL (**B**), and 40 dBSPL (**C**), Significant responses are indicated with an *arrow*. ASSR thresholds are 50, 50, 60 and 60 dB SPL for the left ear and 60, 50, 60, and 60 dB SPL for the right ear for 500, 1000, 2000, and 4000 Hz, respectively.

2000, and 4000 Hz, respectively. For the right ear similar thresholds were obtained, except for 500 Hz, for which a threshold

of 55 dB HL was found. The ASSR thresholds can be interpreted in two ways. First, they can be compared with average ASSR thresholds for normal-hearing babies. In a group of 30 infant ears (corrected age of, on average, 12 days), average ASSR thresholds were found at 37 ± 10, 35 ± 10, 29 ± 10 and 32 ± 9 dB HL for 500, 1000, 2000, and 4000 Hz, respectively (Luts, Desloovere, & Wouters, 2006). When compared with these reference data, the ASSR thresholds of the best ear (left) of the 4-week-old baby indicate a mild hearing loss at the higher frequencies (see Figure 14–4.3A). Second, hearing thresholds can be estimated from average difference scores (ASSR minus behavioural hearing threshold). Ideally, average difference scores for infant ears should be used. The available data set of infant ASSR thresholds with corresponding behavioural thresholds is still limited, however, and the time delay between both tests often is large. Therefore, hearing thresholds are estimated on the basis of average difference scores for adult ears with various degrees of hearing loss for ASSR recordings of 32 sweeps (Luts & Wouters, 2004). Whether or not these values are appropriate for hearing-impaired babies has yet to be determined. The estimated hearing thresholds for the best ear (left) were 25, 37, 46, and 42 dB HL for 500, 1000, 2000, and 4000 Hz, respectively, indicating a mild hearing loss for the lower frequencies and a moderate hearing loss for the higher frequencies.

Outcomes/Management

A conservative approach was taken, and no hearing amplification was prescribed. Follow-up appointments were scheduled regularly (about every 3 months) at the clinic to evaluate the child's hearing status. OAEs remained absent. The mother indicated that several times she had the impression that the child heard well. Findings on behavioural audiometry, first behavioural observation audiometry, and, later, visual reinforcement audiometry (VRA) did not conflict with the ASSR

results. At the age of 14 months, a reliable audiogram was obtained using VRA with warble tones presented in free-field conditions. Because the audiogram had to be assessed in one short test session, no ear-specific information could be obtained. Thresholds were found at 20, 25, 30, and 55 dB HL for 250, 500, 1000, and 4000 Hz, respectively. This corresponds well with the hearing thresholds estimated on the basis of the ASSR recordings (see Figure 14–4.3B).

Comments

Screening and Follow-up of Hearing Loss in Flanders

Flanders was one of the first regions in the world where early auditory screening was systematically offered to all infants, (approximately 60,000 per year). Universal newborn hearing screening has been implemented since 1998. Newborns are screened free of charge by the Flemish organization Kind & Gezin ("Child & Family"), whose purpose is to promote the welfare and health of all children. The screening is carried out at the age of about 4 weeks and is fully integrated into the normal program of basic preventive care.

The ALGO test is used for screening. Clicks of 35 dB nHL are presented at a rate of 37 clicks per second. The device shows a "pass" or "fail" result. If the first ALGO produces a fail result for one or both ears, a second test is performed within 48 hours of the first test. If this second test again shows a fail result, the infant is referred to one of the 22 specialized referral centers in Flanders for further audiological and medical diagnosis within 2 weeks. The audiological

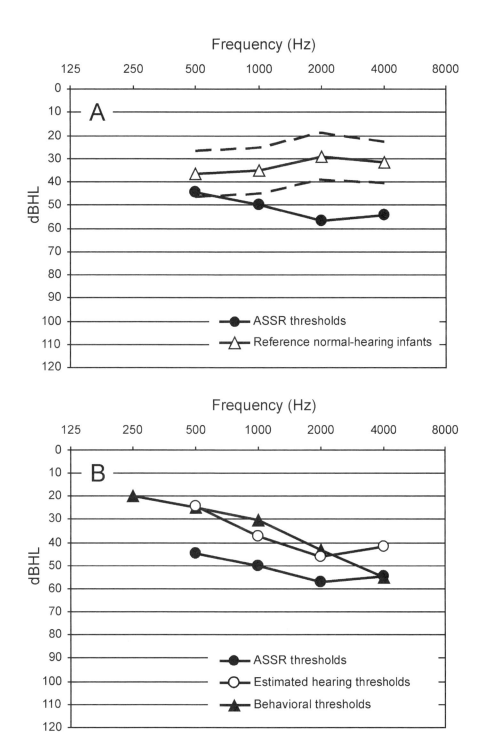

Figure 14–4.3. A, Comparison of the ASSR results obtained in the 4-week-old infant and reference ASSR data for a group of normal-hearing infants (Luts, Desloovere, & Wouters, 2006). The *dashed lines* represent the reference data ± one standard deviation. **B**, Comparison of ASSR thresholds (obtained at the age of 4 weeks), estimated hearing thresholds and behavioural hearing thresholds (obtained at the age of 14 months). Because the behavioural thresholds are not ear-specific, they are compared with the ASSR thresholds of the best ear.

diagnostic test battery at the ENT Department of the University of Leuven consists of 1000-Hz tympanometry, OAEs, and ASSR threshold measurements. If the hearing loss is confirmed, additional specialized tests are carried out in a second phase to define the etiology of the hearing loss. Immediately thereafter, the multidisciplinary rehabilitation begins.

All results of the general screening program are collected in a central database. Referral centers send reports on the diagnostic evaluation and rehabilitation for each patient on regular basis. This centralization of information ensures an optimal circulation of the referred infants through the different stages from screening to rehabilitation and guarantees a very low loss of follow-up. In 2004, screening was offered to 98.7% of the newborns. In 2.1%, a screening test was refused. The referral rate after the second test was 0.3% of the total group of tested infants. The incidence of bilateral hearing loss of more than 40 dB was 0.1% (Van Kerschaver and Stappaerts, 2006).

Difficulties in Differentiating Normal Hearing from Mild Hearing Loss

Mild hearing losses are not often diagnosed in babies, because the screening level is too high. This infant represented a borderline case; one ear passed the hearing screening, and the other ear did not. The ASSR thresholds were compared with reference data obtained in normal-hearing babies. Only at 2000 and 4000 Hz, the thresholds were not within two standard deviations of the mean (a range that should comprise 95% of the data). The large spread of data, which is typical for evoked potential testing, makes

it difficult to differentiate normal hearing and mild hearing loss. However, the same is true for behavioural observation audiometry in young children. Reactions are not always reliable, and thresholds may be elevated, because they are *response* thresholds, rather than hearing thresholds. Assessment of the reliability of the ASSR technique in babies is compromised, because behavioural thresholds cannot be determined at this very young age, and discrepancies between both threshold values can have their origin in the time delay (e.g., acquired hearing loss, middle ear problems, increased ear canal volume). Because of the large spread of data, threshold estimations based on ASSR recordings in babies are not optimal for accurate hearing aid fitting. In my own clinical experience, however, the threshold estimations correspond reasonably well with the hearing thresholds and provide at least a good basis for hearing aid fitting.

In Flanders, babies with a mild hearing loss usually are not referred for early intervention services. They are included in a follow-up program to assess their hearing status on a regular basis. A recent study by Wake and colleagues (2006), however, showed that the phonological short-term memory of children with slight-to-mild bilateral hearing loss was poorer compared with that observed in matched normal-hearing children. Nevertheless, this did not translate into poorer language, reading, behavior, or health-related quality of life.

Bone Conduction ASSR

In infants with a mild to moderate hearing loss according to their ASSR thresholds, possible middle ear involvement is an important concern. In this child, otoscopy at the first consultation suggested middle ear involvement on the right side. At that time, 1000-Hz tympanometry was not yet available. To distinguish between sensorineural and conductive hearing losses, determination of bone conduction ASSR thresholds might have been useful but this is currently not part of the clinical protocol. Although bone conduction ABR in infants has already been investigated extensively (for a review, see Stapells & Oates, 1997), bone conduction ASSR in infants is not that straightforward, because no standardized procedures or normative data are available. Moreover, practical issues arise that compromise the use of bone conduction ASSR. It is already a challenge to assess air conduction ASSR thresholds for four frequencies because of the limited testing time (because the baby needs to sleep). The additional assessment of bone conduction ASSR thresholds requires again a lot of time. Furthermore, the placement of the bone oscillator poses an additional risk for awakening the infant.

Recently, the bone conduction ASSR has been investigated in infants (Small, Hatton, & Stapells, 2007; Small & Stapells, 2006). These studies have shown that handheld coupling of the bone oscillator to the infant's head by a trained assistant is reliable. This coupling method will reduce the risk of waking up the infant. In infants, no difference was found between bone conduction ASSR thresholds obtained with temporal or mastoid oscillator placements. Moreover, the occlusion effect was not observed. ASSR thresholds to multiple bone conduction stimuli were obtained in normal-hearing infants (Small & Stapells, 2006). Before this technique can be implemented in clinical practice, however, normative data will need to be obtained in larger groups of normal-hearing as well as hearing-impaired infants of different ages.

References

John, M. S., & Picton, T. W. (2000). MASTER: A Windows program for recording multiple auditory steady-state responses. *Computer Methods and Programs in Biomedicine, 61,* 125–150.

Luts, H., Desloovere, C., & Wouters, J. (2006). Clinical application of dichotic multiple-stimulus auditory steady-state responses in high-risk newborns and infants. *Audiology and Neuro-Otology, 11,* 24–37.

Luts, H., & Wouters, J. (2004). Hearing assessment by recording multiple auditory steady-state responses: The influence of test duration. *International Journal of Audiology, 43,* 471–478.

Small, S. A., Hatton, J. L., & Stapells, D. R. (2007). Effects of bone oscillator coupling method, placement location, and occlusion on bone-conduction auditory steady-state responses in infants. *Ear and Hearing, 28,* 83–98.

Small, S. A., & Stapells, D. R. (2006). Multiple auditory steady-state response thresholds to bone-conduction stimuli in young infants with normal hearing. *Ear and Hearing, 27,* 219–228.

Stapells, D. R., & Oates, P. (1997) Estimation of the pure-tone audiogram by the auditory brainstem response: A review. *Audiology and Neuro-Otology, 2,* 257–280.

Van Kerschaver, E., & Stappaerts, L. (2006). Gehoorscreening in Vlaanderen 2004: Doelgroepbereik, testresultaten en resultaten van de verwijzingen. Brussels: Kind & Gezin.

Wake, M., Tobin, S., Cone-Wesson, B., Dahl, H. H., Gillam, L., McCormick, L., et al. (2006). Slight/mild sensorineural hearing loss in children. *Pediatrics.* 118, 1842–1851.

Case Study 5
Auditory Steady-State
Response Testing in a
Child with Conductive
Hearing Loss

Authors: Gary Rance and Barbara
Cone-Wesson
Affiliations: University of Melbourne
(Rance); University of Arizona
(Cone-Wesson)

Subject History

Subject C was born at 39 weeks post-conceptual age after a normal pregnancy. He was in good health, but genetic testing revealed abnormality of chromosome 21 (Down Syndrome). Newborn hearing screening (transient evoked otoacoustic emissions) showed no response in either ear.

Results

Diagnostic hearing testing was undertaken at the University of Melbourne School of Audiology Clinic when Subject C was 4 weeks of age. Otoscopy was challenging because of the infant's narrow ear canals, but what could be seen of the tympanic membranes suggested the presence of middle ear effusion bilaterally. Tympanometry also showed type B response patterns, consistent with middle ear pathology in both ears.

Evoked potential testing was carried out using a GSI Audera system in a soundproof room with the child in natural sleep. Air-conducted click–auditory brainstem response (ABR) and auditory steady-state response (ASSR) assessments

were undertaken using the procedures outlined in Case Study 2. The stimuli in this instance were delivered via insert tubephones. Bone conduction ASSR (BC-ASSR) assessment also was attempted. In this case, the setup was as for the air conduction testing, but the transducer was a handheld bone vibrator placed on the (left) mastoid (Small, Hatton, & Stapells, 2007).

Air-conducted click-ABR testing showed repeatable waveforms to stimuli presented at 60 dB nHL (and above) in each ear. This result is broadly consistent with mid- to high-frequency hearing loss of mild-to-moderate degree. Air-conducted ASSR (AC-ASSR) thresholds for a range of carrier frequencies were similarly elevated, suggesting flat configuration losses of approximately 40 to 50 dB HL in each ear (Figure 14–5.1). By contrast, ASSRs to bone-conducted tones were obtained at low presentation levels (1 kHz: 5 dB HL; 4 kHz: 15 dB HL) indicating normal (cochlear level) hearing in at least one ear.

On the basis of these findings, referral to a pediatric ear-nose-and-throat specialist was arranged. The possibility of surgery to insert middle ear ventilation tubes was discussed but not immediately pursued owing to the anesthetic risks related to this child's immaturity and recently identified heart condition. The option of a temporary bone conduction hearing aid fitting also was considered, but the family was not ready for intervention at this stage.

Subject C was mature enough for conditioned audiometric assessment at 8 months of age. Visual reinforcement testing revealed air conduction hearing levels around 40 to 50 dB HL across the audiometric range in each ear and an unmasked bone conduction threshold

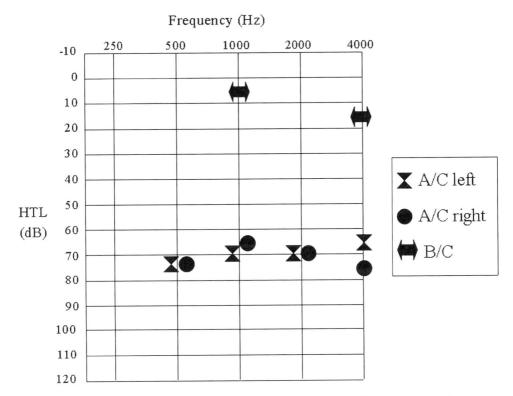

Figure 14–5.1. ASSR thresholds obtained for Subject C at 4 weeks of age.

at 1 kHz of 10 dB HL. At this point, the parents consented to bilateral middle ear surgery.

In conjunction with the fitting of ventilation tubes, pre- and postoperative ASSR assessments were carried out in the operating room (with the patient under general anesthesia).[9] Air conduction thresholds determined before surgery were at levels around 60 to 70 dB HL in each ear, and a 1-kHz bone conduction threshold of 15 dB HL was obtained (Figure 14–5.2). These results were consistent with the behavioural findings from 2 weeks earlier.

Grommets were then inserted and the middle ears cleared of effusion. AC-ASSR testing was repeated, and response thresholds consistent with normal hearing were observed bilaterally (see Figure 14–5.2).

Outcomes

Subject C continues to experience the chronic middle ear problems typical for children with Down syndrome. When his ears are clear, he shows normal hearing thresholds. He has recently been fit with his third set of grommets.

[9]Such testing is not part of our standard clinical protocol for children capable of providing conditioned audiometric results.

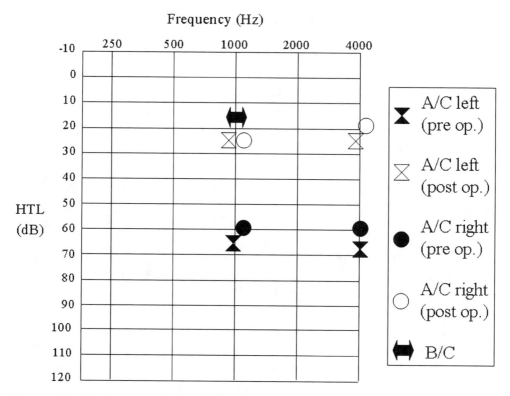

Figure 14–5.2. Preoperative and postoperative ASSR thresholds for Subject C at 9 months of age.

Comments

The BC-ASSR thresholds obtained at 4 weeks of age for Subject C are consistent with normative infant data presented by Small and Stapells (2006). Responses at each of the test frequencies were considerably lower than those expected for AC-ASSR testing in normally hearing babies (Rance & Tomlin, 2006). Furthermore, Subject C's BC-ASSR threshold at 1 kHz (5 dB HL) was lower than expected for adults (tested by bone conduction). These differences probably are related to the way the infant skull (which is smaller and structurally immature) conducts the signals produced by bone vibrators (Small & Stapells, 2006).[10]

The possibility of artifactual response in BC-ASSR recordings is an important consideration in clinical application of the technique. A number of investigators have shown that such responses can be observed for stimuli at reasonably low presentation levels (Jeng, Brown, Johnson, & Vander Werrf, 2004; Small & Stapells, 2004). Various approaches such as modifying the analog-to-digital conversion rate on the electroencephalogram (EEG) to prevent stimulus artifact from "alias-

---

[10]The slight increase in 1-kHz ASSR threshold (10 dB) between the 4-week and 8-month assessments for Subject C may reflect maturation of these anatomical structures.

ing" to the modulation frequency, or employing stimuli with reduced electrical artifact (such as alternating polarity tones), have been used, with some success. Even so, the possibility of spurious response remains, particularly for low-frequency carrier tones at relatively high (50 dB HL or higher) presentation levels (Small & Stapells, 2006).

To date, no normative data describing BC-ASSR artifact levels for the AUDERA system have appeared in the literature. In our laboratory, we tested five profoundly deaf adult subjects and two babies (who subsequently showed) total hearing loss. ASSR responses were obtained in these subjects to bone-conducted stimuli at levels 40 dB HL or greater at the 500-Hz test frequency and 50 dB HL or greater for the 1-kHz and 2-kHz carriers. (No responses were seen at 50 dB HL for the 4-kHz tone.) It seems likely, therefore, that the BC-ASSR thresholds obtained for Subject C (at significantly lower levels) were a true reflection of his auditory function. Assessment of cochlear reserve in patients with sensorineural hearing loss is, however, likely to be challenging.

Clinical Application of the Bone Conduction Masking Method

This case study illustrates that important information can be gained from threshold ASSR tests using both air- and bone-conducted stimuli. There are three critical issues in BC-ASSR tests: first, the issue of what constitutes normal bone conduction thresholds in infants younger than 1 year of age, the correspondence with psychophysical thresholds, and the ever-present problem of artifact. Use of an alternative method for BC-ASSR threshold tests can help to reduce the possibil-

ity of artifact: Bone conduction threshold can be estimated from the effective masking level for bone-conducted noise.

There is a long history of using bone-conducted masking noise (for an air-conducted test stimulus), going back to Rainville (1955, 1959). This researcher determined the effective masking level for bone conduction masking during pure-tone threshold tests. That is, bone-conducted masking noise is used to mask the air-conducted test stimulus. This method was named the *sensorineural acuity level* test (Jerger & Jerger, 1965; Jerger & Tillman, 1960) and, when applied to auditory evoked potential threshold tests, often is referred to as the SAL method. We prefer the term *bone conduction masking method*.

For a person with normal middle ear function, the BC effective masking (BC-EM) level is equal to the AC threshold—there is no difference between AC threshold and BC-EM level. For the person with a conductive component to the hearing loss, the BC-EM level will be equivalent to the bone conduction thresholds. For example, if bone conduction pure-tone thresholds are 30 dB HL and air conduction pure-tone thresholds are at 60 dB HL, the BC-EM level for an air-conducted signal at 60 dB HL is 30 dB EM. There is a 30-dB air-bone gap, and the BC-EM level indicates a mild sensorineural component (30 dB BC-EM = 30 dB BC threshold).

This method has been used for BC-ABR tests (see Cone-Wesson, 1995, for a review) and for ASSR tests (Cone-Wesson et al., 2002). Just as for any bone conduction test, the stimuli must be calibrated. This is done by determining the effective masking levels for noise presented through a bone conduction oscillator, when the test stimulus is presented using insert phones. It is necessary to perform this "biologic" calibration using ASSR tests. The method is as follows:

1. Determine the ASSR threshold for an air-conducted stimulus (eg. 1000-Hz amplitude- and frequency-modulated [AM-FM] tone). In this example, the ASSR threshold in a normal adult is 30 dB HL.

2. Present masking noise through a bone conduction oscillator. Repeat the AC-ASSR test (at 30 dB HL) with masking noise presented simultaneously through the bone conduction oscillator. Bracket the effective masking level as would be done for threshold (e.g., down 10 dB, up 5 dB). The level of masking needed to mask the 30 dB HL stimulus is 30 dB EM.

3. Repeat the procedure using AC stimulus levels of 40, 50, and 60 dB HL. There should be a linear relationship between the BC-EM levels and the air conduction levels.

This method should be determined for 5 to 10 subjects with normal hearing. Although this appears to be somewhat labor-intensive, it is no more so than should be done for any bone conduction test method. That is, it is always necessary to establish threshold electrophysiologically for any stimulus type that is to be used in testing. For this bone conduction masking method, the effective masking levels for air-conducted test stimuli are established. The so called *direct* method (of Small and Stapells, presented in Chapter 11) also requires that threshold be established electrophysiologically for each stimulus used in the ASSR evaluation.

Cone-Wesson and associates (2002) showed that this method could be used to test infants with normal hearing and those at risk for conductive hearing loss. ASSR threshold testing was performed using a 1000-Hz AM-FM tone at 90 Hz. A group of 6- to 8 week-old infants who had normal click-evoked ABR thresholds, normal distortion product otoacoustic emissions, and normal tympanometry (1000-Hz probe tone) served as the control group. In these infants, the AC-ASSR threshold was 27 dB HL, and the BC-EM level was 15 dB, indicating a 12-dB air-bone gap. This result is similar to that found with the direct method: Infants have better bone conduction thresholds than air conduction thresholds. Another group of infants at risk for conductive hearing loss was tested. These infants demonstrated elevated click-ABR thresholds, abnormal tympanometry, and absence of otoacoustic emissions. In these infants, the average 1000-Hz AC-ASSR threshold was 50 dB HL, whereas the BC-EM level was 15 dB, just as in infants with normal ASSR thresholds and middle ear function. This finding was consistent with a conductive hearing loss: normal bone conduction thresholds (15 dB) and elevated AC-ASSR thresholds. Several children with known audiometric configurations also were tested using the bone conduction masking method. In these cases, the BC-EM levels were consistent with the bone conduction pure-tone thresholds, and the AC-ASSR thresholds were consistent with the pure-tone AC thresholds.

The bone conduction masking method has limitations similar to those observed with the direct method. First, BC-EM levels are much lower in infants younger than 1 year of age than in older infants with more adult-like skull properties. Both the bone conduction masking method and the direct method are likely to indicate an air-bone gap in infants younger than1 year of age, even when middle ear function is normal. Another limitation is that there are output limitations to the BC oscillator and EM levels are limited to 70 dB. A third limitation is the error of the EM estimate, which is approximately ±10 dB, as is the direct threshold estimate. This means that BC tests, and the estimate of the air-bone gap, will be best for subjects with moderate or greater hearing losses. The mixed loss with a 15- to 20-dB air-bone gap could be missed.

Several advantages are recognized for the bone conduction masking method. First, the same stimulus is used for the air conduction and bone conduction test: an air-conducted (modulated) tone. Second, there is no problem with "crossover": If the masking noise crosses over to the non-test ear, it is of no consequence. Third, the artifact from the bone conduction oscillator is noise, and averaging will reduce the artifact, rather than enhancing it.

Given the good test performance of the bone conduction masking method for BC-ABR tests (Janssen et al., 1993; Ysunza & Cone-Wesson, 1987) and the published results for applying the technique for ASSR (Cone-Wesson et al., 2002), the technique offers a viable alternative to BC-ASSR testing for those clinicians who cannot manipulate the analog-to-digital rate for their signal averagers, or who have concerns about the artifact for bone conduction tests at higher levels.

References

Cone-Wesson, B. (1995). Bone-conduction ABR tests. *American Journal of Audiology*, *4*, 14–19.

Cone-Wesson, B., Rickards, F., Poulis, C., Parker, J., Tan, L., & Pollard, J. (2002). The auditory steady-state response: Clinical observations and applications in infants and children. *Journal of the American Academy of Audiology*, *13*, 270–282.

Janssen, E. A., Borcaar, M. P., & Van Zanten, G. A. (1993). The masked threshold to noise ratio in brainstem electric response. *Audiology*, *32*, 153–163.

Jeng, F.-C., Brown, C. J., Johnson, T. A., & Vander Werff, K. R (2004). Estimating air-bone gaps using auditory steady-state responses. *Journal of the American Academy of Audiology*, *15*, 67–78.

Jerger, J., & Jerger, S. (1965). Critical evaluation of SAL audiometry. *Journal of Speech and Hearing Research*, *8*, 103–127.

Jerger, J., & Tillman, T. (1960). A new method for the clinical determination of sensorineural acuity level (SAL). *Archives of Otolaryngology*, *71*, 948–955.

Rainville, M. J. (1955). Nouvelle method d'assourdissement pour le releve des courbes de conduction osseuse. *Journal Fr Otolrhino-Laryngol*, *4*(8), 851–858.

Rainville, M. J. (1959). New method of masking for the determination of bone conduction curves. *Translations Beltone Institute for Hearing Research*, *No. 11*.

Rance, G., & Tomlin, D. (2006). Maturation of auditory steady-state responses in normal babies. *Ear and Hearing*, *27*, 20–29.

Small, S. A., Hatton, J. L., & Stapells, D. R. (2007). Effects of bone oscillator coupling method, placement location, and occlusion on bone-conduction auditory steady-state responses in infants. *Ear and Hearing*, *28*, 83–98.

Small, S. A., & Stapells, D. R. (2004). Artifactual responses when recording auditory steady-state responses. *Ear and Hearing*, *25*, 611–623.

Small, S. A., & Stapells, D. R. (2006). Multiple auditory steady-state response thresholds to bone-conduction stimuli in young infants with normal hearing. *Ear and Hearing*, *27*, 219–228.

Ysunza, A., & Cone-Wesson, B. (1987). Bone conduction masking for brainstem auditory evoked potentials (BAEP) in pediatric audiological evaluations. Validation of the test. *International Journal of Pediatric Otorhinolaryngology*, *12*, 291–302.

Case Study 6
Use of Auditory Evoked Potentials in Workers' Compensation Cases

Author: Anna Van Maanen
Affiliations: University of British Columbia, Vancouver; WorkSafeBC (formerly Workers' Compensation Board of British Columbia), Richmond, British Columbia, Canada

Background

At the British Columbia WorkSafeBC Audiology Unit, it is standard practice for all workers who are potentially eligible for monetary compensation to have behavioural hearing test results confirmed with an auditory evoked potential (AEP). Behavioral test protocols are designed to detect nonorganic hearing loss (e.g., ascending pure-tone testing).

At the WorkSafeBC Audiology Unit, 6% to 8% of clients evaluated demonstrate some degree of nonorganic hearing loss (sometimes referred to as functional hearing loss, or pseudohypacusis) (Adelman & Van Maanen, 2001); this figure is consistent with those from other studies (e.g., Alberti, Hyde, & Riko, 1987). Most clients provide consistent, reliable, and accurate behavioural results. Nevertheless the behavioural test protocols used by WorkSafeBC are designed to look for consistency of test results. Behavioural test protocols include conducting speech testing before pure-tone testing and the use of an ascending stimulus presentation technique when obtaining speech and pure-tone thresholds. Despite the effectiveness of these protocols for ascertaining the presence of nonorganic hearing loss, hearing thresholds may remain undetermined. If reliable behavioural results cannot be obtained for any WorkSafeBC client, AEP testing is required to estimate hearing thresholds.

For the passively or actively alert adult population, the *slow cortical potential* (SCP), sometimes referred to as the slow vertex potential, the cortical auditory evoked potential, or the late vertex response, has been considered to be the AEP measure of choice for threshold estimation (Hyde, 1994; Lightfoot & Kennedy, 2006; Stach, Jerger, & Penn, 1994; Stapells, 2002). This is due in part to the good frequency specificity of the response and its robust nature in alert adults (Picton, 1991). The SCP has been used successfully for medicolegal and compensation cases (Adelman & Van Maanen, 2001; Alberti et al., 1987; Bonvier, 2002; Coles & Mason, 1984; Tsui, Wong, & Wong, 2002).

The auditory steady-state response (ASSR) and its use for threshold estimation have been investigated for many years, since the 40-Hz work of Galambos, Makieg, and Talmachoff (1981). Interest in the ASSR has increased since research has shown that both single ASSR and multiple ASSR testing using approximately 80-Hz modulation frequencies is an accurate means of estimating hearing thresholds for infants and adults (for a review, see Picton, John, Dimitrijevic, & Purcell, 2003). Another area of potential clinical interest is the estimation of threshold for adults using an approximately 40-Hz response to multiple stimuli. It has long been known that 40-Hz ASSR is not ideal for infants or sleeping subjects (Stapells, Galambos, Costello, & Makeig, 1988); however, previous research suggests that using the 40-Hz modulation frequency is optimal in awake adults for evoking an ASSR (e.g., Galambos et al., 1981; Levi, Folsom, & Dobie, 1993; Picton et al., 2003). An objective technique for threshold estimation in cooperatively alert, passive adults, in whom multiple frequencies could be obtained at once, would be a welcome addition to the clinical armamentarium for clinicians involved in medicolegal or compensation cases. Multiple ASSRs are analyzed in the frequency domain by fast fourier transform (FFT), and presence or absence of responses is determined by statistical analyses using the amplitude of the response relative to surrounding noise or phase variability (see Picton et al., 2003). An advantage to assessing multiple ASSRs over other AEPs is that no clinical judgement is required for determination of the presence or absence of a response.

Van Maanen and Stapells (2005) compared the multiple ASSR at approximately 80 Hz, 40 Hz, and the SCP. Multiple ASSRs were obtained using the MASTER research system (John & Picton, 2000). Starting intensity was randomly selected at 40 or 60 dBHL. A bracketing procedure with a 10-dB final step size was used. SCP testing was conducted using the Intelligent Hearing Systems Smart-EP. Frequencies tested were, in order, 0.5, 1, and 2 kHz (use of these frequencies is specified by the Workers' Compensation Act of British Columbia). A bracketing procedure with a 5-dB final step size was used.

Results indicate that multiple ASSRs and SCPs provide good estimates of the configuration of the pure-tone audiogram. 40-Hz ASSR showed the best accuracy, however. Recording times were estimated on the basis of collection of thresholds for four frequencies (for one ear). The mean time required to estimate four thresholds for one ear was 36 minutes

for the 80-Hz multiple ASSR, 21 minutes for the 40-Hz multiple ASSR, and 15 minutes for the SCP. Despite obtaining four frequencies at once with multiple ASSR, the SCP was the fastest. Clearly, if one is to consider ASSR for threshold estimation in adults, a 40-Hz, rather than a 80-Hz, modulation frequency is the best choice. The results suggested that in view of the objectivity of response determination of the ASSR, the difficulty in obtaining training and experience with SCP testing, and the potential need for multiple AEP thresholds for each ear, the 40-Hz multiple ASSR is a potentially a better choice than the SCP.

Since then, Tomlin, Rance, Graydon, and Tsialios (2006) compared 40-Hz ASSR (single stimulus) and SCPs at 500 and 4000 Hz. Their results suggested that the SCP may provide a more reliable estimate of hearing in awake adults. However, single-stimulus ASSRs were obtained with a maximum recording time of 90 seconds, and longer recording periods would be expected to result in lower ASSR thresholds (Picton, Dimitrijevic, Perez-Abalo, & Van Roon, 2005).

WorkSafeBC has not yet incorporated 40-Hz multiple ASSR testing into the standard test protocol and continues to use the SCP to verify behavioural threshold or, in cases of nonorganic hearing loss, as the best representation of true hearing threshold, but is investigating it for possible future use.

Subject History

A 70-year old client (E.R.) applied for an occupational noise–induced hearing loss claim with WorkSafeBC. He had a significant history of hazardous noise exposure including 3 years as a general laborer in construction (Lex of 91dBA) and 27 years as a ramp attendant at a busy international airport (Lex of 90dBA). He had retired approximately 5 years before filing his claim.

The client reported a history of a heart attack, for which he was on medication, but had no other significant medical or otological history.

As part of WorkSafeBC's occupational health and safety regulation requirements, the client had had screening audiograms done at work for 6 consecutive years. All audiograms showed high-frequency hearing loss above 2000 Hz; however, the last audiogram was at least a decade before the client's last hazardous noise exposure, and a diagnostic audiologic assessment at the WorkSafeBC Audiology Unit was recommended.

Results

Behavioural test results indicated mild-to-severe sensorineural hearing loss bilaterally. Acoustic immittance testing indicated limited compliance of the tympanic membrane, but ipsilateral and contralateral acoustic reflexes were within normal limits. Behavioural results were confirmed by SCP testing (performed blind). In addition to the SCP testing, 40-Hz multiple ASSR testing was undertaken as part of the study by Van Maanen and Stapells (2005).

Figure 14–6.1 shows SCP, 40-Hz ASSR, and behavioural hearing thresholds for Subject E.R. These findings are typical of the results from the subjects in this study (Van Maanen & Stapells, 2005), showing good AEP correlation with overall hearing thresholds and audiogram configuration.

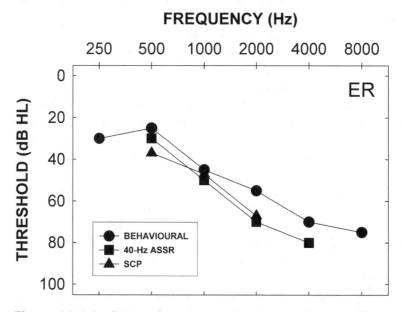

Figure 14–6.1. Behavioural thresholds from 250 to 8000 Hz; approximately 40-Hz multiple ASSR thresholds for 500, 1000, 2000, and 4000 Hz; and SCP thresholds from 500, 1000, and 2000 Hz.

Outcomes

As a result of all test results (behavioural confirmed by AEP tests) showing hearing loss consistent with the client's history of hazardous noise exposure, this particular client's claim was accepted. Under the Workers' Compensation Act, he was entitled to coverage of amplification (for life) and monetary compensation.

Comments

Medicolegal cases require a unique approach to testing. Modified behavioural test protocols should be used to detect nonorganic hearing loss. As part of the test battery, an objective method to confirm behavioural results is recommended. AEP testing is the preferred method. If ASSR is to be considered for threshold estimation in adults, a 40-Hz, rather than 80-Hz, modulation frequency is the best choice. WorkSafeBC uses the SCP as the preferred method of verification of behavioural threshold but is investigating the 40-Hz multiple ASSR for possible use in the future.

Acknowledgments. Thanks to David R. Stapells for his assistance with this case study.

References

Adelman, S., & Van Maanen, A. (2001 July). Use of SVP for threshold estimation in WCB claimants. Poster presented at the 17th meeting of the International Evoked Response Audiometry Study Group Symposium, Vancouver, Canada.

Alberti, P., Hyde, M., & Riko, K. (1987). Exaggerated hearing loss in compensation claimants. *Journal of Otolaryngology*, *16*, 362–366.

Bonvier, R. (2002). Slow auditory evoked potentials: The end of malingering in audiology. *International Tinnitus Journal*, *8*, 58–61.

Coles, R. R. A., & Mason, S. M. (1984). The results of cortical electric response audiometry in medico-legal investigations. *British Journal of Audiology*, *18*, 71–78.

Hyde, M. L. (1994). The slow vertex potential: Properties and clinical applications. In J. T. Jacobson (Ed.), *Principles and applications in auditory evoked potentials* (pp. 179–218). Boston: Allyn & Bacon.

Galambos, R., Makeig, S., & Talmachoff, P. J. (1981). A 40-Hz auditory potential recorded from the human scalp. *Proceedings of the National Academy of Science of the United States of America*, *78*, 2643–2647.

Levi, E. C., Folsom, R. C., & Dobie, R. A. (1993). Amplitude-modulation following response (AMFR): Effects of modulation rate, carrier frequency, age, and state. *Hearing Research*, *68*, 42–52.

Lightfoot, G., & Kennedy, V. (2006). Cortical electric response audiometry hearing threshold estimation: Accuracy, speed and the effects of stimulus presentation features. *Ear and Hearing*, *27*, 443–456.

Picton, T. W. (1991). Clinical usefulness of auditory evoked potentials: A critical evaluation. *Journal of Speech-Language Pathology and Audiology*, *15*, 3–16.

Picton, T. W., Dimitrijevic, A., Perez-Abablo, M. C., & Van Roon, P. (2005). Estimating audiometric thresholds using auditory steady-state responses. *Journal of the American Academy of Audiology*, *16*, 140–156.

Picton, T. W., John, M. S., Dimitrijevic, A., & Purcell, D. (2003). Human auditory steady-state responses. *International Journal of Audiology*, *42*, 177–219.

Stach, B. A., Jerger, J. F., & Penn, T. O. (1994). In J. T. Jacobson (Ed.), *Principles and applications in auditory evoked potentials. Chapter 21—Auditory evoked potential testing strategies.* (pp. 541–560). Boston: Allyn & Bacon.

Stapells, D. R. (2002). Cortical event-related potentials to auditory stimuli. In J. Katz (Ed.), *Handbook of clinical audiology* (pp. 378–406). Baltimore: Lippincott Williams & Wilkins.

Stapells, D. R., Galambos, R., Costello, J. A., & Makeig, S. (1988). Inconsistency of auditory middle latency and steady-state responses in infants. *Electroencephalography and Clinical Neurophysiology*, 71, 289–295.

Tomlin, D., Rance, G., Graydon, K., & Tsialios, I. (2006). A comparison of 40 Hz auditory steady-state response (ASSR) and cortical auditory evoked potential (CAEP) thresholds in awake adult subjects. *International Journal of Audiology*, 45, 580–588.

Tsui, B., Wong, L., & Wong, E. (2002). Accuracy of the cortical evoked response audiometry in the identification of nonorganic hearing loss. *International Journal of Audiology*, 41, 330–333.

Van Maanen, A., & Stapells, D. R. (2005). Comparison of multiple auditory steady-state responses (80 vs. 40 Hz) and slow cortical potentials for threshold estimation in hearing-impaired adults. *International Journal of Audiology*, 44, 613–624.

Case Study 7
Auditory Steady-State Responses in a Child with Auditory Neuropathy/Dyssynchrony

Author: Gary Rance
Affiliation: University of Melbourne

History

Subject A was born at 33 weeks gestation weighing 2.05 kg. Her mother initially was well during the pregnancy but suffered severe preeclampsia in the third trimester. Despite her prematurity, the infant presented with no neonatal risk factors for permanent hearing loss apart from hyperbilirubinemia (peak serum bilirubin level of 415 mol/l), for which she received blood transfusion.

Newborn hearing screening assessment by automated auditory brainstem response (ABR) at discharge from the special care unit (at 38 weeks postconceptual age) and again at 41 weeks postconceptual age showed no response in either ear. Transient otoacoustic emission (TEOAE) responses were present bilaterally when sought on the second of these occasions.

Findings

The family was referred to the University of Melbourne School of Audiology Clinic, where Subject A underwent diagnostic testing at 44 weeks postconceptual age. Evoked potential assessment was carried out with the child in natural sleep on the mother's lap using the GSI Audera system. Multiple-probe tone tympanometry and otoscopic examination yielded normal results; there was no evidence of peripheral (ear canal or middle ear) abnormality.[11]

Auditory steady-state response (ASSR) thresholds to amplitude- and frequency-modulated (AM/FM) tones at octave frequencies between 250 Hz and 4 kHz were obtained between 75 and 105 dB HL in both ears (Figure 14–7.1). In a baby with sensorineural hearing loss, these findings would be consistent with hearing impairment in the severe-to-profound

---

[11]Tests of middle ear function were carried out and showed normal results on each of the test occasions described in this case study.

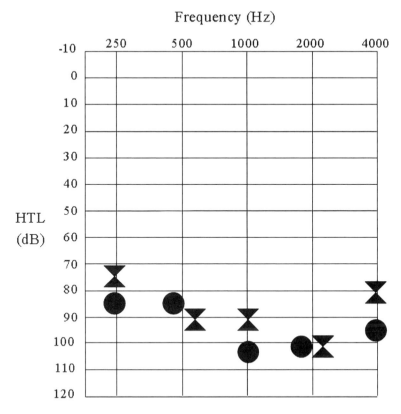

Figure 14–7.1. ASSR thresholds (dB HL) obtained at the age of 1 month (corrected). *Filled circles* represent the findings for the right ear, and *filled crosses* represent data for the left ear.

range (Rance & Rickards, 2002). ABR testing did, however, reveal the presence of auditory pathway disorder (rather than "typical" cochlear hearing loss) in this case.

Click-evoked ABR assessment was carried out in the manner described by Rance and colleagues (1999). Figure 14–7.2 shows the results obtained for Subject A's right ear. (Findings were identical on the left side.) The top tracing shows no identifiable waveform in response to acoustic clicks presented at 100 dB nHL. This result, in a child with peripheral or cochlear hearing loss, would indicate that the stimulus was not loud enough to elicit sufficient electrical activity in the auditory pathway to produce an ABR

and would be consistent with severe-to-profound hearing loss. An ear with this degree of loss would, however, typically show no response from the cochlear hair cells, yet Subject A demonstrated repeatable cochlear microphonic responses to unipolar stimuli at 80 dB nHL (middle tracings in Figure 14–7.2). The presence of this preneural activity, together with the absence of recordable neural response from the brainstem, is indicative of an auditory pathway abnormality termed *auditory neuropathy/dyssynchrony* (AN/AD) (Berlin, Hood, & Rose, 2001; Starr, Picton, Sininger, Hood, & Berlin, 1996). Further evidence of preneural response and hence AN/AD type hearing loss was provided by a repeat

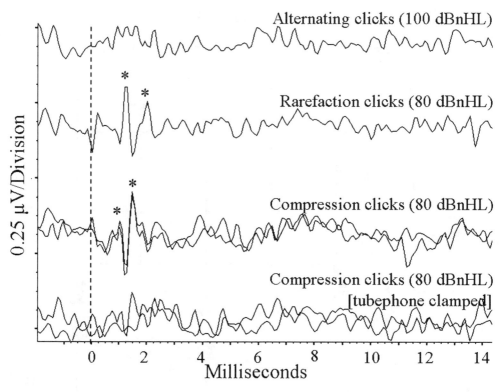

Figure 14–7.2. Averaged EEG tracings obtained for Subject A's right ear. The *dotted line* represents the point at which the stimulus was generated (at the transducer). The *top tracings* show no recordable potentials in response to alternating acoustic clicks presented at 100 dB nHL. The *middle tracings* show repeatable cochlear microphonic responses but absence of ABRs to unipolar stimuli at 80 dB nHL. *Asterisks* denote the positive peaks in the CM waveform. The *bottom tracings* were obtained to compression clicks presented with the tubephone clamped.

otoacoustic emission assessment. Clear responses (greater than 10 dB) at octave frequencies between 1 and 4 kHz confirmed the presence of the cochlear active process in each ear.

On the basis of these findings, when the child was 1 month of age, the family was referred for early intervention support. Amplification was not offered at this point, because it is not possible to predict the audiogram of babies with AN/AD type hearing loss from auditory evoked potential findings (Rance et al., 1999).

Conditioned behavioural hearing testing proved a challenge in the early period, but a reliable audiogram showing hearing levels in the mild-to-moderate range was obtained when the child was 10 months of age. Figure 14–7.3 shows the hearing thresholds for each ear.[12] Also shown are the earlier ASSR findings. The

[12]The predominantly low-frequency hearing loss in this case is another feature typical of AN/AD (Rance, 2005).

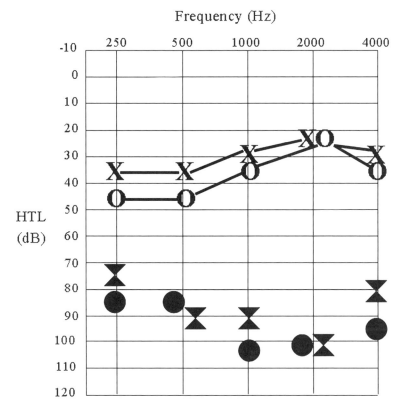

Figure 14–7.3. Behavioural hearing thresholds established at the age of 10 months (*open symbols*) and ASSR thresholds obtained at the age of 1 month (*filled symbols*).

incompatibility between evoked potential and behavioural results (with ASSR responses only recordable at high sensation levels) in this case is consistent with previously reported findings for children with AN/AD (Rance & Briggs, 2002).

Behind-the-ear hearing aids were fit to Subject A at 11 months of age. These devices were configured to match the degree and audiometric pattern of her loss and afforded complete access to the speech spectrum at normal levels.

Through the preschool years, Subject A showed a relatively normal developmental course. She met all of her physical milestones at expected times, and a Kaufman Brief Intelligence Test (K-BIT) conducted

at the age of 4 years 6 months revealed age-appropriate (nonverbal) cognitive development. She did, however, experience significant auditory perceptual problems and mildly delayed speech and language development, as is typical of many children with AN/AD-type hearing loss (Rance et al., 2007; Rance, et al., (2007).

At 5 years of age, Subject A was enrolled in a research project conducted at the University of Melbourne. ASSR assessment of the right ear was carried out with the child awake but reading quietly. Responses to tones amplitude-modulated at two rates (40 Hz and 90 Hz) were sought. As can be seen in Figure 14–7.4, ASSRs at both modulation

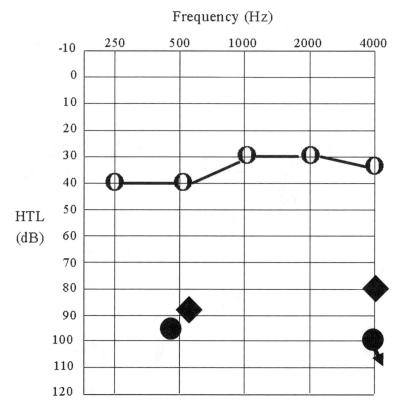

Figure 14–7.4. ASSR and behavioural thresholds for the right ear at the age of 5 years. 40-Hz ASSR thresholds are represented by *filled diamonds*, 90-Hz ASSR thresholds are represented by *filled circles*, and behavioural hearing levels are represented by *open circles*.

rates could be detected, but only at sensation levels much higher than would be expected for sensorineural type hearing loss.

A possible explanation for these abnormal ASSR findings can be found in the psychophysical profile obtained for Subject A. Disruption of timing-related information appears to be the major way in which auditory perception is distorted in patients with AN/AD type hearing loss (Rance, McKay, & Graydon, 2004; Zeng, Oba, Garde, Sininger, & Starr, 1999).

Unlike their sensorineural counterparts, who typically present with normal

temporal resolution, subjects with AN/AD have shown severely impaired performance on a range of perceptual tasks based on the processing of timing cues. One such measure is the *temporal modulation transfer function* (TMTF), which requires that the subject detect sinusoidal amplitude fluctuations in the level of a steady-state signal. (In this regard, the stimuli resemble the signals used to elicit the ASSR.) Figure 14–7.5 shows TMTF findings for a group of school-aged children with sensorineural hearing loss (filled circles). In these subjects, the ability to detect amplitude modulation at

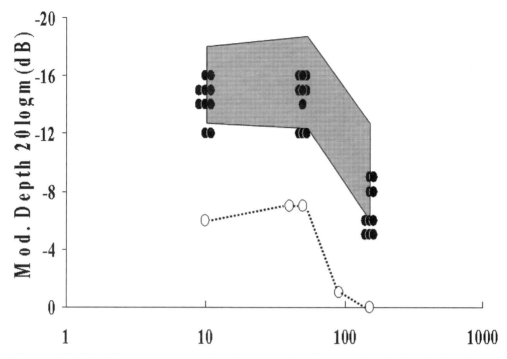

Figure 14–7.5. Temporal modulation transfer function results for Subject A (*open circles*). The *filled points* represent data from a control group of children with sensorineural-type hearing loss, and the *shaded area* represents the performance range (mean ± 2 standard deviations) for a cohort of normally hearing subjects. (From Rance, McKay, & Graydon, 2004.)

10-, 50-, and 150 Hz was broadly equivalent to the performance range for for normally hearing subjects (represented by the shaded area). By contrast, modulation detection limits for Subject A (open circles) at these rates (plus 2 others, 40 and 90 Hz, selected to match the modulation frequencies used in the ASSR assessment) were significantly worse. This was particularly the case at the higher rates (90 and 150 Hz), when amplitude changes of close to 0 dB (100%) were required before the fluctuations could be perceived. Although the ASSR stimuli used in this study (and in most clinical systems) were amplitude-modulated at a depth of 100%, the psychophysical find-

ings for Subject A point to a reduced capacity of her auditory system to accurately encode rapid amplitude changes, potentially explaining explain its impaired ability to produce steady-state responses to stimuli modulated at high rates.

Comments

In summary, the results presented in this study support the conclusion that auditory evoked potentials, or at least those generated in the region of the auditory brainstem such as the ABR and high-rate ASSR, cannot be used to predict hearing levels in children with AN/AD. In this child with only mild-to-moderate hearing loss, the ABR was absent to clicks at maximum presentation levels, and ASSRs were present only to modulated tones at high sensation levels. It is noteworthy that the latter response could be obtained at all in this child, suggesting that measurement of the ASSR may be less dependent on precise synchrony of neural firing in the auditory pathway. Thus, the ASSR may offer an objective measure of the degree of dyssynchrony. Further investigation into the effects of stimulus modulation rate and perhaps modulation depth on the response in affected ears may allow insight into the auditory pathway's ability to encode rapidly changing signals and could provide an indicator of the level of temporal disruption suffered by an individual subject. This may in turn inform management choices for affected children.

In the clinical context, AN/AD, which accounts for approximately 10% of cases of permanent hearing loss in children (Rance, 2005), poses significant challenges for auditory clinicians. One particular limitation of the ASSR technique in this population is that it cannot differentiate between cochlear hearing loss and hearing impairment that is the result of neural transmission disorder. Transient evoked potential techniques such as ABR testing can make this distinction based on the presence or absence of the preneural, cochlear microphonic response. ASSR testing, on the other hand, involves analysis in the frequency rather than the time domain and is unable to distinguish between preneural and neural elements within the electroencephalogram (EEG). Accordingly, it is important in clinical practice to use the ABR and ASSR techniques in concert for diagnostic assessment of hearing in young children.

References

Berlin, C. I., Hood, L .J., & Rose, K. (2001). On renaming auditory neuropathy as auditory dys-synchrony. *Audiology Today*, *13*, 15-17.

Rance, G. (2005). Auditory neuropathy/dys-synchrony and its perceptual consequences. *Trends in Amplification*, *9*(1), 1-43.

Rance, G. , Barker, E., Mok, M., Dowell, R., Rincon, A., & Garratt, R. (2007). Speech perception in noise for children with auditory neuropathy/dys-synchrony type hearing loss. *Ear and Hearing*, *28*(3), 351-360.

Rance, G., Barker, E.J., Sarant, J.Z. & Ching T. (2007). Spoken Language Abilities in Children with Auditory Neuropathy/Dys-Synchrony Type Hearing Loss. *Ear & Hearing*, *28*(5), 694-702.

Rance, G., Beer, D. E., Cone-Wesson, B., Shepherd, R. K., King, A., Rickards, F. W., et al. (1999). Clinical findings for a group of infants and young children with auditory neuropathy. *Ear and Hearing*, *20*(3), 238-252.

Rance, G., & Briggs, R.J.S. (2002). Assessment of hearing level in infants with significant hearing loss: The Melbourne experience with steady-state evoked potential threshold testing. *Annals of Otology, Rhinology, and Laryngology*, *111*(5), 22-28.

Rance, G., McKay, C., & Grayden, D. (2004). Perceptual characterisation of children with auditory neuropathy. *Ear and Hearing*, *25*, 34-46.

Rance, G., & Rickards, F. W. (2002). Prediction of hearing threshold in infants using auditory steady-state evoked potentials. *Journal of the American Academy of Audiology*, *13*, 236-245.

Starr, A., Picton, T. W., Sininger, Y. S., Hood, L. J., & Berlin, C. I. (1996). Auditory Neuropathy. *Brain*, *119*(3), 741-753.

Zeng, F.-G., Oba, S., Garde, S., Sininger, Y., & Starr, A. (1999). Temporal and speech processing deficits in auditory neuropathy. *Neuroreport*, *10*(16), 3429-3435.

Case Study 8
Free-Field Auditory
Steady-State Response
Testing for Assessment of
Hearing Aid Function
in an Infant

Authors: Gary Rance and Alison King
Affiliations: University of Melbourne
(Rance); Australian Hearing (King)

Subject History

Subject H was a 6-week-old, full-term infant when first seen at the University of Melbourne School of Audiology Clinic. He had presented with an enlarged liver and spleen when assessed by his pediatrician at 2 weeks of age and was referred for hearing assessment and blood tests, which subsequently proved positive for cytomegalovirus (CMV) antibodies.

Click-evoked auditory brainstem response (ABR) assessment was carried out at the Monash Medical Centre at the age of 3 weeks. A response threshold of 80 dB nHL, consistent with the presence of severe hearing loss in the mid- to high-frequency range, was obtained for the right ear (Stapells, Picton, & Durieux-Smith, 1994). No repeatable waveforms were observed to clicks at the maximum presentation level, in the left ear suggesting at least severe-to-profound hearing loss (Rance, Dowell, Beer, Rickards, & Clark, 1998)[13] (Figure 14–8.1). Impedance audiometry showed Type A tympanograms at the 220-, 660-, and 1000-Hz test frequencies. Hence, there was no evidence of middle ear abnormality. Behavioural testing showed no response to noisemakers at maximum presentation levels (90 to 100 dBA). Therefore, significant bilateral sensorineural hearing loss was indicated, and Subject H was referred for auditory steady-state response (ASSR) assessment as a prelude to hearing aid fitting.

Auditory Steady-State Response Testing

Each of the ASSR assessments were carried out using a custom-built evoked potential system that employed an IBM-compatible XT-type microcomputer to generate stimuli and analyze responses in the manner described by Cohen, Rickards, and Clark (1991).[14] The test stimuli were 250-, 500-, 1000-, 2000-, and 4000-Hz tones, amplitude- and frequency-modulated at a rate of 90 Hz. ASSR thresholds were established for each of these signals using a presentation step size of 5 dB. All evoked potential testing was carried out in a sound-treated room with the child in natural sleep. Test procedures for the unaided ASSR assessments were as described by Rance and associates (1998). The stimuli in this case were presented to each ear individually through mu-metal–shielded TDH 39 headphones, which allowed maximum presentation levels of 104 dB HL for the 250-Hz stimulus and 120 dB HL for the higher test frequencies.

ASSR assessment of hearing aid function was undertaken with the child lying

[13]Assessment with unipolar clicks also showed no cochlear microphonic response, suggesting peripheral, rather than auditory neuropathy/dyssynchrony-type hearing loss.

[14]The testing in fact took place in 1991 and so predated the release of commercial ASSR systems.

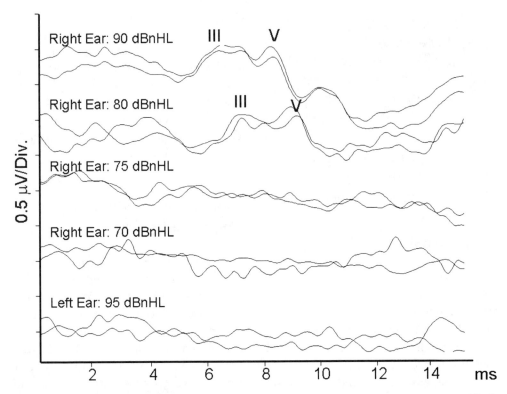

Figure 14–8.1. Averaged EEG tracings obtained after acoustic clicks presented individually to the left and right ears.

across the mother's lap as she sat in an armchair in the center of the test room. The child's better-hearing ear (the right) faced a loudspeaker situated at a distance of approximately 1.25 meters. The non-test ear was occluded with a foam plug throughout the assessment. The free-field stimuli were calibrated at a point as close as practical to the child's ear, using a Bruel and Kjaer sound level meter. Maximum presentation level was limited to 80 dB SPL at each of the test frequencies.

A clinical trial had previously been carried out using the free-field setup in a small group (N = 5) of normally hearing adult subjects to establish that results could be reliably obtained. ASSR thresh-

olds to stimuli presented by means of the loudspeaker were not significantly different from those obtained under headphones in these individuals.

Results

Unaided ASSR testing was undertaken when the child was 6 weeks of age. Assessment at octave frequencies between 250 Hz and 4 kHz showed threshold levels ranging from 70 to 115 dB HL in each ear (Figure 14–8.2). Thus, these results were broadly consistent with the earlier click-ABR findings.

Bilateral behind-the-ear hearing aids (Phonak PicoForte PPSC) were subse-

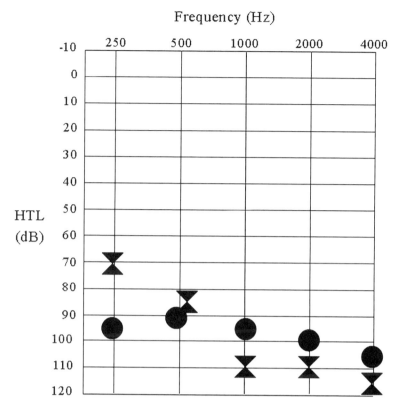

Figure 14–8.2. ASSR thresholds (dB HL) obtained at the age of 6 weeks. *Filled circles* represent response thresholds for the right ear, and *filled crosses* are for the left ear.

quently fit to this child. The aids were configured according to the National Acoustics Laboratories (N.A.L.) prescription (Byrne & Dillon, 1986; Byrne, Parkinson, & Newell, 1991), assuming behavioural hearing levels 10 dB lower than the ASSR thresholds. (As can be seen in Figure 14-8.4, this assumption was later shown to be essentially correct.)

Aided ASSR assessment was attempted at 10 weeks of age because the child's mother was concerned by his general lack of auditory responsiveness. Subject H wore his hearing aid on the settings prescribed by the audiologist, and battery and listening checks were carried out before testing. Figure 14-8.3 shows the N.A.L. "required aided thresholds" (unfilled circles) based on his assumed hearing levels and on the amount of amplification provided. Also shown are the child's aided ASSR thresholds (dBSPL). These values are close to the required thresholds and represent reasonable access to the normal 70 dB SPL speech spectrum (shaded). The difference between unaided and aided threshold offers a measure of the functional gain afforded by the hearing aid. In this case, the evoked potential threshold improvement closely matched the amount of amplification provided.

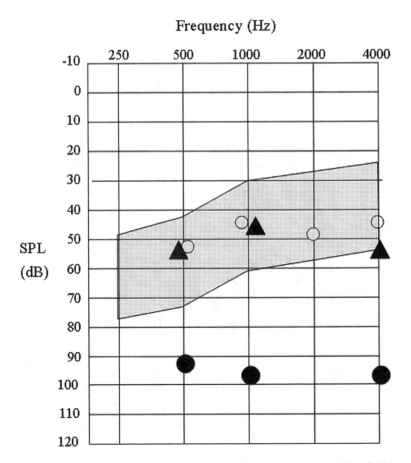

Figure 14–8.3. Free-field aided ASSR thresholds (dB SPL) obtained at the age of 10 weeks for the right ear (*filled triangles*) and unaided ASSR thresholds (dB SPL) for the right ear obtained at 6 weeks (*filled circles*). *Open circles* represent required aided threshold targets based on the National Acoustics Laboratories aiding prescription.

Behavioural hearing assessment using conditioned audiometric techniques (visual reinforcement audiometry) was possible in this child from 7 months of age and reliable from 8 months. Figure 14–8.4A and B shows his hearing threshold levels for each ear. It is clear from these data that ASSR results (obtained at the age of 6 weeks) reflected both the degree and the configuration of the hear-

ing loss. Figure 14–8.5 shows a similar correlation between behavioural and ASSR threshold levels obtained through the hearing aid.

Outcomes

Consistent hearing aid use was established for Subject H at a young age. He

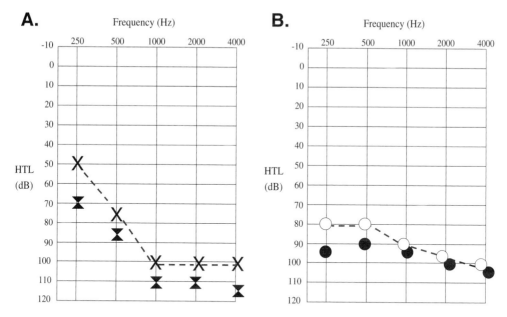

Figure 14–8.4. A, Behavioural and ASSR threshold levels for the left ear. ASSR assessment was conducted at the age of 6 weeks, and behavioural hearing levels were established at 8 months. **B,** Behavioural and ASSR threshold levels for the right ear. ASSR assessment was performed at the age of 6 weeks, and behavioural hearing levels were established at the age of 8 months.

initially was enrolled in an early intervention program that supported an oral-aural communication strategy. His subsequent educational placements all have been in mainstream schools.

Speech and language development has never been a concern for this child. Figure 14–8.6 shows receptive language scores obtained on the Peabody Picture Vocabulary Test from 2.5 to 9 years of age. The data in this case show receptive vocabulary acquisition at levels expected for normally hearing children.

Comments

This case study, in concert with data presented by Picton and coworkers (1998), suggests that it is possible to measure aided ASSR thresholds that correlate with behavioural aided thresholds. The stimuli used to elicit ASSR (continuous modulated tones) are better suited to objective assessment of aided hearing than the brief signals required to elicit the ABR. We now need to consider the application of aided threshold assessment within a pediatric hearing aid fitting program. What purpose do aided hearing thresholds serve in current clinical practice and with nonlinear hearing aids?

Verification

Aided hearing thresholds are no longer recommended for verifying that hearing aid prescriptive targets have been achieved. Real-ear measures of hearing

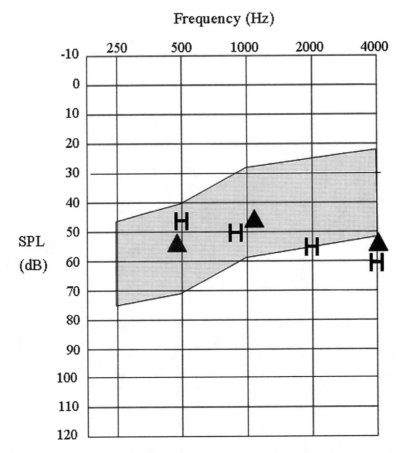

Figure 14–8.5. Aided thresholds established using free-field ASSR testing (at the age of 10 weeks) and conditioned audiometric assessment (at 8 months).

aid output provide the most accurate means of verifying that the hearing aid prescription has been matched for varying levels of input. In infants, the technique of *real-ear aided gain* (REAG) measures using either measured or age-averaged real-ear to coupler differences is recommended (Ching, Britton, Dillon, & Agung, 2002; Munro (2004); Seewald, (1995). This technique enables prescriptive targets to be matched quickly and to a high degree of accuracy, (within 2 to 3 dB, according to Ching and colleagues). Aided threshold ASSR assessment will be

less accurate than REAG measures for several reasons. Aided thresholds assess the gain of the hearing aid at discrete frequencies and a fixed input level, whereas REAG measures enable the gain of the aid to be evaluated over the entire frequency range and at different input levels. In nonlinear aids, the level at which an aided threshold is recorded is determined by overall gain, compression thresholds, and ratios, so it is not possible to infer which type of adjustment would be most appropriate if the aided threshold differs from the expected value (Dillon, 2001).

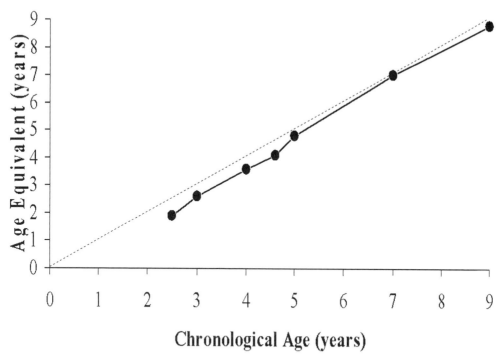

Figure 14–8.6. Peabody Picture Vocabulary Test (PPVT) results obtained over a 6-year period (2.5 to 9 years). Chronological age is plotted against equivalent language age at each data collection point.

Furthermore, the measurement errors inherent in ASSR testing, and practical clinical considerations mean that it is not realistic to measure aided thresholds in steps smaller than 5 dB.

Parent Information/Education

Aided ASSR assessment does offer an objective indication of the levels at which a baby's auditory system is responding to amplified sound. Thus, the results can be used to confirm that the aids are improving the child's sound detection ability. This can be particularly reassuring to parents of infants because the behavioural signs of hearing in very young children can be subtle and are highly dependent on the infant's state of arousal. In this case study, the results of the aided ASSR test helped the mother to have faith that the aids were making reasonably low-level sounds audible to her son.

Nonlinear Amplification

It should be noted that the devices worn by the child in this example were linear aids. With use of ASSR to measure aided thresholds in children wearing nonlinear hearing aids, it is essential to take into account the possible effects of signal processing features of the aids on the amplification provided to a continuous modulated tone.

Caution should be exercised in interpreting the results of any aided testing (behavioural or electrophysiological) with nonlinear hearing aids. The response of the hearing aid to a stimulus that has its energy concentrated in a narrow frequency band will be quite different from the way the aid processes the complex, varying input of running speech. Although aided thresholds can be used to indicate improved detection, more detailed explanations of the impact of improved audibility on speech perception will be best undertaken using visual representations of the amplified speech signal. See, for example, the work of Ching and associates (2002), Seewald (1995), and Stelmachowicz, Lewis, and Creutz (2007).

Conclusion

Although aided ASSR assessment is not accurate enough to be used in hearing aid verification, it can play a role in evaluating the response of the infant auditory system to amplified sound and in the education of parents. Research in this area is ongoing, but for the moment at least, the most useful way in which ASSR findings can inform the intervention process is by providing accurate estimates of (unaided) hearing levels on which the amplification prescriptions can be based.

References

Byrne, D., & Dillon, H. (1986). The National Acoustics Laboratories (N.A.L.) new procedure for selecting the gain and frequency response of a hearing aid. *Ear and Hearing*, 7, 257–265.

Byrne, D., Parkinson, A., & Newell, P. (1991). Modified hearing aid selection procedures for severe-profound hearing losses. In G. A. Studebaker, F. H. Bess, & L. B. Beck (Eds.), *The Vanderbilt hearing aid report II* (pp. 295–300). Parkton, Md., York Press.

Cohen, L. T., Rickards, F. W., & Clark, G. M. (1991). A comparison of steady-state evoked potentials to modulated tones in awake and sleeping humans. *Journal of the Acoustical Society of America*, 90, 2467–2479.

Ching, T. Y. C., Britton, L., Dillon, H., & Agung, K. (2002). RECD, REAG, NAL-NL1: Accurate and practical methods for fitting non-linear hearing aids to infants and children. *Hearing Review*, 9(8), 12–20, 52.

Dillon, H. (2001). *Hearing aids* (p. 419). Sydney: Boomerang Press. (Also distributed by Thieme, New York & Stuttgart)

Picton, T. W., Durieux-Smith, A., Champagne, S. C., Whittingham, J. A., Moran, L. M., Giguère, C., et al. (1998). Objective evaluation of aided thresholds using auditory steady-state responses. *Journal of the American Academy of Audiology*, 9, 315–331.

Rance, G., Dowell, R. C., Beer, D. E., Rickards, F. W., & Clark, G. M. (1998). Steady-state evoked potential and behavioural hearing thresholds in a group of children with absent click-evoked auditory brain stem response. *Ear and Hearing*, 19, 48–61.

Scollie, S. D., & Seewald, R. C. (2001). Electroacoustic verification measures with modern hearing instrument technology. A sound foundation through early amplification 2001. In R. C. Seewald & S. Gravel (Eds.), *Proceedings of the Second International Conference* (pp. 121–138). Phonak AG 2002. Published by Immediate Proceedings Limited, manufactured in Great Britain by St Edmundsbury Press.

Seewald, R. (1995). *The desired sensation level method for hearing aid fitting in infants and children, Phonak Focus 20*. Accessed via http://www.phonak.com/com_028-0598-xx_focus_20.pdf

Stapells, D. R., Picton, T. W., & Durieux-Smith, A. (1994). Electrophysiologic measures of frequency-specific auditory function. In J. T. Jacobsen (Ed.), *Principles and applications in auditory evoked potentials* (pp. 251–283). Boston: Allyn & Bacon.

Stelmachowitz, P., Lewis, D., & Creutz, T. (n.d.). *Situational Hearing-Aid Response Profile* (SHARP, version 6.0). Boys Town National Research Hospital. Accessed June 13, 2007, at www.boystownhospital.org/

CHAPTER 15

Summary and Future Directions

GARY RANCE
SASHA JOHN

The foregoing chapters have sought to summarize the findings generated by a sustained international research effort spanning more than 25 years. Over that time, the nature of the auditory steady-state response (ASSR) and its physiological generators has been reasonably well explored. We now have a detailed understanding of the various factors that affect this type of evoked potential and a clear picture of the ways in which the response can be efficiently elicited and recorded (at least in adult subjects and children over the age of 12 months).

Further research and development will continue to augment the strength of this technique in a number of ways. The next generation of ASSR test modules will provide several novel features that should allow much more powerful and efficient testing. An expected benefit is greater freedom in the ASSR testing protocols. Audiologists using the multiple-simultaneous-stimuli technique, for example, will be able to independently control the intensity of the individual frequencies so that those modulated carriers that have already elicited significant ASSRs can be decreased, while those that have not yet resulted in detectable ASSRs can be tested at the same intensity or even a higher intensity. Audiologists will also be able to better adjust the test protocol in accordance with automatically calculated indices that use estimates of ASSR amplitude and noise levels from earlier in the testing period, to estimate the amount of remaining time that may be needed for subsequently tested ASSRs to become detected. The test modules will allow for mixing stimuli that have been shown to be best for different frequency regions and age groups. For example, exponential stimuli can be used to test for the 500-Hz and 4000-Hz responses, whereas mixed-modulation stimuli are used to test at the 1- to 2-kHz range. Statistics that have been designed to detect ASSRs using multiple harmonics in the amplitude spectrum (Cebulla, Sturzebecher, & Elberling, 2006), or that have been designed using resampling methods, rather than making assumptions about the structure of the noise, also seem promising. Furthermore, in all likelihood, ASSRs will begin to be used both for screening (e.g., using click or chirp stimuli) and for providing a new type of "frequency-based screening" using band-limited noise or band-limited chirps designed to at least provide a low-frequency estimate (e.g., 135 to 1500 Hz) and a high-frequency hearing estimate (1500 to 8000) (Cebulla, Sturzebecher, Elberling, & Wafaa, 2007; Elberling, Don, Cebulla, & Sturzebecher, 2007) Further, new types of testing procedures in which the intensities of the stimuli continuously ramp over time seem promising (Delgado, Acikgoz, Hood, Ozdamar, Bohorquez, 2007; Picton, Van Roon, & John, 2007).

Auditory Steady-State Responses in the Clinic: Current Practice and Future Applications

As illustrated in the preceding chapters, ASSR-based techniques are currently being used in a clinical context. Estimating the audiogram of patients (typically children) with normal hearing or sensorineural hearing loss is an obvious application that has already found a role in audiology clinics worldwide.

Also identified are the areas of weakness that currently limit clinical use of the ASSR. Some of these shortcomings may be inherent in the technique. Analysis of the response in the frequency domain, for example, has a number of advantages in most circumstances, but in some contexts (such as the assessment of cases with auditory pathway disorder) the ability to separate preneural and neural responses in the time domain is essential. On the other hand, some of the concerns currently limiting the scope of clinical ASSR application are likely to be addressed with further research and experience.

Chapter 6 outlined some of the prerequisites for successful clinical application of the ASSR. In these concluding paragraphs, it seems appropriate to use this list of questions as a framework to consider the current situation and research imperatives for the future.

■ Can the ASSR be reliably recorded in subjects of all ages?

■ What effect does auditory pathway maturation have on the ASSR and what is the time course of developmental effects?

It is now well established that ASSRs can be recorded in subjects of all ages including neonates. Response amplitudes are, however, relatively low and response thresholds comparatively high in young babies, and infants show slightly more interstimulus interaction than that observed in adults (Hatton & Stapells, 2007). Accordingly, a significant research objective is to optimize signal to noise ratios in this population. This may be achieved through the development of analysis techniques that minimize background EEG levels, and with the use of stimuli (such as tones with rapid onset and offset envelopes or modulated noise) that maximize the ASSR.

Determining the maturational course of the response and the potential effects that this might have on threshold estimation in the first year of life is another important research objective. The results of this investigation will have an impact on the way ASSRs are used to diagnose hearing loss in the early period and on the possibility of ASSR application as a tool for infant hearing screening (see Chapters 9 and 10 for details).

■ How does subject state affect the response?

■ What are the optimal test parameters for response generation in different subject groups?

The effects of the various test parameters and the ways in which they interact with subject response state are reasonably well understood (at least for adult subjects and older children). The 40-Hz ASSR, which is robust in awake subjects, shows significant amplitude reductions (by greater than 50%) in natural sleep and is further attenuated in general anesthesia. (Accordingly, it has been investigated for medical applications as an indicator of consciousness.) High-rate ASSRs (elicited by presentation or modulation rates greater than70 Hz), by contrast, are relatively stable in both natural and sedated sleep and with general anesthesia. The (limited) available data suggest that threshold sensation levels for the high-

rate ASSR are equivalent across subject states or even slightly lower in sedated or unconscious subjects (as a result of the comparatively low activity levels in the electroencephalogram [EEG]).

High-rate ASSRs have emerged as the optimal responses for assessment of children, for two main reasons: First, obtaining acceptably low noise levels requires that the child be asleep or sedated. Second, the 40-Hz ASSR is immature in infancy and does not in fact become adult-like until adolescence. The 40-Hz ASSR is, however, preferable for assessment of cooperative adult subjects (who can sit quietly and be tested awake) due to its relatively high signal-to-noise ratio. The application of this response for medicolegal assessment is currently an area of investigation. The transient cortical auditory evoked potential (CAEP) is presently the "gold standard" in this field, but the possibility of objective response detection afforded by the 40-Hz ASSR makes it an appealing option.

■ What is the most reliable way to predict hearing threshold from ASSR findings?

■ What is the relationship between ASSR findings and behavioural hearing levels in normally hearing adult subjects?

■ Is this relationship different in hearing-impaired subjects and does the accuracy of hearing level estimation vary with degree and type of hearing loss?

There is now a large body of data relating to the use of ASSRs for hearing level prediction in normally hearing adult subjects and those with sensorineural hearing loss (see Chapter 7 for details). Overall, the results indicate that bracketing techniques (i.e., determining the softest presentation level that elicits an ASSR) can be used to accurately predict hearing levels. This is particularly the case in ears with significant hearing loss, where a "recruitment-like" phenomenon produces recordable responses at consistently low sensation levels.

The advent of newborn hearing screening has shifted the time frame for diagnostic infant hearing assessment into the first few weeks of life. Although it appears that reliable ASSRs can be obtained at low sensation levels in neonates with sensorineural hearing loss (for the reasons just described), more data are certainly required before hearing level predictions can be confidently made in this subject group.

The use of bone-conducted stimuli to distinguish between conductive and sensorineural type hearing loss is one of the cornerstones of audiometric assessment. The development of ASSR testing to bone-conducted signals has had a rocky course, with initial concerns about the generation of artifactual responses. Technical advances have, however, allayed these fears (at least for stimuli at low presentation levels), and normative data for normally hearing adult and infant subjects have been generated (see Chapter 11 for details). The next step toward clinical implementation of the bone conduction (BC)-ASSR technique will involve assessment of subjects with conductive, sensorineural, and mixed hearing loss.

■ Can reliable results be obtained within a manageable test time?

Overall, it is clear that information comprehensive enough to produce an accurate estimate of the behavioural audiogram (in both ears) can be obtained within a clinically viable test period (45 to 60 minutes). Optimizing test times for clinical ASSR assessment is, however, an issue yet to be resolved. This is primarily a reflection of the fact that conventions for clinical ASSR testing currently do not exist. Commercial devices vary widely in their stimulus and recording parameters: Some, for example, use single stimuli presented monaurally, whereas others use multiple simultaneous tones assessing both ears at the same time. Test run times also vary considerably, with some systems testing at each presentation level for less than 90 seconds and others for greater than 10 to 20 minutes.

Optimal run time is likely to vary with test circumstance. A test period of 90 seconds for example may serve well for detecting higher degree hearing losses. Much more time is needed, however, for differentiation between normal hearing and mild-to-moderate hearing loss, particularly in infant subjects. For example, initial reports suggesting criteria for "normal hearing thresholds" have found that run times of approximately 10 minutes would be required for 80% of babies to show responses to stimuli at 40 to 50 dB HL (Stapells & Van Maanen, 2007).

Studies of this type offer an important step toward the development of test protocols for the widespread use of ASSR-based assessment techniques in young infants. Further normative work (involving large numbers of both normal and hearing-impaired babies) is, however, warranted.

■ What factors apart from hearing level (such as site of lesion) may potentially affect the ASSR–hearing threshold relationship?

■ Does the ASSR have any neuro-diagnostic value for identification of central auditory pathway disorders?

The possible effects of central auditory pathway disorder on ASSR threshold levels are yet to be fully investigated. Results in children with auditory neuropathy/dys-synchrony type hearing loss (who typically show responses only at high sensation levels) do, however, illustrate the potential problems. Similar results (threshold elevation) have also been demonstrated in a small number of adults with confirmed neurologic lesions and in premature babies at high risk for auditory pathway impairment. Further research into the effects of central disorders on the ASSR is clearly warranted to inform the hearing level estimation process (allowing better interpretation of threshold results in at-risk subjects). Furthermore, ASSR assessment may eventually allow insights into the function of patients with central auditory pathway disorder.

■ Can the ASSR be used for auditory processing applications?

As discussed in Chapter 12, assessment of auditory processing abilities using the ASSR is an area with clear potential for clinical application. In the future, ASSRs evoked from both the auditory brainstem and cortex by a variety of stimuli such as tones, noise, and speech, and modulated at a range of frequencies (including rates less than 20 Hz), may offer a measure of the underlying neural integrity for basic feature-level processing (such as temporal resolution) and more complex processing such as is required for speech understanding.

Several studies in this area have investigated different aspects of the ASSR that show promise specifically related to speech understanding. For example, ASSRs evoked by amplitude and frequency modulation that simultaneously occur at independent rates have been shown to be correlated with speech recognition abilities (e.g., Dimitrijevic, John, & Picton, 2004). Additionally, investigations that have varied the percentage of frequency or amplitude modulation of the steady-state stimuli have shown a relationship between response amplitudes and speech disorders. Furthermore, using spectrogram analysis, studies have begun to examine envelope following responses in the time-frequency domain, rather than simply the time domain, and have shown correlations between the evoked responses and the slow-frequency speech envelopes (e.g., Aiken & Picton, 2006). Interestingly, the phase locking of ASSRs has been shown to be worse in elderly than in younger listeners and also to be correlated with speech perception abilities (Leigh-Paffenroth & Fowler, 2006).

Conclusion

ASSR technology has developed to the point where it has found a place in the clinical audiology armamentarium. The ability to provide objective, frequency-specific estimates of hearing level in young children make it an obvious diagnostic tool for assessment of babies identified through newborn hearing screening. Future technical developments and greater experience will no doubt open up opportunities for further insights into auditory pathway function and new possibilities for clinical application.

References

Aiken, S. J., & Picton, T. W. (2006). Envelope following responses to natural vowels. *Audiology and Neurotology, 11*, 213–232.

Cebulla, M., Stfirzebecher, E., & Elberling, C. (2006). Objective detection of auditory steady-state responses: Comparison of one-sample and q-sample tests. *Journal of the American Academy of Audiology, 17*(2), 93–103.

Cebulla, M., Sturzebecher, E., Elberling, C., & Wafaa, S. D. (2007). *New chirp stimuli for hearing screening.* International Evoked Response Audiometry Study Group (IERASG). IERASG XX Meeting, Bled, Slovenia.

Delgado, R. E., Acikgoz, N., Hood, L., Ozdamar O., & Bohorquez J. (2007). Fast infant audiogram determination using an intensity-ramping ASSR technique International Evoked Response Audiometry Study Group (IERASG). IERASG XX Meeting, Bled, Slovenia.

Dimitrijevic, A., John, M. S., & Picton, T. W. (2004). Auditory steady-state responses and word recognition scores in normal-hearing and hearing-impaired adults. *Ear and Hearing, 25*(1), 68–84.

Elberling, C., Don, M., Cebulla, M., & Sturzebecher, E., (2007). *Chirp stimuli based on Cochlear Traveling Wave Delay.* International Evoked Response Audiometry Study Group (IERASG) XX Meeting, Bled, Slovenia.

Hatton, J., Stapells D., (2007). *Effects of single- vs multiple-stimulus presentation on 80 Hz ASSR amplitude and threshold: Results in young infants.* International Evoked Response Audiometry Study Group (IERASG). XX Meeting, Bled, Slovenia.

Leigh-Paffenroth, E. D., & Fowler, C. G. (2006). Amplitude-modulated auditory steady-state responses in younger and older listeners. *Journal of the American Academy of Audiology, 17*(8), 582–597.

Picton, T. W., van Roon, P., & John, M. S. (2007). Human auditory steady-state responses during sweeps of intensity. *Ear and Hearing, 28*(4), 542–557.

Stapells D., Van Maanen A. (2007). *ASSRs to multiple simultaneous air-conducted stimuli: Criteria for normal hearing in infants.* International Evoked Response Audiometry Study Group (IERASG) XX Meeting, Bled, Slovenia.

APPENDIX

Commercial Instruments for Auditory Steady-State Response Tests

BARBARA CONE-WESSON*

Clinical research with auditory steady-state responses (ASSRs) was limited during the 1990s and early 2000s because of the lack of availability of commercial instruments. The foundational work in ASSRs was completed using laboratory-based instrumentation that was developed for specific research applications. As an outgrowth of that research, four systems for ASSR testing are now commercially available.

There are some commonalities among the instruments. First, they all have mod-ules or programs for performing transient evoked potential test such as auditory brainstem response (ABR). Stimuli can be presented through insert phones, headphones, loudspeakers, or a bone conduction oscillator. They all have two-channel inputs from the physiologic amplifier to permit ipsi-lateral and con-tralateral recordings. (In the case of Viasys-Audera, this is available only for transient evoked potentials, not ASSR.) The systems can be interfaced with a laptop computer for portability. All of

Author's note: I have used both the Audera and the SmartEP-ASSR systems in my research and clinical work. I receive a portion of patent royalties from the University of Melbourne based on sales of the Audera. I also serve on the Viasys speakers bureau and receive honoraria from Viasys for some sponsored lectures and workshops. In addition, I received an equipment grant from Intelligent Hearing Systems.

the systems have received approval from the U.S. Food and Drug Administration (FDA) or its European equivalent (CE mark). The instruments are in worldwide distribution.

The first ASSR system to be brought to the marketplace (around 1997) was the *The Audix* by Neuronic, SA (www.neuronicsa.com). Up to four amplitude-modulated carriers can be presented to each ear simultaneously. The software uses two different statistics (including a spectral analysis algorithm) for detection of the ASSR (i.e., detection of brain electrical activity that is significantly different from background "noise" on the electroencephalogram [EEG]). The Audix provides online displays of the EEG and the response spectrum. The test protocols can be automated, and estimations of behavioural hearing threshold from ASSR thresholds are provided. The limitation of the system is that the carriers are limited to amplitude-modulated tones; mixed modulation (amplitude modulation plus frequency modulation [AM+FM]) or modulated noise is not available. The Audix is used in South America, South Africa, and China and in other countries in which the U.S. trade embargo with Cuba is not observed.

At approximately the same time as that when the Audix was marketed, ERA Systems, Pty Ltd, Australia, commercialized the ERA System, an instrument for performing ASSR test based on the work of Lawrence T. Cohen, Field W. Rickards, and Gary Rance at the University of Melbourne, Australia. The instrument was sold within Australia and also in Hong Kong and throughout Europe. U.S. and worldwide distribution was made possible when the technology was transferred to Grason-Stadler Instruments (GSI)–Nicolet Instruments (Madison, Wiscon-

sin), which further developed and refined the concept and marketed it as the *Audera*. (GSI-Nicolet was subsequently bought by Viasys, and the Audera is now part of the Viasys product line [http://www.viasyshealthcare.com].) Unlike the other instruments, the Audera tests only one carrier modulation frequency at a time. The carrier can be any frequency from 250 to 8000 Hz, and the modulator can be varied from 1 to 250 Hz. It is possible to create stimuli that vary with respect to modulation depth and modulation type (AM, FM, or AM+FM). A phase coherence-squared statistic is used to determine when a response has occurred. An ASSR time-domain waveform is not provided; however, a frequency domain representation is. This is a polar plot that shows the phase angle of each sample's vector. The statistical significance of the phase clustering is tracked in real time and also is displayed. Test protocols can be automated, and estimation of behavioural hearing threshold from the ASSR thresholds is provided. A limitation of the Audera is that the sampling (averaging) time of the responses cannot be extended. This means that for a "noisy" subject, the test must be discontinued and restarted once the subject is in an appropriate response state. The Audera uses a strict criterion for determining when the ongoing EEG is noisy and will reflect that condition in the ongoing polar plot and on the statistical significance graph. ASSR thresholds cannot be determined when the outcome of this algorithm is "noise," rather than "phase-locked" (response present) or "random" (response absent).

The *M-A-S-T-E-R* (*m*ultiple *a*uditory *s*teady-state *r*esponse) system was the outgrowth of a systematic research program undertaken by M. Sasha John and

Terence Picton and their colleagues at the Rotman Research Institute of Baycrest Centre in Toronto, Canada. It is available as a component of the BioLogic Navigator-Pro evoked potential system (now a part of Natus [www.natus.com]), and a research instrument also is available (http://www.mastersystem.ca). It is the only commercially available instrument that incorporates technology that has undergone peer review in scientific journals. Design features that were reviewed include the choice and design of stimuli (including AM, FM, AM+FM, and exponential modulation envelopes) and signal processing including weighted averaging. These features increase the efficiency and accuracy of ASSR testing. Like the Audix, the MASTER allows for the presentation of up to four stimuli per ear and dichotic testing, so that eight frequencies can be tested simultaneously. The ASSR detection algorithm is based on the response spectrum analysis, and the system also provides an online display of the "noise floor" and the response amplitude so that the audiologist can make clinical judgments about when to extend the averaging time. A majority of clinically oriented (peer-reviewed) ASSR research studies have been completed using the MASTER system. Selected research papers supporting the methods and the technology of MASTER can be found at http://master system.ca.

Intelligent Hearing Systems (http://www.ihsys.com) offers the *SmartEP-ASSR* system. One of the differentiating features of the system is its facility for creating stimuli with a number of different modulation functions. This feature can be advantageous in research. The "default" stimuli for the SmartEP-ASSR system are tone bursts, similar in duration and rise time to those used for ABR tests. They are presented in trains of approximately 1 s in duration. It also is possible to use click stimuli and analyze the results by means of spectral analysis methods. "Ramped stimuli" also are implemented, in which the stimulus level is steadily increased or decreased until response threshold is found. The SmartEP-ASSR analysis of the response is in the frequency domain, using spectral analysis methods (F-test). Also, analysis of response phase and amplitude is provided. It is possible to present up to eight stimuli monaurally, or four in each ear, dichotically. Software routines are available for stimulus calibration (used in conjunction with a sound pressure level meter).

Index

A

Acoustics, ear canal, 244
Adults
    behavioral threshold relationships in,
        126–130
    state of consciousness of, 109–111
AEPs (Auditory evoked potentials), 2
    80-Hz auditory steady-state response
        compared with, 149–157
        brainstem response, 150–153
Aliased energy, 27
AMFR (Amplitude modulated frequency
    response), 5
Amplitude
    development in infants, 165
    versus phase-based statistical methods,
        30–33
Amplitude modulated frequency response
    (AMFR), 5
Amplitude projection procedure (APP),
    hearing devices and, 244–245
Amplitude spectrum, ASSR sweep, 28
Analog-to-digital conversion, 12
Anesthesia, effects of, 113–114
APP (Amplitude projection procedure),
    hearing devices and, 244–245
Apparent latency, 42
Artifacts
    bone conduction and, 207–210
        clinical implications, 209–210
    of, 46–49
ASSEP (Auditory steady-state evoked
    potential), 5

ASSR (Auditory steady-state response)
    40-Hz auditory, reset mechanism, 98
    amplitude spectrum at, 28
    behavioral threshold estimation and,
        126–133, 138–142
    bone conduction, 201–225
        hearing loss and, 221–222
        normal hearing, 202–207
    child with auditory
        neuropathy/desynchronize,
        302–308
    child with conductive hearing loss,
        292–297
    clinical application of, 119–122,
        178–180
    clinical protocols, 133–135
    comparison of 80-Hz and 40Hz, 153–155
    continuously distributed, 101–102
    described, 1
    developmental mechanisms affecting,
        169–172
    effect of test parameters, 135–138
    effects of age on, 114
    electrically evoked, fitting hearing aids
        and, 259–262
    fitting hearing aids and, 241–258
        loudness, 246–251
    free field, infant testing for assessment
        of hearing aid function in,
        309–316
    future directions of, 319–323
    hearing impaired infants, 175–176
    hearing-impaired infants, testing time
        requirements, 190–194

ASSR *(continued)*
   hearing level prediction using, 175
   hearing screening and, 185–196
      automated, 194–195
   historical perspective of, 2–8
   ipsilateral/contralateral asymmetries in
      bone conduction, 220–222
   neonates/infants responses in
      detection of, 165–167
      hearing-impaired, 189–194
      in normal, 163–165, 186–187
   neural generators of, 83–103
   premature babies and, 176–178
   response testing, 44–45
   responses for steady-state vowels,
      230–231
   rules pertaining to, 20
   slow cortical potential comparison
      with, 155–156
      high-level processing and, 156–157
   stimulus-response relationship, 55–76
      binaural processing testing, 70–77
      carrier frequency, 68–69
      modulation depth, 67–68
      modulation rate, 56–64
      single/multiple stimuli and, 69–70
      stimulus intensity, 64–66
      stimulus type and, 66–67
   subject variables in, 109–115
   technology, 195–196
   testing as a screening tool, 187–189
   testing techniques, 12–16
      with different audiometric
         configurations, 49
   tone burst-evoked auditory, in
      neonates/infants, 172–174
Audiometer threshold, pure-tone
   establishment and, 242–243
Audiometry, speech, 229–231
Auditory ability, suprathreshold tests of,
   229–238
Auditory evoked potential Auditory
   evoked potentials (AEPs), 2
   80-Hz auditory steady-state response
      compared with, 149–157
      brainstem response, 150–153
   applications of in hearing devices,
      244–246

      assessment, case studies, child with
         multiple disabilities, 265–271
   pure-tone establishment and, 242–243
   workers' compensation cases, case
      study of, 298–302
Auditory middle-latency response,
   sources of, 91–92
Auditory processing, 122
Auditory steady-state evoked potential
   (ASSEP), 5
Auditory steady-state evoked response, 5
Auditory steady-state response (ASSR)
   40-Hz auditory, reset mechanism, 98
   80-Hz, 84–90
   amplitude spectrum at, 28
   behavioral threshold estimation and,
      126–133, 138–142
   bone conduction, 201–225
      normal hearing, 202–207
   bone conduction and, hearing loss and,
      221–222
   child with auditory
      neuropathy/dyssynchrony, case
      study of, 302–308
   child with conductive hearing loss,
      case study of, 292–297
   clinical application of, 119–122
   clinical protocols, 133–135
   comparison of 80-Hz and 40Hz,
      153–155
   continuously distributed, 101–102
   described, 1
   developmental mechanisms affecting,
      169–172
   effect of test parameters, 135–138
   effects of age on, 114
   electrically evoked, fitting hearing aids
      and, 259–262
   fitting hearing aids and, 241–258
      loudness, 246–251
   free field, infant testing for assessment
      of hearing aid function in, 309–316
   future directions of, 319–323
   hearing impaired infants, 175–176
      testing time requirements, 190–194
   hearing level prediction using, 175
   hearing screening and, 185–196
      automated, 194–195

historical perspective of, 2–8
ipsilateral/contralateral asymmetries in
      bone conduction, 220–222
neonates/infants responses in, 161–180
   detection of, 165–167
      hearing-impaired, 189–194
      in normal, 163–165, 186–187
neural generators of, 83–103
premature babies and, 176–178
response testing, 44–45
responses for steady-state vowels,
      230–231
rules pertaining to, 20
slow cortical potential comparison
      with, 155–156
      high-level processing and, 156–157
stimulus-response relationship, 55–76
   binaural processing testing, 70–77
   carrier frequency, 68–69
   modulation depth, 67–68
   modulation rate, 56–64
   single/multiple stimuli and, 69–70
   stimulus intensity, 64–66
   stimulus type and, 66–67
subject variables in, 109–115
suprathreshold tests of auditory ability,
      229–238
technology, 195–196
testing as a screening tool, 187–189
testing techniques, 12–16
   with different audiometric
      configurations, 49
tone burst-evoked auditory, in
      neonates/infants, 172–174
Auditory steady-state stimuli
   calibration of, 21–22
   creation of, 16–21

B

Babies
   amplitude development in, 165
   auditory steady-state response (ASSR)
      development in normal, 163–165
      detection of, 165–167
      developmental mechanisms
         affecting, 169–172
      in hearing-impaired, 189–194

hearing level prediction, 175
      responses, 161–180
      tone burst-evoked auditory, 172–174
   with mild hearing loss, hearing
      screening and, 286–291
   sensorineural hearing loss following
      meningitis, case study of, 271–278
   state of consciousness of, 111–113
   with steeply sloping high-frequency
      hearing loss, case study of,
      278–285
Behavioral threshold estimation, 125–142
   ASSR (Auditory steady-state response),
      126–133, 138–142
   history of, 126
BIC (Binaural interaction component),
      71–72
Binaural interaction component (BIC),
      71–72
Binaural processing, tests of, 70–77
Bone conduction, 201–225
   artifact, 207–209
      clinical implications, 209–210
   bone oscillator
      dynamic range, 210
      placement location, 215–216
   brainstem responses, clinical
      implications, 207
   calibration of stimuli, 216
   conduction thresholds, estimation of
      direct/indirect, 217–219
   dynamic range, 210
      clinical implications, 210
   hearing loss and, 221–222
   interaural attenuation to stimuli in
      dB IIL, 217
   ipsilateral/contralateral asymmetries in,
      220–222
   normal hearing, 202–207
   oscillator coupling method, 211–213
   recommendations for, 222–224
   test ear isolation, 219–221
   unoccluded vs. occluded ears, 215–216
Bone oscillator
   coupling method, 211–213
   placement location, 213–215
Brainstem responses, 150–153
   bone conduction and, 205–207

C

Calibration, of auditory steady-state
   stimuli, 21–22
Carrier frequency, 56
   stimulus-response relationship, 68–69
Case studies
   auditory evoked potential assessment,
      child with multiple disabilities,
      265–271
   auditory neuropathy/dyssynchrony,
      child with, 302–308
   auditory steady-state response (ASSR)
      testing in hearing loss, child with
      conductive hearing loss, 292–297
   free-field auditory steady-state
      response, infant testing for
      assessment of hearing aid function
      in, 309–316
   hearing screening, infant with mild
      hearing loss, 286–291
   high-frequency hearing loss, infant with
      steeply sloping, 278–285
   sensorineural hearing loss following
      meningitis, infant with, 271–278
   use of auditory evoked potentials,
      workers' compensation cases,
      298–302
Children
   behavioral threshold relationships in,
      130–133
   with conductive hearing loss, case
      study of, 292–297
   with multiple disabilities, case study of,
      265–271
Clark, Graeme, 2
Clinical protocols, auditory steady-state
   response (ASSR), 133–135
CNV (Contingent negative variation), 2
Cochlear multichannel implant, 2
Contingent negative variation (CNV), 2
Conventional AM stimuli, 16
Conversion, time-to-frequency, 22–26
Correction vs. regression techniques,
   140–142

D

Differential diagnosis, 121–122
Digital-to-analog conversion, 12

Dipole source analysis, 88
   auditory steady-state response
      localization, 99
Discontinuities, 20
   dissociation between steady-state
      responses and, 94–98

E

Ear canal acoustics, 244
EEG signal, 14
EFR (Envelope following response), 5,
   237
Electrodes, scalp, EEG signal and, 14
Electromagnetic energy, 27
Electrophysiological gain verification,
   hearing devices and, 245–246
Energy, measuring, at modulation
   frequency, 28–30
Envelope following response (EFR), 5, 237
Exponential AM stimuli, 16–17

F

F-ratio, 15, 61
Fast fourier transform (FFT), 24–25, 39
Feature detectors, 3
FFT (Fast fourier transform), 24–25, 39
Field potentials, 4
Fourier transforms, 22
Free-field auditory steady-state response,
   infant testing for assessment of
   hearing aid function in, case study
   of, 309–316
Frequency modulation, modeled speech
   and, 232–235
Frequency specificity, hearing aids, 243
Functional magnetic resonance imaging,
   90

H

Harmonics, measuring modulation
   frequency at, 30
Hearing aids
   amplitude projection procedure and,
      244–245
   applications of audio evoked
      potentials, 244–246

dynamic range, 252
electrophysiological gain verification
    and, 245–246
fitting
    audio steady-state responses in,
        241–258
    loudness, 246–251
    using electrically evoked auditory
        steady-state responses, 259–262
    frequency specificity, 243
    gain/compression factor, 252
    Maximum power output (MPO), 252
    pure-tone establishment and, 242–243
    selection of, 251–252
    stimulus calibration, 243
Hearing level prediction, infants, 175
Hearing loss
    bone conduction and, 221–222
    high-frequency, infant with steeply
        sloping, 278–285
Hearing screening
    auditory steady-state response (ASSR)
        and, 185–196
        automation of, 194–195
    infant with mild hearing loss, case
        study of, 286–291
Hearing threshold, estimation of,
    119–121
Hypothesis of intrinsic oscillations, in
    neural networks, 92–93

I

ILDs (Interaural level differences), 71
Independent amplitude, modeled speech
    and, 232–235
Infants
    amplitude development in, 165
    auditory steady-state response (ASSR)
        development in normal, 163–165
        detection of, 165–167
        developmental mechanisms
            affecting, 169–172
        in hearing-impaired, 189–194
        hearing level prediction, 175
        responses, 161–180
        tone burst-evoked auditory, 172–174
    with mild hearing loss, hearing
        screening and, 286–291

sensorineural hearing loss following
    meningitis, case study of, 271–278
    state of consciousness of, 111–113
    with steeply sloping high-frequency
        hearing loss, case study of,
        278–285
Information-processing channels, 3
Intensity, 56
Interaural level differences (ILDs), 71
Interaural phase differences (IPDs), 71
Interaural time differences (ITDs), 71
IPDs (Interaural phase differences), 71
ITDs (Interaural time differences), 71

K

Ketamine-induced anesthesia, 113

L

Latency
    calculations of, 39–43
    estimates, 88
Long-term average speech spectrum
    (LTASS), 251
LTASS (Long-term average speech
    spectrum), 251

M

Magnetic resonance imaging, functional,
    90
MASTER (Multiple auditory steady-state
    response), 12
Maximum power output (MPO), 251
Middle-latency response, sources of
    auditory, 91–92
Mixed modulation (MM) stimulus, 16–18
Modeled speech, 232–235
Modulation depth, stimulus-response
    relationship, 67–68
Modulation envelope, 18
Modulation frequency, 56
    energy sources at, 26–28
    measuring energy at, 28–30
    measuring responses at harmonics of,
        30
Modulation rate, 56–64
    stimulus-response relationship, 56–64

MPO (Maximum power output), 251
Multiple ASSR, 12
Multiple auditory steady-state response
    (MASTER), 12
Multiple auditory steady-state stimuli,
    switching between single and,
    38–39
Multiple-frequency ASSR, 12
Muscle responses, 27

N

Neonates
    auditory steady-state response (ASSR)
        responses, 161–180
        detection of, 165–167
    auditory steady-state response (ASSR),
        tone burst-evoked auditory,
        172–174
    auditory steady-state responses (ASSR),
        in hearing-impaired, 189–194
Neural generators, 83–103
Neural networks, hypothesis of intrinsic
    oscillations in, 92–93
Newborns, state of consciousness of, 112
Noise, 14
    energy, 28–30

O

Oscillatory networks, significance of
    40-Hz, 93

P

Perceptual responses, described, 2
Phase ambiguity, 42
Phase calculations, 39–43
Phase circularity, 42
Phase delay, calculations of, 39–43
Phase variability, 32
Phased-based, versus amplitude statistical
    methods, 30–33
Physiologically based
    evoked energy, 27
    noise, 26–27
Polar plot, 15
Postauricular muscle response, 27
Posterior neck muscle response, 27

Preceding cycle technique, 42
Premature babies, auditory steady-state
    response (ASSR) and, 176–178

R

Regression vs. correction techniques,
    140–142
Response detection, strategies of, 33–38

S

Scalp electrodes, EEG signal and, 14
SCP (Slow cortical potential) testing, 153
    ASSR (Auditory steady-state response)
        compared with, 155–156
Screening tools, ASSR (Auditory steady-
        state response) as, 187–189
Sensorineural hearing loss, following
        meningitis, case study of, 271–278
Signal, 14
Single auditory steady-state stimuli,
        switching between multiple and,
        38–39
Sinusoidally amplitude-modulated (AM)
        stimuli, 16
Slow cortical potential (SCP) testing, 153
    ASSR (Auditory steady-state response)
        compared with, 155–156
SOC (Superior olivary complex), 71
Somatosensory steady-state potentials, 3
Spectral analysis, 22–26
Speech audiometry, 229–231
State of consciousness
    adults, 109–111
    infants, 111–113
Steady-state potentials, visual/
        somatosensory, 3
Steady-state responses
    40-Hz auditory, 90–103
    80-Hz auditory, 84–90
        audio evoked potentials compared
            with, 149–157
        latency estimates, 88
    dissociation between transient and,
        94–98
Sternocleidomastoid response, 27
Stimuli, creation of, auditory steady-state,
        16–21

Stimulus intensity, 64–66
  stimulus-response relationship, 67–68
Superimposition hypothesis, 90–91
  probing the, 93–94
Superior olivary complex (SOC), 71
Suprathreshold tests of auditory ability,
      229–238
Sustained responses, described, 2

T

Temporal processing, 236–238
Test ear, isolation of, 219–221
Test parameters, effects of, 135–138
Testing techniques, auditory steady-state
      response (ASSR), 12–16
tGBR (Transient gamma band response),
      94
Threshold, defined, 133
Time-to-frequency conversion, 22–26
Transient gamma band response (tGBR),
      94
Transient responses, described, 2

Transients, 20
  dissociation between steady-state
      responses and, 94–98

U

Universal newborn hearing screening
      (UNHS), 8, 185
University of Melbourne, Department of
      Otolaryngology founded, 2
Unoccluded vs. occluded ears, 215–216

V

Visual steady-state potentials, 3
Vowels, steady-state, 230–231

W

Wilson, Orile, 8
Workers' compensation cases, use of
      auditory evoked potentials, case
      study of, 298–302